Assessing and Diagnosing Young Children with Neurodevelopmental Disorders

Now in its second edition, this practical handbook assesses global developmental delay and other neurodevelopmental disorders in young children. Explaining diagnostic, support, and treatment services available for children and their families, this volume clarifies psychological and medical terminology, and global legislative and societal factors relating to assessment. Fully updated, this new edition incorporates the transition from DSM-5 to DSM-5-TR and has an increased emphasis on cross-cultural and ethnic diversity aspects of assessing and diagnosing neurodevelopmental disorders in young children.

Designed as a comprehensive compendium for student and practicing psychologists, it offers an introduction to historical perspectives around child development and developmental disorders, and how these have affected our understanding of neurodevelopmental disorders. It explains professional and ethical considerations surrounding the clinical practice of developmental assessments and focuses on the crucial importance of understanding and supporting the parental experience of assessment and diagnosis. Key topics covered include definitions and descriptions of genetic and chromosomal disorders and neurodevelopmental disorders; eligibility criteria for support and assistance; the Griffiths Scales, Bayley Scales, and other notable assessments for young children; autism spectrum disorder; the process of assessment and diagnosis, diagnostic tools, and report writing.

Including a chapter on illustrative case studies of children with developmental disorders, this book is essential reading for educational, clinical, and developmental psychologists working with children and their families, as well as postgraduate students training in the field.

Neil Nicoll is a Fellow of the Australian Psychological Society College of Educational and Developmental Psychologists, providing services for children with developmental delays and disorders, training programmes for psychologists and paediatricians, and presentations at international conferences.

Assessing and Diagnosing Young Children with Neurodevelopmental Disorders

A DSM-5-TR Compliant Guide

Second Edition

Neil Nicoll

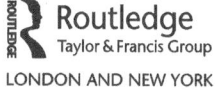

LONDON AND NEW YORK

Cover image: Tetiana Lazunova via Getty Images

Second edition published 2025
by Routledge
4 Park Square, Milton Park, Abingdon, Oxon, OX14 4RN

and by Routledge
605 Third Avenue, New York, NY 10158

Routledge is an imprint of the Taylor & Francis Group, an informa business

© 2025 Neil Nicoll

The right of Neil Nicoll to be identified as author of this work has been asserted in accordance with sections 77 and 78 of the Copyright, Designs and Patents Act 1988.

All rights reserved. No part of this book may be reprinted or reproduced or utilised in any form or by any electronic, mechanical, or other means, now known or hereafter invented, including photocopying and recording, or in any information storage or retrieval system, without permission in writing from the publishers.

Trademark notice: Product or corporate names may be trademarks or registered trademarks, and are used only for identification and explanation without intent to infringe.

First edition published by Routledge 2022

British Library Cataloguing-in-Publication Data
A catalogue record for this book is available from the British Library

ISBN: 978-1-032-93311-5 (hbk)
ISBN: 978-1-032-93310-8 (pbk)
ISBN: 978-1-003-56533-8 (ebk)

DOI: 10.4324/9781003565338

Typeset in Sabon
by KnowledgeWorks Global Ltd.

Contents

List of figures and tables	*vii*
Acknowledgements	*ix*
Introduction to the second edition	1

PART I
Historical overview of neurodevelopmental disorders in young children   7

 1 Historical overview of neurodevelopmental disorders in young children   9
 2 What is a neurodevelopmental disorder?   21
 3 Genetic and chromosomal disorders   40
 4 Selected genetic and chromosomal disorders   49
 5 Population demographics   68

PART II
Why do we assess and diagnose neurodevelopmental disorders?   73

 6 Why do we assess young children?   75
 7 Parental experience of assessment and diagnosis   84
 8 Systemic reasons to assess and diagnose childhood disorders   96

PART III
The assessment and diagnostic process   109

 9 Psychometric assessment of childhood development   111
10 The griffiths scales of mental development   125
11 Bayley scales of infant and child development   130
12 Mullen scales of early learning (Eileen M. Mullen)   133
13 Other notable assessments for young children: The McCarthy scales and the Miller scales   135

14	Checklist and questionnaire-based assessments	138
15	Cross-cultural adaptations of developmental assessments	149
16	Assessing autism spectrum disorder in young children	161
17	Cross-cultural assessment and diagnosis of autism spectrum disorder	173

PART IV
From theory to practice — 183

18	From theory to clinical practice	185
19	Pre-assessment preparation	187
20	The assessment process	193
21	"Driving" the test: The 75-25 rule and its application	200
22	Remote and online assessments	211
23	Scoring developmental tests	214
24	Giving feedback	216
25	Intervention strategies	221
26	Diagnostic considerations and formulation	227

PART V
Report writing and case studies — 239

27	Report writing	241
28	Case studies and reports	252

PART VI
Follow-up — 297

29	Follow-up and support	299

PART VII
Pondering the future — 303

30	Pondering the future of neurodevelopmental disorders	305

Appendices	*310*
Glossary of terms	*346*
Index	*351*

Figures and tables

Figures

1.1	The "Wild Boy of Aveyron"	10
1.2	Sample of Binet and Simon's 1909 test items	12
1.3	Australian Disability Services Act, National Standards	17
3.1	The normal sequence of chromosomes	42
3.2	Down Syndrome Association of N.S.W. fridge magnet	43
3.3	The path to genetic assessment	46
4.1	Clear evidence of Trisomy 21	50
4.2	Schematic diagram of velocardiofacial syndrome	54
4.3	Cardiac anomalies in 22q11.2 syndrome	55
4.4	Schematic representation of Fragile X syndrome	61
5.1	Incidence of childhood disability per 100,000 population as measured by the socio-demographic index (SDI)	69
5.2	Sub-Saharan "less developed" countries	71
7.1	The cycle of grief	91
9.1	John Dewey's reference to intelligence testing	112
9.2	The normal or Gaussian curve	113
9.3	Rates of developmental growth by level of developmental delay	118
9.4	Examples of the sequence of gross motor skills	120
9.5	Examples of the sequence for fine motor skills	121
10.1	Griffiths' original "Avenues of Learning"	126
10.2	Griffiths III "Avenues of Learning"	128
15.1	Equality and equity	150
19.1	Suggested assessment room layout	190
21.1	The "75%-25%" rule of assessment	200
24.1	Providing feedback to families	217
26.1	"From referral to diagnosis to action" flow chart	228
27.1	The components of communication	244
27.2	A "common language" for discussing and reporting	245
27.3	Summary of suggested report structure	250
27.4	Sample graphic representations of psychometric data	250

Tables

0.1	Timeline of significant events	4
1.1	Factors underlying neurodevelopmental disorders	19

2.1	Changes in diagnostic criteria for autism spectrum disorder, 1943–2023	26
3.1	Timeline of genetic discoveries: National Human Genome Research Institute	40
4.1	Comorbidity with various genetic disorders	49
4.2	Incidence by maternal age of Down syndrome	50
4.3	Rates of psychiatric disorder in studies of vcfs	56
4.4	Behavioural symptoms in Smith-Magenis syndrome	57
4.5	Diagnostic criteria for fetal alcohol spectrum disorder	65
4.6	Incidence of fetal alcohol spectrum disorder by geographic zone	66
8.1	Summary of Global Statistics on financial support schemes	97
8.2	Australian Centrelink Carers Allowance Eligibility Evidence	98
9.1	Standard scores, percentiles and standard deviations	114
9.2	Standardisation sample demographics	117
14.1	Vineland-III assessment domains	142
14.2	ABAS 3 assessment domains	144
15.1	Substitute test items from Malawi	152
16.1	Diagnostic statement, Autism Spectrum Rating Scale	166
21.1	Qualitative descriptions of test items passed	204
21.2	Pass/fail and qualitative descriptions of item attempts	205
21.3	American Psychological Association test adaptation guidelines	206
25.1	Selected medications used with neurodevelopmental disorders	224
25.2	Sample medication side effect chart	225
26.1	DSM-5-TR criteria, global developmental delay	232
28.1	Mullen scales programme intake and exit results	293
28.2	Pre- and post-test results, Vineland Adaptive Behaviour Scale	294
30.1	Percentage of Gross Domestic Product expenditure on disability benefits	307
30.2	Percentage of gross national income (GNI) expenditure on overseas aid	308
A.1	Global disability laws, acts and legislations	310
A.4	Selected national disability service programs	317
A.10	DSM-5-TR levels of intellectual disability	327
A.11	DSM-5-TR levels of support, autism spectrum disorder	330
A.14	Fine motor skills developmental sequence	335
A.15	Sequence of gross motor skills	337
A.16	Language development sequence	339
A.17	United Nations "Less Developed Countries" 2024	341
A.19	Adapted and "new assessment tools for specific cultures"	343
A.20	Screening tests for general population usage	345

Acknowledgements

Although one author is responsible for the writing of this book, it must be emphasised that it also embodies the cumulative interactions and collaborations with other psychologists, paediatricians, psychiatrists and geneticists over many years. Particular gratitude is also given to those professionals who reviewed this book and supported the development and publishing of the Second Edition. I am indebted to Professor Melissa Gladstone from the University of Liverpool in the United Kingdom for sharing her considerable experience in and commitment to the process of adapting standardised "western" assessment tools and protocols for use in lesser developed countries. Finally, this book would not have been possible without the ongoing support of Routledge Publishing, through Doctor Helen Pritt (the Editor of the first edition), and Doctor Molly Helen Selby, Editor of the second edition and the team from Routledge Publishing.

Introduction to the second edition

There are many reasons to write a book about the process of assessing young children for possible neurodevelopmental disorders, and it is hoped that this book may clarify many of the issues associated with such assessments in a manner which will assist other psychologists in their journey towards careers in early childhood assessments. This second edition of this book addresses historical, cultural, theoretical, professional and ethical considerations surrounding the clinical practice of developmental assessments, as well as the sometimes complex bureaucratic and systemic requirements associated with eligibility criteria for support and assistance. As with its predecessor, this book is not intended to be a dogmatic, prescriptive or definitive description of the skills required, the processes to adhere to, the tests to use or the outcomes to be expected from developmental assessments. It is intended to be a practical "Users' Guide" for students studying Developmental Psychology or commencing their careers "in the field". The need for a book such as this stems from several motivations and sources:

- The differences in education and training opportunities and standards for developmental psychology across countries, states, counties and jurisdictions.
- Changing employment opportunities for psychologists that have occurred over recent years, particularly for educational and developmental psychologists.
- Ongoing research into the understanding of child development, particularly in the ever-expanding knowledge base around genetic factors – the "building blocks" of child development.
- The introduction or expansion of support programmes for children with delayed or disordered development, and the subsequent need for accurate and timely diagnosis for service eligibility and treatment.
- The need to understand and consider the differing cultural and ethnic values, beliefs, customs, languages and idioms, which may be encountered in everyday psychological practice.
- The need to illustrate the processes by which psychological and psychometric assessments have been and can be adapted to ensure that they are as aligned as possible to these cultural diversities which define and enrich our world.
- The need to help psychologists best support young children with developmental concerns and support their families in a manner sympathetic and appropriate to their needs.

The last point should resonate the loudest. It reflects the privilege and responsibility which come from engagement with young children and their families, when they are perhaps at their most vulnerable. Parents need to know how to help their children when there may be a reason for concern. They need to know if their children are developing appropriately, and if not, why not. They need to know if their children have a clearly definable "diagnosis", and if there are appropriate therapeutic and educational programmes to assist them. They need to know how and where to seek help, and they need to know how successful such treatments will ultimately be.

It is not that psychologists can answer all these questions. However, the role of the psychologist is vital in assisting families through what can be an arduous and confusing "journey". The birth of a child always brings a complex array of emotions and expectations: Excitement, love, fear, hopes, dreams and goals. When a young child is seen to be "lagging behind", or manifesting unusual or concerning behaviours, parents can be thrown into a state of turmoil: "Is it my fault?" "What did I do wrong?" "Does this mean I am not a good parent?" "What do I do now?" "Will it get better?" "What if it does not?" These, and many other mixed emotions are very likely to occur when concerns arise about a young child.

In 2004, I was privileged to be part of a writing project with journalist Cindy Dowling and publisher Bernadette Thomas, both of whom are also the parents of children with disabilities. The aim of the project was to give parents free voice and opportunity to "tell their stories" about their journey through the process of raising children with developmental disorders, genetic and physical disabilities, and chronic medical conditions: From early suspicions, through the often torturous route of assessment and diagnosis, seeking assistance and clarity, support and advocacy. Many families never have the opportunity to tell their stories.

Released in Australia and Japan under the title "Lessons from my Child", and in America as "A Different Kind of Perfect", the book chronicled the fact that no two families experience these journeys the same way, and that it is inherent in the role of professionals such as medical practitioners, psychologists, therapists and educators, to appreciate and accommodate these individual experiences. The term "lessons" is therefore entirely appropriate, not just for parents but also for professionals.

A point stressed frequently in this publication is that the assessment and diagnostic process in the realm of young children requires considerable patience, flexibility and adaptability, but it is equally true that these qualities are best learned when professionals have a solid grounding in the basic theories, knowledge base, genetic underpinnings, professional and bureaucratic requirements surrounding the domain of assessment and diagnosis, service provision and support, when young children present with potentially significant genetic or neurodevelopmental disorders.

Although this book is intended for students of psychology, or "early career" psychologists with particular interest in young children with neurodevelopmental disorders, such professionals generally do not work alone in this domain. The role of Paediatricians, Neurologists, General Practitioners, Social Workers, Community Nurses, Speech Pathologists, Occupational Therapists, Physiotherapists and Early Childhood Teachers must be acknowledged and valued as well through their vital roles assisting parents through their "journeys" along the disability pathway.

Educational and Developmental Psychologists, Clinical Psychologists, Neuropsychologists and Generalist Psychologists often find themselves working in partnership with these professionals, either on an ongoing basis, or as part of a temporary "support team". Understanding the contribution and expertise of these professionals should be part and parcel of the role of psychologists in complementing and shadowing their roles. Respectful and amicable sharing of information, expertise and knowledge is always to

Introduction to the second edition 3

the benefit of families and to young children with neurodevelopmental disorders, genetic disorders or simple developmental concerns.

This book attempts to illustrate some of the following:

- The historical perspectives around child development and developmental disorders, and how these have affected our understanding of neurodevelopmental disorders.
- The current status of neurodevelopmental disorders, their classification, causation and diagnostic criteria.
- Classificatory descriptions and definitions of genetic disorders, and the relationships between these and neurodevelopmental disorders.
- Parental expectations of assessment and diagnostic services and processes.
- The various ethnic and cultural belief systems, values, social mores, languages and customs, which need to be appreciated when supporting families in our rich and diverse world.
- Current methodologies around assessment and diagnosis of developmental delays and disorders, including specific assessment tests – the tools of trade for psychologists, and adaptations made to such assessments to accommodate as far as possible differing cultural needs.
- Best practice procedures in assessment and diagnostic services, including diagnostic formulations, parental feedback, report writing and other follow-up services.
- Useful professional resources such as relevant textbooks and references.
- Ethical considerations for the role of psychologists, such as those embodied in the various international Psychological Society' Codes of Ethics and Guidelines.

This book makes a number of assumptions about the knowledge base of psychologists and other professionals who may choose to read it. It assumes an understanding of psychometric assessment procedures and basic statistical knowledge around assessment processes. It assumes adequate knowledge of diagnostic classificatory systems, particularly the Diagnostic and Statistical Manual 5th Edition Text Revision (DSM-5-TR), but also the International Classification of Diseases 11th Edition (ICD-11).

This book follows the historical path of neurodevelopmental disorders in young children through the research and development of theories and models of child development, methods of assessing, measuring and categorising developmental skills and deficits in young children, the medical and scientific advances which unlocked many of the mysteries of child development and deviation from the norm, and the role played by political and statutory forces in influencing societal attitudes towards disability and disorders, and the manner in which these in turn drove the improved provision of services for young children with disabilities and their families.

A "timeline" of significant aspects of this journey follows as a prelude to the written history. It reflects that in the context of medical science, psychological theory and practice, change can be incremental and gradual, and sometimes radical. If there is one "lesson" to stem from this publication, it is that change is the only certainty in these matters. The ability to adapt to change was never so crucial as during the 2020 coronavirus pandemic. Psychology as a profession was not immune from the need to adapt and change, to meet new challenges, to learn from the past, to rediscover previously used and sometimes discarded methodologies, and to devise and trial new and untested methods. History will look back with interest upon these times, but the profession of psychology continues to adapt to a complex and changing world.

Notes on the second edition

The first edition of this book was published in 2021 when the Diagnostic and Statistical Manual 5th edition (DSM 5) was the most recent iteration of that manual. In 2022, DSM 5 was superseded by DSM-5-TR, and at the same time, the diagnostic criteria and coding for ICD 11 were finalised and released. For neurodevelopmental disorders such as intellectual disability, autism spectrum disorder, attention deficit hyperactivity disorder and global developmental delay, the changes to DSM-5-TR were insignificant. What was significant was that for the first time in their respective histories, the diagnostic criteria and coding protocol for both DSM-5-TR and ICD 11 were effectively synchronised.

A second edition of "Assessing and Diagnosing Young Children with Neurodevelopmental Disorders" was therefore necessary for the sake of accuracy, but this updated edition also provided an opportunity to update other elements and content. Specifically:

- "New" genetic disorders implicated in neurodevelopmental disorders were announced to the scientific community.
- Ongoing research into neurodevelopmental disorders continues to enlighten and clarify assessment protocols, aetiology, characteristics, treatment and outcomes associated with neurodevelopmental disorders.
- Attention could be focussed upon the disparity between the "developed", western world and underdeveloped or developing countries where child development outcomes can be suboptimal due to socioeconomic, medical and cultural factors.

In respect to this final point, the work of Professor Melissa Gladstone from the University of Liverpool in the United Kingdom is gratefully acknowledged, as it opened the way to a greater understanding of the conditions for young children and their families in sub-Saharan Africa, the Subcontinent, South East Asia, remote areas of Australia and other places where accurate and timely assessment, diagnosis and management of neurodevelopmental disorders cannot be readily assumed to occur, where attitudes and beliefs about childhood disability may be at variance to those of developed nations, and where there is a need to adapt, adjust or event replace the standard means of assessing neurodevelopmental disorders in young children (Table 0.1).

Timeline

Table 0.1 Timeline of significant events

1805?	Jean Marc Gaspard Itard studies "the Wild Boy of Averyon"
1866	John Langdon Down and Eduard Seguin describe Down syndrome
1898	Bertillon Classification of Causes of Death (later to become the International Classification of Disease, or ICD) adopted by American Public Health Association, to be reviewed every 10 years
1905	Simon and Binet's "Metric Scale of Intelligence"
1908	Dr Eugen Bleuler introduces the term "autism"
1931	Merrill-Palmer Scale of Mental Tests
1933	California First Year Mental Scale (Bayley)
1936	Vineland Social Maturity Scale (Edgar Doll)
1940	Minnesota Preschool Scale (Goodenough)
1943	Leo Kanner describes Autism

(Continued)

Table 0.1 (Continued)

1944	Hans Asperger describes mild Autism
1949	ICD-6 released
1952	DSM first published (DSM-I)
1954	Griffith's "Abilities of Babies" 0–2 years test published
1955	ICD-7 released
1959	Genetic proof of Down syndrome (Lejeune)
1964	US Child Health and Mental Retardation Act
1965	ICD-8a released
1968	DSM II published
1969	Bayley Scales of Infant Development published
1970	Griffiths "Abilities of Young Children" and 0–8 years Test published
	US Developmental Disability Facilities and Construction Amendment
1971	UN Declaration of Rights of Persons with Mental Retardation
1975	UN Declaration of Rights of disabled persons
	US Public Law 94-142
	ICD-9 released
1980	DSM III released
1986	US Public Law 99-457
1987	DSM III-R released
1988	Childhood Autism Rating Scale (CARS) (Schopler) published
1990	ICD-10 released
1994	DSM IV released
1995	Mullen Scales of Early Learning published
1996	Revised Griffiths Scales (Rutter) published
1999	Autism Diagnostic Observation Schedule-Generic published
2000	DSM IV-TR released
2006	Second revision of Griffiths Scales (Luiz) published
	Bayley-3 published
2009	Childhood Autism Rating Scale-2 (CARS 2) published
2012	ADOS-2 published
2013	DSM 5 released
2016	Griffiths III published
2020	Bayley-4 published
	ICD-11 released
2022	DSM-5-TR released

Part I
Historical overview of neurodevelopmental disorders in young children

Part I explores the historical, social, scientific and political influences which defined and categorised neurodevelopmental disorders in young children and led to coherent and systematic approaches to assessment, diagnosis, treatment, education and support for young children with disordered or delayed development. Part I then explores the two universally accepted classificatory systems for defining the various neurodevelopmental disorders:

- The Diagnostic and Statistical Manual (DSM), currently DSM-5-TR.
- The International Classification of Diseases (ICD), currently ICD 11.

This part also outlines basic concepts of genetic disorders and syndromes and provides descriptions and historical perspectives on a range of such disorders and syndromes.

1 Historical overview of neurodevelopmental disorders in young children

Introduction

Children are born every minute of every day in every corner of the world, to a multitude of different families from differing ethnic origins, social and socio-economic circumstances. There is a universal expectation that newborn children will grow, develop, thrive and mature to become healthy and well, able and productive, independent and inquisitive, social and, in a vast variety of ways, successful, regardless of how those outcomes and virtues are defined in different cultures and peoples. However, for many families, these dreams and expectations are challenged and changed from an early age, sometimes from the point of birth or even during gestation, when their beloved and cherished offspring do not develop in the manner anticipated.

They may be born with genetic defects or anomalies, congenital medical conditions or predispositions. Or they may initially appear to be following expected growth and developmental trajectories only to experience unexplained delays, regressions or deviations in their progress. Or difficulty for many families in social and financial disadvantage, their children may be born into an expectation of struggle and difficulty. Children who experience and manifest these atypical developmental patterns are frequently referred to as having "neurodevelopmental disorders", whether arising from genetic inheritance or anomalies, medical conditions or through unknown aetiology.

Nowadays, such children can be "assessed", "diagnosed" and categorised through a plethora of sophisticated processes:

- Genetic tests, both in utero and in early life.
- MRI and CT scans.
- Blood and metabolic analyses.
- Systematic observation, measurement and assessment processes, including psychometric testing of developmental milestones, intelligence and social/emotional functioning and status.

In "developed" countries, access to these services is taken for granted, as are follow-up programmes, therapies and teaching/learning strategies specifically designed to "intervene early" in the difficulties and deficits arising from these various conditions. In "lesser developed countries", these services may not be readily available or even assumed to exist, and it cannot even be assumed that there is an equivalent level of understanding of childhood disability, delay or disorder.

DOI: 10.4324/9781003565338-3

10 *Diagnosing Young Children with Neurodevelopmental Disorders*

In advantaged, "developed" nations, there is an increasing expectation that such assessment, diagnostic and "early intervention" services will be available and financed at least in part through the public purse. Government-supported assessment, diagnostic and intervention programmes now proliferate in most developed nations as a matter of social health and welfare policy. The prognoses for children with chronic health and medical conditions, developmental delays and disorders in the Western world are now better than ever, but this has not always been the case, and it is valuable to revisit the historical journey that our understanding and acceptance of neurodevelopmental disorders has taken, both for general interest and to establish the lessons learned along the way.

Individual observations

The history of progression towards "scientific methods" of assessment and diagnosis, treatment and care, along with the assumption of responsibility by nation states and governments for these advances and services, can tell vital stories and teach important lessons.

The "story" of these trends can perhaps be seen to begin in the 18th century. Society has always had an interest in observing the behaviours of others, particularly when behavioural traits would appear to be "different", "unusual" or maladaptive. However, the application of "scientific method" to such observations of human behaviours, abilities and foibles is a relatively recent historical phenomenon. Individual case studies through detailed observation reflected the growing curiosity in natural variation, and perhaps the most famous illustration of early "one-to-one" observational practice is embodied in the story of the "Wild Boy of Aveyron" (Figure 1.1).

Victor of Aveyron was a French "feral child" who was found at around the age of twelve. Upon his discovery, he was given to many people to stay with but continually ran away. Eventually, his case was taken up by a young physician, Jean Marc Gaspard Itard, who worked with the boy for five years, giving him the name Victor. Itard was interested in determining what Victor could learn and devised various methods to teach the boy words and record his progress, including the equivalent to modern-day "flashcards".

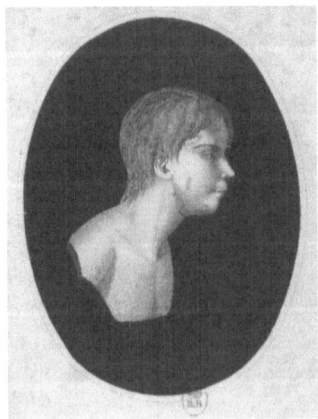

Figure 1.1 The "Wild Boy of Aveyron"

Victor is estimated to have been born around 1788, a normal child at birth, but neglected by his alcoholic parents from an early age. He then left civilisation and fended for himself in the wild. On January 8, 1800, he emerged from the forests on his own. His lack of speech, his food preferences and the numerous scars on his body suggested that he had been in the wild for most of his life.

A local abbot and biology professor examined him. The local government commissioner also observed the boy and wrote there was "something extraordinary in his behaviour, which makes him seem close to the state of wild animals". Despite his diligent efforts, Itard could not teach Victor to speak. He wondered why Victor would choose to remain silent when he was not deaf. Victor also did not understand tones of voice. Itard proclaimed, "Victor was the mental and psychological equivalent of someone born deaf-and-dumb".

Today, there are hypotheses that Victor, though born normal, developed a serious mental or psychological disturbance before his abandonment. Precocious schizophrenia, infantile psychosis or autism are amongst the technical terms that have been suggested as retrospective diagnoses. Victor's story was alluded to in the French television series "The Forest".

The development of scientific models

The 19th century was a time of great and sometimes controversial scientific progress and discovery, and never so much as in the growing exploration of the nature of humanity itself. Charles Darwin's "On the Origin of Species" was published in 1859 and sent shock waves through the scientific and religious orthodoxy. Particularly contentious was the proposition that humans evolved from other animal life forms such as apes, rather than springing into existence *de novo* by divine creation.

Humans and animals were increasingly the subject of scientific scrutiny, and in 1866, Doctor John Langdon Down, an English physician, wrote a paper entitled "Observations on the Ethnic Classification of Idiots", in which he described the characteristics of a condition which came to be known as Down syndrome. Genetic science and testing were not advanced at that point in history, and so Down's descriptions were mainly associated with the physical and behavioural characteristics of his subjects.

He made the observation, in language and idiom consistent with the times, that people with Down syndrome were displaying a "reversion to a primitive Mongolian ethnic stock". This inappropriate characterisation unfortunately came into common usage and led pejoratively to the syndrome being called "mongolism" for quite some time, before the term was repudiated by amongst others Reginald Down, John Langdon Down's son.

However, the significance of Down's work was that perhaps for the first time, significant human "difference" and dysfunction were able to be ascribed directly to evolutionary and developmental anomalies and not to cultural or religious myths, beliefs or legends. It was perhaps also the first time a developmental "phenotype" was described. John Langdon Down was also the first person to describe what is now known as Prader–Willi syndrome, which he called "polysarcia".

The rise of psychometrics

The 19th century also witnessed increasing interest in the notion of "generalised intelligence" and its measurement. Francis Galton was a scholar and researcher who obtained permission to establish an "anthropometric laboratory" at an international health exhibition. It was originally intended to refer to the management of physical characteristics but was equally interested in the measurement of psychological performance. This intersected with the work of American student, James Cattell, and together, they began to investigate variations in performance across different people.

Cattell subsequently established a psychological laboratory at the University of Pennsylvania to research "mental tests and measurements", but the American Psychological Association could not reach consensus about the best focus of standardised tests. British psychologist Charles Spearman claimed in 1904 that performance on specific tests depended upon both "general intelligence" and other specific traits or factors. Meanwhile, Alfred Binet and Victor Henri proposed an "individual psychology" where differences in "higher" mental functions such as memory and comprehension could be measured similarly to traits such as sensory processes.

In 1905, Binet and Simon introduced a "metric scale of intelligence" which differentiated between "idiocy", "imbecility" and "feeblemindedness". Binet's 1905 scale was able to measure intelligence in children from 3 to 15 years. It is interesting to review selected test items from this scale for the age range of 3–6 years and to compare these with the tasks now inherent in modern assessments of developmental skills in young children (Figure 1.2):

Although ostensibly theorising about human intelligence, Binet's work also illustrated the nexus between typically developing skills in childhood and "normal" development as a function of age. It is also worth noting however that much of the early research and development of standardised assessment tools was related not to children or their care and education, but to the more unsavoury task of "screening" immigrants arriving in New York Harbor at Ellis Island.

Any tourist visiting this facility cannot help but be moved by the stories of families being separated through "assessment" techniques based upon individual immigration officials' opinion of one's physical and mental aptitudes, and this remained the status quo until the pioneering works of Howard Knox, superintendent of Ellis Island in the early 20th century,

---

Three years

- Point to the nose, the eyes and the mouth.
- Name the objects in a picture.
- Repeat a sentence containing six syllables.
- Give one's family name.

Four years

- Give one's gender.
- Name a key, a knife and simple coinage.
- Repeat three digits.
- Compare two lines of different length.

Five years

- Compare two boxes of different weights.
- Copy a square.
- Repeat a sentence containing 10 syllables.
- Count four "pennies".
- Put together two triangles to make a rectangle.

Figure 1.2 Sample of Binet and Simon's 1909 test items

and psychologist Henry H. Goddard. There was an economic imperative for accurate "assessment and screening", with individual American states not wanting to be encumbered with "inappropriate labour" or "imbeciles". This was impressed upon the American federal government, and once the seed of formalised assessment was sown, it blossomed, and Knox's work added to the foundations laid by Binet, Cattell, Spearman, Galton and others. It was perhaps the first known instance of "eligibility criteria" being used.

Concurrently, interest was blossoming into aspects of the human condition such as mood and behaviour. Paul Eugen Bleuler was a Swiss psychiatrist who added much to the early understanding of psychiatric illness. He is noted for introducing such terms as "schizophrenia", as opposed to "dementia praecox" as was the practice of the day, as well as schizoid characteristics. In 1908, he referred to "abnormal associations", "autistic behaviour and thinking", abnormal affect and ambivalence.

This early usage of the term "autistic" was not as we would know it today, rather a description of some of the disconnection and remoteness that can accompany mental illness, and it was not until the early 1940s that Professor Leo Kanner and Doctor Hans Asperger made the first definitive descriptions of autism as we understand it today. Their personal stories and contributions to the science of psychology are compelling but in some respects controversial and will be the subject of a later chapter.

The early decades of the 20th century witnessed a veritable explosion in knowledge about child development, assessment and categorisation. By 1925, Gesell had compiled an item database of approximately 150 skills for his developmental schedule, encompassing motor skills, language skills, adaptive behaviour skills and personal-social skills. In 1931 came the Merrill-Palmer Scale of Mental Tests; in 1933 the California First-Year Mental Scale, with the involvement of a young Nancy Bayley; and in 1936 the Iowa Tests for Young Children. And in 1940, before the interruption caused by World War II, there was the Minnesota Preschool Scale, which included contributions by Florence Goodenough, later to develop the Goodenough–Harris "Draw-A-Man" test.

Meanwhile, in the United Kingdom, a young psychologist Doctor Ruth Griffiths began to formulate her interpretation of child developmental stages and skills, which she eventually called the "Avenues of Learning". Thus, at least 80 years ago, the foundations were laid for systematic psychometric assessment of the abilities of young children. Even at this early juncture, concerns were expressed about the core difficulties associated with assessing children so young-test reliability, predictive validity and score stability.

And it was not simply "performance-related" assessment tools that were developing during this period. Screening questionnaires for learning and adaptive behaviour skills came into being in the 1930s, including the original Vineland Social Maturity Scales as pioneered by Edgar Doll.

The social context

Knowledge of, and attitudes towards, people with disabilities have also changed over time, reflecting broader social beliefs, understandings, myths and falsehoods and also a gradual development of tolerance, understanding, insight and acceptance of people who were perceived as "different". The usage of terminology such as "mental defectives", "idiots" and "imbeciles" was often reflected in segregation of people with disabilities from broader society. Institutions were often established by both governments and religious institutions, and even if these were well intentioned, they were often examples of "good ideas and bad institutions".

Specific legislation and Acts of Parliament began to be passed in support of people with disabling conditions. In the United Kingdom, for example, the 1920 Blind Persons Act came into being, bringing forward access to the pension for people with visual impairments. But this trend was not helped by the rise of the Eugenics movement and the increasing use of IQ testing. People described as "feeble minded" were described as potentially "diluting the genetic pool", and as having the "prolific breeding habits of 'inferiors'". In Australia, for example, a 1929 Act of Parliament, fortunately never enacted, recommended the sterilisation of people with intellectual disabilities. The rise of Nazi Germany during the 1930s and 1940s was very much associated with the belief that the German "Aryan race" was "pure" and must in no way be diluted or compromised by any other "inferior" bloodline.

The immediate post–World War II period after 1945 witnessed a surge of compassion and energy focused upon the welfare of children, whether they were socially or financially disadvantaged, orphaned or disabled. Church and charity-administered schools and institutions were established for children with sensory disorders such as deafness and blindness and physical disabilities such as cerebral palsy. Many of these schools were eventually supported financially through government grants, and many in fact were subsumed into government services. Research blossomed into such conditions as phenylketonuria (PKU). The Oslo breakfast programme, first pioneered in Norway in 1932, spread to other European nations mindful of the plight of many children through the privations of war. In Australia, the "school milk" programme was introduced, providing a small bottle every day.

The development of disability rights and responsibilities

The progression towards care for people with disabilities gradually entered into legislation and "state" responsibility, for example the United Kingdom's Disabled Persons Employment Act of 1944 and the Chronically Sick and Disabled Persons Act of 1970. This move towards legislated support for people disabilities was driven significantly by movements in the United States. In fact, the 1960s in the United States of America came to be regarded as "the golden age" in the understanding of childhood developmental issues and the provision of appropriate services, as evidenced by:

- In 1964, the United States Government ratified the Child Health and Mental Retardation Act.
- Early intervention programmes such as Head Start and Follow Through commenced.
- The children's television programme Sesame Street, itself a direct outcome from such programmes, first aired in the United States in 1969.

At the same time, there was a resurgence of research into assessments for young children. It is estimated that at least 120 individual tests were subject to development and review during this period, comprising over 630 individual subtests. Again, much of the focus of research was related to issues of predictive validity and reliability. Amongst those achieving positive reviews at that time were tests devised by McCarthy, Kaufmann and Vineland.

The conceptualisation of childhood development was changing and growing, and this increased knowledge needed to be reflected in the structure and layout of assessments, for example, the growing understanding of the vital developmental changes, which occurred in young children at approximately 18 months of age. In particular, the shift towards symbolic thought processes ("cognitive revelation") and problem-solving skills was recognised. For individual item development and selection, this meant that emphasis could not merely focus upon psychomotor skills, although these were seen as the "easiest" to measure accurately.

Global socio-political forces were also at work and influential in changes to both attitudes and practices in disability services. In 1968, the International League of Societies for the Mentally Retarded produced a statement of rights for people with intellectual disabilities, and this was followed in short order by two statements by the United Nations:

- The 1971 United Nations declaration of the rights of persons with mental retardation.
- The 1975 United Nations declaration of rights of disabled persons.

The impact of these declarations was profound, and in 1975, the understanding of developmental delays and disorders took on an entirely new dimension in the United States with the ratification of Public Law 94-142. Public Laws in the United States are emblematic of the complex relationship between the Federal Government and individual state jurisdictions. Public Laws lay down overarching policies and goals and broad parameters around attaining these goals. To an extent, Public Laws dictate what individual states are required to undertake and to achieve, but not necessarily how to do so. There is however a clear nexus between the parameters of the individual Public Laws and the granting of Federal funds to individual states to comply with these.

Passed in 1975, Public Law 94-142 guaranteed a free appropriate public education to each and every child with a disability. This law had a dramatic, positive impact on countless numbers of children in every state and local community across the country. The four purposes of the law articulated a compelling national mission to improve access to education for children with disabilities. Changes implicit in the law included efforts to

a Improve how children with disabilities were identified and educated.
b Evaluate the success of these efforts.
c Provide due process protections for children and families.
d In addition, the law authorised financial incentives to enable states and localities to comply with Public Law 94-142. The four purposes are detailed as follows:

- To assure that all children with disabilities have available to them a free appropriate public education, which emphasises special education and related services designed to meet their unique needs.
- To assure that the rights of children with disabilities and their parents are protected.
- To assist states and localities to provide for the education of all children with disabilities.
- To assess and assure the effectiveness of efforts to educate all children with disabilities.

In other words, individual states and school boards were required to provide equal educational opportunities for all children of school age, including those with disabilities. Preschool-aged children did not factor into these provisions until 1986 and the enactment of Public Law 99-457. This law necessitated individual states to make available appropriate and free public education to children ages 3 through 5 who were disabled. The law made a requirement for states that offered interdisciplinary educational services to disabled toddlers, infants and their families, to receive financial grants.

These financial grants acted as incentives for states to provide for children from birth to age 2 with disabilities. Public Law 99-457 also stimulated, and to a degree stipulated, the development and validation of infant development schedules and tests. For example, developmental tests were required to produce not just scores and/or diagnoses but also recommendations for education and "remediation".

The global context

Although there is not a direct correlation between the United States Public Laws mandating services for children with disabilities and events which occurred elsewhere, there are of course similarities. Australia, for example, progressed through the following legislations and acts:

- The Commonwealth Government Handicapped Persons Assistance Act of 1974.
- The 1992 Disability Discrimination Act.
- The 1994 disability services standards for services funded under the Commonwealth Disability Services Act of 1986.
- The Disability Services Act of 1996.

Similarly in the United Kingdom, came:

- The Disability Discrimination Act 1995 (amended in 2005).
- The Special Educational Needs and Disability Act 2001.
- The Equality Act 2010.

In South Africa, support legislation for people with disabilities was a complex process, tied to the long and bitter struggle towards unification and the end of apartheid. Under that policy, the inequalities and divisions between people prevented black people from accessing many basic rights. In 1981, the government established a committee called the Inter-departmental Co-ordinating Committee on Disability (ICCD), which was tasked with advising the government on policy reform in response to the World Programme of Action Concerning Disabled Persons (1982).

Nelson Mandela, the first black president of South Africa from 1994 to 1996 following the country's first fully representative election, set about the task of dismantling the policies associated with apartheid, and the new constitution and associated legislative changes recognised the need to address the disadvantages that particular groups of people had experienced in the past. This new constitution included the provision that no unfair discrimination could occur on the basis of disability.

In November 1997, a White Paper on an Integrated National Disability Strategy, known as INDS, was implemented. The INDS provided guidelines to promote non-discriminatory development planning, programme implementation and service delivery. There were also a "White Paper" on Special Needs Education provision and amendments to existing legislation to expand the scope of the Social Assistance Act of 1992, introducing child support grants, which eventually included specific grants for children with disabilities.

Canada progressed from a nation which legislated in favour of legal sterilisation of people with mental health disabilities in the 1930s (legal in the provinces of Alberta and British Columbia until the 1970s), through deinstitutionalisation in the 1950s and 1960s, to the Canadian Human Rights Act and the Employment Equity Act in the 1980s. The

1. **Rights:** The service promotes individual rights to freedom of expression, self-determination and decision-making and actively prevents abuse, harm, neglect and violence.

2. **Participation and Inclusion:** The service works with individuals and families, friends and carers to promote opportunities for meaningful participation and active inclusion in society.

3. **Individual Outcomes:** Services and supports are assessed, planned, delivered and reviewed to build on individual strengths and enable individuals to reach their goals.

4. **Feedback and Complaints:** Regular feedback is sought and used to inform individual and organisation-wide service reviews and improvement.

5. **Service Access:** The service manages access, commencement and leaving a service in a transparent, fair, equal and responsive way.

6. **Service Management:** The service has effective and accountable service management and leadership to maximise outcomes for individuals.

Figure 1.3 Australian Disability Services Act, National Standards

discrimination against people with disabilities is prohibited by the Canadian Human Rights Act of 1985, and this along with the Charter of Rights and Freedoms, enacted in 1982, guarantees that persons with disabilities are protected by and will receive the same benefits under the law as any other Canadian.

This is in contrast to Australia, which does not have in its constitution a Bill of Rights for citizens. However, the set of "Disability Service Standards", first created in 1993 and fully adopted in 2014, laid out very clearly the role of service providers for people with disabilities and what people with disabilities should be able to expect and assume. They are universal (Figure 1.3).

There is now universal recognition of the rights of people with disabilities to live as normal and unrestricted a life as possible, and that governments of all persuasions have an undeniable responsibility to ensure as far as possible that these rights are protected and realised. The manner in which these lofty goals are achieved varies from country to country, state to state, regime to regime and culture to culture, reflecting various factors:

- The centralised or decentralised nature of governance.
- The relationship between central government and state, provincial, regional or local management of human affairs.
- The economic and financial circumstances of individual nations and the manner in which these impact upon the distribution and provision of appropriate support, facilities and services.

There are many and various examples of how disability support provisions are provided across the globe, particularly for young children with neurodevelopmental disorders. There are government and non-government early intervention and specialist school programmes, therapy services, medical and paediatric assessment and diagnostic services. These must be crafted to suit the specific cultural, economic and logistic factors of individual nations, but the "bottom line" remains the same.

Such services come at a considerable cost, either to individual families or to national, state or local governments. Financial support programmes have proliferated to help families defray the costs of assessments, treatments, programmes, therapies and specific technologies and equipment. The sheer numbers involved are worth considering.

Latest research suggests that globally, approximately 53 million children under the age of 5 years have developmental disorders. Of these, some 2.7 million live in "high-income" countries, while the other 95% reside in "less developed nations" (LDNs). This significant imbalance in the global distribution of neurodevelopmental disorders is the subject of a later chapter. But wherever such disability occurs, it is increasingly the responsibility of governments not only to provide services for these children, either directly or indirectly, but also to fund either in part or *in toto* the associated costs.

Not surprisingly, governments endeavour to "manage" these financial and logistical aspirational as best they can, and specifying "eligibility criteria" is a natural and logical response. Accurate diagnostic assessment therefore serves not only clinical goals and outcomes, but also "systems-orientated" needs such as management and distribution of services, budgetary restrictions and "down-stream" service provision.

Thus, there have been both "push and pull" factors associated with the ongoing development of assessment tools and service provision for young children. There has been a growing knowledge base of the type, frequency and causation of developmental delays and disorders in young children, and a need to quantify these, and at the same time a clearly mandated legislative requirement to provide accurate comprehensive assessments so that appropriate early intervention services can be provided but within the financial capacities of families and governments.

The changing knowledge of neurodevelopmental disorders

We live in a time of great scientific enlightenment, and through this, medical science can explain and prove many of the underlying causes and "risk factors" associated with developmental delays and disorders. Reference is made to "biological risk", "established risk" and "environmental risk". Gone from the "developed" world are notions of witchcraft, changelings, divine retribution and "bad" parenting, and instead, we have scientifically based and demonstrable causative factors such as prenatal, perinatal and postnatal events and circumstances. Of course, there are always disbelievers and cynics, and "mysteries" do occur. To this day, for example, there is no clear view as to the cause of autism spectrum disorder (Table 1.1).

The concept of a "developmental disability" gained legal status in the United States through the 1970 Developmental Disabilities and Facilities Construction Amendment, and the nomenclature was eventually adopted in other countries. For example, in Australia, the New South Wales Health Commission changed its "Division of Mental Retardation" to "Division of Developmental Disability". Changes in nomenclature highlighted the need of government to support all disabilities and not just intellectual disability.

These factors are increasingly incorporated into the successive editions of the DSM and the ICD. These two classificatory systems are currently referred to as DSM-5-TR and ICD 11, and in recent years, efforts have been made to "synchronise" the nomenclature and coding systems for most neurodevelopmental disorders. A thorough understanding of the diagnostic criteria for developmental disorders and disabilities as defined in these classificatory systems is imperative for the process of making timely, accurate and appropriate diagnoses of disabling conditions in young children.

Table 1.1 Factors underlying neurodevelopmental disorders

Prenatal	Perinatal	Postnatal
Chromosomal disorders	Intrauterine disorders	Head injuries
Syndrome disorders	Neonatal disorders	Infections
Inborn metabolism errors		Demyelinating disorders
Disorders of brain formation		Degenerative disorders
Environmental influences		Seizure disorders
Other non-specific influences		Toxic-metabolic disorders
		Malnutrition
		Environmental deprivation
		Hypoconnection syndromes

Today, children can be assessed as necessary from the moment of birth, in fact before in some circumstances. There are *in utero* genetic tests such as amniocenteses and detailed measures taken at birth such as APGAR scores. Children born significantly prematurely and underweight ("small for dates") are closely monitored in neonatal intensive care units and receive follow-up reviews and assessments in their formative years.

Early childhood intervention programmes proliferate to assist young children with delayed or problematic developmental histories or neurodevelopmental or genetic disorders. National, state and local governments have realised the importance of early intervention support for children and families, both through direct service provision and funding support to families.

The foundation to utilising these services remains the timely, systematic and accurate appraisal of young children, accomplished by the various professions working together. The role of psychologists in this process is fundamental in its value and purpose.

Bibliography

American Psychiatric Association (2022), Diagnostic and Statistical Manual (5th Edition, Text Revision; DSM-5-TR), American Psychiatric Association.
Ashok, A. H., Baugh, J., and Yeragani, V. (2012), "Paul Eugen Bleuler and the Origin of the Term Schizophrenia", Indian Journal of Psychiatry, 54(1), pp 95–96.
Asperger, H. (1944), "Die Autistischen Psychpathen in Kindersalter", Archiv Fur Psychiatrie und Nervenkrankheiten, 117, pp 76–136.
Bolajoko, O., et al. (2018), "Developmental Disabilities Among Children Younger than 5 years in 195 Countries and Territories, 1990–2016: A Systematic Analysis for the Global Burden of Disease Study 2016", The Lancet, 6(10), pp E100–E1121.
Cocks, E. (1998), An Introduction to Intellectual Disability in Australia. Australian Institute on Intellectual Disability.
Down, J. L. (1866), "Observations on an Ethnic Classification of Idiots", London Hospital Reports, 3, pp 259–262.
Galer, D. (2015), Disability Rights Movement in Canada, The Canadian Encyclopedia.
Goddard, H. H. (1917), "Mental Tests and the Immigrant", Journal of Delinquency, 2(5), pp 243–277.
Griffiths, R. (1970), The Abilities of Young Children: A Comprehensive System of Mental Measurement for the First Eight Years of Life, ARICD and University of London Press.
Individuals with Disabilities Education Act (2024), "A History of the Individuals With Disabilities Education Act". https://www.ed.gov/laws-and-policy/individuals-disabilities/idea#:~:text=The%20 Individuals%20with%20Disabilities%20Education,for%20infants%20and%20toddlers%20and.
Jarrett, S. (2023), A History of Disability in England, Liverpool University Press.
Jones, L. V., and Thissen, D. (2007), "A History and Overview of Psychometrics", In Rao, C. R. and Sinharay, S. (Eds.), Handbook of Statistics (Vol. 26), Elsevier, pp 1–27.

Kanner, L. (1943), "Autistic Disturbances of Affective Contact", Nervous Child, 2, pp 217–250.

Lane, H. (1976), The Wild Boy of Aveyron. Harvard University Press.

Meisels, S. (1984), "Prediction, Prevention and Developmental Screening in the EPSDS Program", In Stevenson, H. W. and Siegel, A. E. (Eds.), Child Development Research and Social Policy, University of Chicago Press.

Meisels, S., and Atkins-Burnett, B. (2005), Developmental Screening in Early Childhood: A Guide (5th Edition), National Association for the Education of Young Children.

Moodley, S. (2021), "Children with Disabilities in South Africa: Policies for Early Identification and Education", In Pearson Jr., W. and Reddy, V. (Eds.), Social Justice in the 21st Century: Research from South Africa and USA, Springer, pp 95–112.

OECD Family Database, Social Policy Division (2022), "Child Disability", in Disability, Work and Inclusion, OECD. https://www.oecd.org/en/topics/policy-issues/social-policy.html.

Reed, G. M., et al. (2019), "Innovations and Changes in the ICD-11 Classification of Mental, Behavioural and Neurodevelopmental Disorders", World Psychiatry, 18(1), pp 3–19.

Richardson, J. T. (2011), "Howard Andrew Knox: Pioneer of Intelligence Testing at Ellis Island", Columbia University Press.

Selikowitz, M. (2008), Down Syndrome, Oxford University Press.

United Nations Department of Economic and Social Affairs Disability and Development Report (2018). https://social.desa.un.org/publications/un-flagship-report-on-disability-and-development-2024.

Ward, O. C. (1999), "John Langton Down: The Man and the Message", Down Syndrome Research and Practice, 6(1), pp 19–24.

World Health Organisation (2015), International Statistical Classification of Diseases and Related Health Problems Volume 11, World Health Organisation. https://www.who.int/standards/classifications/classification-of-diseases.

2 What is a neurodevelopmental disorder?

To understand this terminology, psychologists should be familiar with two systems of categorisation for disorders of development in young children: The Diagnostic and Statistical Manual (DSM) and the International Classification of Diseases (ICD). DSM-5-TR (Text Revision) is the current edition of the former, having superseded the previous DSM 5 in 2022, whilst the latter, originally known as the "Bertillon Classification of Causes of Death", is currently referred to as ICD-11. DSM has generally been the more popular classificatory "system of choice", for psychologists, but the similarities and subtle differences between their perspectives on developmental disorders in children are important. For the most recent iterations of both, there has been a concerted effort to "harmonise" DSM-5-TR and ICD-11 diagnostic classifications, criteria and codes.

DSM as a diagnostic manual had its origins in the early 1800s in the United States through concerns as to how to classify such conditions known then as "idiocy" and "insanity". In 1921, the American Medico-Psychological Association became the American Psychiatric Association (APA) and developed the "American Medical Association's Standard Classified Nomenclature of Disease". Following the inclusion of selected mental disorders in ICD-6 after World War II and the deleterious impact of battle upon servicemen and women, the APA developed its own version, DSM-I, in 1952. DSM-I was the first official manual and glossary of mental disorders with a focus on clinical use. Subsequent editions of DSM took an "agnostic approach" to the aetiology of mental disorders, focusing on explicit diagnostic criteria. DSM-III is regarded as heralding the start of "modern psychiatric diagnosis".

DSM-5-TR refers to a cluster of conditions known as "neurodevelopmental disorders". These by necessity feature onset in the early developmental period and are characterised by "developmental deficits that produce impairments of personal, social, academic, or occupational functioning, ranging from highly specific limitations of function to global impairment". This category includes:

- Intellectual disabilities (including global developmental delay).
- Communication disorders.
- Autism spectrum disorder.
- Attention deficit hyperactivity disorder.
- Specific learning disorder.
- Motor disorders.
- Tic disorders.
- Other neurodevelopmental disorders.

DOI: 10.4324/9781003565338-4

Specific neurodevelopmental disorders often "co-exist", referred to as "co-morbidity", and may be characterised by symptoms ranging from "excesses" of certain behaviours and features to deficits and delays in others. Over the course of the various iterations of DSM, most of the above diagnoses have been included, but with changes in nomenclature, sub-categorisation and descriptive breadth, through DSM III, DSM III R, DSM IV, DSM IV TR (Text Revision), DSM 5 and now DSM-5-TR. The one notable exception was the inclusion of Global Developmental Delay in DSM 5, the first edition to have defined this disorder. As well as diagnostic criteria, DSM-5-TR includes "specifiers" to delineate clearly between conditions, to clarify clinical features such as the age of onset or level of severity of symptoms, and to highlight possible associations with known medical or genetic conditions or disorders.

A thorough reading and understanding of both DSM-5-TR and ICD-11 is important for psychologists engaged in child development assessments and diagnoses. Although psychologists are not medical practitioners, they should also have some understanding of the "three-tiered categorisation system" of possible causes of neurodevelopmental disorders:

- Prenatal, perinatal and postnatal causative factors such as birth history and complications.
- Genetic influences such as known genetic and chromosomal anomalies.
- Environmental influences such as socio-economic factors, substance use and abuse and acquired injury.

This descriptive schema frequently refers to conditions with relatively clear medical, genetic or environmental causation factors, and as such, many do not appear in DSM-5-TR but in medical and scientific literature. There have been massive advances in the science of genetic assessment and diagnosis, leading to greatly enhanced accuracy and conceptualisation. Paediatricians, particularly in the "developed" world, have at their disposal excellent training and experience, along with extensive texts and medical resources about such conditions, their causation, prognoses and impacts. Psychologists should continue to develop their understanding of these conditions, because even though they are not medical practitioners, they benefit from a grounding in the theories and practices of medical science to understand the issues associated with the referrals they will receive and the families they will become involved with.

This is particularly important in understanding that children with clearly diagnosed medical or genetic diagnoses can, but not necessarily will, experience developmental delays and disorders. Sometimes the interactions between known medical and genetic conditions and neurodevelopmental disorders will lead to complex behavioural, developmental and diagnostic presentations, requiring careful consideration in the formulation of diagnostic hypotheses.

Neurodevelopmental disorders defined by DSM-5-TR

- Intellectual development disorder (intellectual disability) (ICD-11 code 6A00).
- Unspecified intellectual disorder (Intellectual disability) (ICD-11 code 6A00).
- Global developmental delay (ICD-11 code 6A00).
- Language disorder (ICD-11, Developmental Language Disorder Code 6A01.2).

- Autism spectrum disorder (ICD-11 code 6A02).
- Attention deficit/Hyperactivity disorder (ICD-11 code 6A05).
- Other specified attention-deficit/Hyperactivity disorder (ICD-11 code 6A05).
- Unspecified attention-deficit hyperactivity disorder (ICD-11 code 6A05.Z).
- Specific learning disorder.
- Developmental coordination disorder (ICD-11 code 6A04).
- Stereotypic movement disorder (ICD-11 code 8A0Z).
- Tic Disorders 307.20 (ICD code 8A05).
  - Tourette's disorder (ICD-11 code 8A05.00).
  - Persistent (Chronic) motor or vocal Tic disorder (ICD-11 codes 8A05.1 and 8A05.2).

These disorders have been described and conceptualised differently over successive iterations of DSM and ICD, as knowledge and understanding of these conditions have expanded, and it is a valuable exercise to follow the historical course and formulation of some of these diagnoses, through successive editions of DSM and ICD.

DSM-5-TR intellectual developmental disorder (intellectual disability)

Intellectual developmental disorder (intellectual disability) is defined as "a disorder with onset during the developmental period that includes both intellectual and adaptive functioning deficits in conceptual, social, and practical domains". There must be

- Deficits in intellectual functions confirmed by both clinical assessment and individualised standardised intelligence testing.
- Deficits in adaptive functioning that result in failure to meet developmental and sociocultural standards, with onset occurring during the developmental period.

Levels of severity are specified, ranging from profound through to mild, with reference to specific conceptual, social and practical skills at different age levels:

F70: Mild.
F71: Moderate.
F72: Severe.
F73: Profound.

The importance of these criteria is that it is often aligned to the philosophical basis of support funding schemes, with their emphasis upon developing increased functionality and independence over time, through specific therapeutic, educational and medical supports and treatments. Access to such support funding can in some instances be dependent on evidence of such progress.

ICD-11 intellectual development disorder (6A00.2)

A major change in ICD-11 is the change from reference to "mental retardation", to its current "disorders of intellectual development". These continue to be defined on the basis of significant limitations in intellectual functioning and adaptive behaviour, determined by individualised standardised testing, but with specific reference to the fact that in some countries, cultures and circumstances, such assessments may not be possible.

Global developmental delay

DSM-5-TR stipulates that:

> This diagnosis is reserved for individuals under the age of five years when the clinical severity level cannot be reliably assessed during early childhood. This category is diagnosed when an individual fails to meet expected milestones in several areas of intellectual functioning and applies to individuals who are unable to undergo systematic assessments of intellectual functioning, including children who are too young to participate in standardised testing. This category requires reassessment after a period of time.

DSM 5, released in 2013, marked the first appearance of global developmental delay as a discrete diagnosis. Psychologists engaged in assessments of children under the age of five years, using psychometric assessments tools such as Griffiths III or Bayley-4, may rightly be concerned about this diagnostic criterion. Assessments of developmental delay, using developmental tests such as Griffiths or Bayley, are by definition conducted "thorough systematic, standardised testing".

This begs the question as to how, without such assessments, it could accurately be determined whether a child is failing to meet "expected milestones" in several areas of functioning. This is the primary purpose of such assessments. It should also be noted that DSM-5-TR makes no reference through specifiers, to levels of global developmental delay, whether profound, severe, moderate or mild. It is essentially a matter of the psychologist's clinical judgement to make such determinations on the basis of assessment results and clinical expertise.

Unspecified intellectual developmental disorder (intellectual disability) F79

New to DSM-5-TR, this is defined as referring to:

> Individuals over the age of 5 years when assessment of the degree of intellectual developmental disorder (intellectual disability) by means of locally available procedures is rendered difficult or impossible because of associated sensory or physical impairments, as in blindness or prelingual deafness; locomotor disability; or presence of severe problem behaviours or co-occurring mental disorder. This category should only be used in exceptional circumstances and requires reassessment after a period of time.

By comparison, ICD-11 describes "Mental, behavioural or neurodevelopmental disorders, unspecified" (code 6E8Z).

Language disorder F80.2

A number of specific disorders of language are specified in DSM-5-TR covering expressive and receptive language, stuttering and fluency and speech sound disorders. These are of great interest but are more germane to the skills and roles of speech pathologists. However, one specific category is of importance to psychologists-social (pragmatic) communication disorder (F80.82), defined as:

- "Deficits in using communication for social purposes".
- "Impairment of the ability to change communication to match context".
- "Difficulties following rules for conversation and storytelling".
- "Difficulties understanding what is not explicitly stated".

During the 1990s, there was considerable professional debate around the possible term "Semantic Pragmatic Disorder". Such a diagnosis did not eventuate, but social (pragmatic) communication disorder may have risen from the ashes of those deliberations when it first appeared in DSM 5 in 2013, as the criteria relate closely to the semantic and pragmatic skills required to initiate and sustain effective social communication.

Impairment of such skills needs to be considered in any assessment of mild autism spectrum disorder, as there are obvious parallels with some of the traits described therein. Whether social (pragmatic) communication disorder is a valid or useful description for preschool-aged children is debatable.

Autism spectrum disorder F84.0

The 2013 DSM 5 categorisation of autism spectrum disorder marked a major conceptual shift from previous descriptions. It referred to "Persistent deficits" in social communication and social interaction across multiple contexts, i.e.

1 Deficits in social-emotional reciprocity.
2 Deficits in nonverbal communicative behaviours.
3 Deficits in developing, maintaining and understanding relationships.

Restricted, repetitive patterns of behaviour, interests or activities, i.e.

1 Stereotyped or repetitive motor movements, use of objects or speech.
2 Insistence on sameness, inflexible adherence to routines or ritualised patterns of verbal or nonverbal behaviour.
3 Highly restricted, fixated interests that are abnormal in intensity or focus.
4 Hyper, or hyporeactivity to sensory input or unusual interest in sensory aspects of the environment.

The understanding of autism spectrum disorder, as reflected in sequential iterations of DSM and ICD, has changed significantly over the last 30 years.

DSM III-R detailed "Infantile Autism", whilst DSM-IV described "Pervasive Developmental Disorders" such as Autistic Disorder, Asperger's Disorder, Rett's Syndrome, Childhood Disintegrative Disorder and Pervasive Developmental Disorder (Not Otherwise Specified). Similarly, ICD-10 referred to "Childhood Autism", "Atypical Autism", "Rett's Syndrome", Asperger's Syndrome and "Pervasive Developmental Disorder, Unspecified". These changes reflect a gradual broadening of the "Autism Spectrum" and an appreciation of its complex and varied presentation.

Prior to any DSM or ICD definitions, less scientific and considered descriptors were applied to those who would appear to have had autism spectrum disorder. Reference has already been made to "Victor" the wild boy of Averyon, but other children were referred to as "wolf children", "aliens" or "changelings". Doctor Eugen Bleuler, when introducing the term "autism" to the field of psychiatry in 1908, linked it to behaviours associated with schizophrenia.

Freudian influence at the turn of the 20th century also spoke of "childhood mania" and eventually "childhood schizophrenia", but it was not until Professor Leo Kanner's breakthrough publication in 1943 that the word "Autism" gained respected currency (Table 2.1).

Table 2.1 Changes in diagnostic criteria for autism spectrum disorder, 1943–2023

	KANNER 1943	DSM III 1980	DSM-IV 1994	DSM-5-TR 2013
NAME	Extreme Autistic Loneliness	Infantile Autism	Autistic Disorder, within PDD Category	Autism Spectrum Disorder
PREVALENCE		1/10,000	10–15/10,000	1/100 Approx.
ONSET		Before 30 months	Prior to age 3	Symptoms noted in second year of life
SOCIAL	• Avoidance of eye contact • Lack of visual/auditory response to others • Socially aloof	• Pervasive lack of response to other people	• Qualitative impairment in reciprocal social interaction	• Deficits in social-emotional reciprocity • Deficits in developing, maintaining and understanding relationships
COMMUNICATION	• Non-initiation of sounds or gestures • Failure to use speech for communication	• Gross deficits in language, and peculiar speech patterns	• Qualitative impairment in communication	• Deficits in social communication across multiple contexts
OTHER	• Sameness seeking • Abnormal mannerisms • Evidence of normal to superior intelligence	• Bizarre responses to various aspects of the environment	• Restricted and stereotyped patterns of behaviour, interests and activities	• Restricted, repetitive patterns of behaviour, interests and activities • Stereotyped or repetitive motor movements • Insistence on sameness and rigid routines • Highly restricted, fixated interests • Hyper- or hyporeactivity to sensory input
RELATED DISORDERS	• Heller's syndrome (Childhood disintegrative disorder)	• Disintegrative psychosis	• Rett's, Childhood Disintegrative Disorder, Asperger's Disorder, PDD (NOS)	• Rett syndrome • Selective mutism • Language disorders • Intellectual disability • Stereotypic movement disorder

There are two people stand out in the history and understanding of autism spectrum disorder, both psychiatrists: Leo Kanner and Hans Asperger. Their stories could not be more different.

Leo Kanner

Leo Kanner was an Austrian-American psychiatrist, physician and social activist. He was originally trained as a cardiologist and worked in Berlin before moving to the United States to escape the crippling economic circumstances that bedevilled post-World War I Germany. Based in South Dakota, he studied paediatrics and entered the field of psychiatry on a scholarship. His social activism and concern for the mentally ill led to improvements in the treatment of individuals with mental health issues, most notably when a group of men in and around Baltimore, previously institutionalised with mental health disorders, were "released" into the community to be used as servants and domestics without pay. The publicity that Kanner generated in support of these men and their rights was instrumental in leading to significant changes in support for people with such disorders. Kanner also helped rescue hundreds of Jewish physicians from Nazi Germany before and during World War II, assisting in relocating them to work in the United States.

Starting in 1938, Kanner began observing a group of eleven of his young in-patients and in 1943 wrote his seminal paper "Autistic Disturbances of Affective Contact". Each one of the eleven were individually named and described in detail. Kanner later served as the Chief of Child Psychiatry at Johns Hopkins University until his retirement in 1959. He continued to publish papers on autism until 1973. He died in 1981. Not shy of publicity, Kanner can still be seen being interviewed for television on video clips available online.

When first defined in 1943 by Professor Leo Kanner as "Extreme Autistic Aloneness" or "Extreme Autistic Aloofness", the emphasis was on severe autism. There was an abiding lack of social and communication behaviours and skills, and at the same time an excessive presence of abnormal mannerisms.

Hans Asperger

Hans Asperger was an Austrian physician known for his early studies of atypical neurology in young children. He studied medicine at the University of Vienna and became director of the special education section at the university's children's clinic in 1932. According to his daughter, two events greatly affected Hans Asperger between 1931 and 1945, the development of "curative education" (Heilpädagogik) and the ideology of National Socialism. Curative education is an interdisciplinary approach to providing holistic support to individuals with "significant challenges" to their development. It is often linked to educational philosophies such as the Rudoph Steiner methods.

Although there is no direct evidence that Asperger was ever a formal member of the Nazi Party, he was described as having relationships Nazi ideologues and sympathisers. During World War II, Asperger was a medical officer, serving in the Axis occupation of Yugoslavia. Near the end of the war, Asperger opened a school for children, but this was bombed and destroyed, and much of Asperger's early work was lost. Controversy surrounds more recent archival discoveries concerning Asperger's role in sending children with disabilities to the notorious "Am Spiegelgrund" Clinic in Vienna, where many were simply euthanised. He also made decisions as to the fate of young children who were deemed "uneducable". The suggestion is made that although Asperger did not necessarily support or recommend euthanasia, nor did he openly object to it. Asperger returned to his academic career after the end of World War II and eventually died in 1980.

In 1944, Hans Asperger reported his observations of individuals with milder traits of Autism than described by Kanner, describing an "autistic psychopathy of childhood". He identified in over 200 children a pattern of behaviour and skills, including "lack of empathy, poor ability to make friends, unidirectional conversation, strong preoccupation with special interests, and awkward movements". Asperger referred to these boys as "little teachers" because of their ability to talk about their favourite subject in great detail. His works, originally written in German, were finally and definitively translated into English in 1991 by the Developmental Psychologist Uta Frith. Prior to this, interest in his research and writing had been rekindled by English researcher Lorna Wing who in 1981 wrote in support of his findings. Although Asperger's work was obscure to the broader western world for some decades, the concept of "eccentric men" was culturally understood in literature and film of the day. For example, the 1953 movie "Time Bomb" featured the train obsessed savant "old Charlie".

The formalisation and acceptance of "Autistic conditions" began with DSM III, which referred to "Infantile Autism", characterised by "a serious lack of social response", "gross language deficit", "bizarre features of speech", "excessively disturbed social and emotional relationships", "oddities of motor movements" and self-mutilation. By the mid-1970s, Professor Michael Rutter was referring to "impaired social development", "delayed and deviant" language development and "insistence on sameness". DSM III-R described autistic disorder as a pervasive developmental disorder, with such symptoms as a lack of empathy, aloofness, a lack of imitation, no or abnormal social play and a lack of friendships. By the publication of DSM IV in 1994 and then DSM IV-TR, the emphasis was upon "qualitative impairments" in social and communicative skills, and "restricted and stereotyped" patterns of behaviour and interests. Reference was made to the "Triad of Impairments"-Communication, Social and Behaviour.

Formal criteria for the diagnosis of Aspergers Disorder first appeared in DSM-IV at this time. Perhaps the most significant conceptual change occurring between DSM IV-TR and DSM 5 was the removal of individual "subtypes" of autism, replaced instead by an overarching "Autism Spectrum Disorder" label. DSM IV-TR included Autistic Disorder; Asperger's Disorder; Rett Syndrome; Childhood Disintegrative Disorder; and Pervasive Developmental Disorder (not otherwise specified). The removal of Rett syndrome is easily understood. Evidencing the ongoing research into genetic disorders, Rett syndrome was found to be the direct result of a genetic mutation, and therefore inappropriate for DSM classification.

The removal of Asperger's disorder marked the conclusion of a long-running debate about what Professor Hans Asperger actually said and meant, and how this was interpreted over time. He described a cohort of individuals less severely affected, with a probable "organic basis" to the disorder, and a familial tendency. Although his descriptions and perceptions of such individuals were detailed and vivid, he did not provide clear diagnostic criteria. He did however make specific note of the gender imbalance in the prevalence of this behavioural constellation, referring to his observed subjects as "the extreme manifestation of the male personality". When Asperger's disorder was later described in DSM IV, males were said to outnumber females 10:1.

After a considerable period of neglect, the 1980s and 1990s saw international research interest return to Asperger's work and findings, most notably driven by Doctors Christopher Gilberg, Michael Rutter, Peter Szatmari and Tony Attwood. Formal adoption of the term

Asperger's Disorder occurred in DSM IV and generated considerable debate as to whether it may in fact be a separate and discrete condition or simply part of a broad spectrum of autistic disorders. These deliberations were long and drawn-out, but by the release of DSM 5 in 2013, it was determined that Asperger himself was right: His descriptions were of a mild variant of autism, and therefore consistent with a "spectrum" of autistic disorders.

Similarly, there was insufficient evidence to suggest that childhood disintegrative disorder constituted a valid and sustainable diagnostic classification, but the removal of pervasive developmental disorder (not otherwise specified) (PDD-NOS) has for some been problematic. This diagnosis was often reserved for cases of very young children, (particularly younger than 30 months), where there was some but not sufficient "autistic" symptomatology to confirm a diagnosis of autistic disorder, and when the child by virtue of his/her age was not yet able to engage in formal preschool programmes or therapeutic interventions. This diagnosis was sometimes referred to colloquially as "Atypical Autism" or the "wait and see" diagnosis. The latter term is reflective of the rapid changes in development, which can occur in young children after 30 months of age.

It is therefore of interest to note that the current "gold standard" for assessment and diagnosis of autism spectrum disorder, the Autism Diagnostic Observation Schedule 2 (ADOS 2) includes a "Toddler's Module" for children aged 12–30 months. Specific diagnoses of autism spectrum disorder do not eventuate through this module, rather there is a relative rating as to the "Range of Concern" about possible autism spectrum disorder.

The changes in the conceptualisation from DSM-IV-TR to DSM 5 may be one of the factors leading to the increase in reported incidence of autism spectrum disorder, with the various "subtypes" of autism being subsumed under one universal "label". It also illustrates the growing understanding of the condition itself, its range and complexity, differing presentations and increased community awareness and acceptance of "difference". There is now considerable interest in and acceptance of "neurodiversity", a term which began to gain currency in the 1990s. Sometimes attributed to Australian sociologist Judy Singer in 1998, but also to journalist Harvey Blume in 1997, the term referred to the notion that everyone's brain develops in a unique way.

Blume in particular wrote of "neurological pluralism" and neurological diversity but described his ideas as having emanated from an online discussion group of individuals with autism spectrum disorder. And in some cultures, this pluralism was described as an example of "border children", not clearly meeting diagnostic criteria for autism spectrum disorder but presenting with some traits that may have been associated with autism spectrum disorder without many of the attendant pervasive problems.

The release of DSM-5-TR sees two minor but important amendments to the DSM-5 criteria for autism spectrum disorder. Firstly, in relation to "persistent deficits in communication and social interaction", there must be evidence of **ALL** of the following:

- Deficits in social-emotional reciprocity.
- Deficits in nonverbal communication behaviours.
- Deficits in developing, maintaining and understanding relationships.

The second subtle but important amendment relates to the presence of comorbid conditions such as attention deficit hyperactivity in the profile of many children with autism spectrum disorder. Where previously it had been necessary to "codify" any such comorbid conditions by DSM 5 criteria, under DSM-5-TR, it is merely required that reference be made to the presence of "problems" relating to other possible DSM-5-TR coded conditions.

DSM 5 and DSM-5-TR criteria for autism spectrum disorder both provide "specifiers" related to severity levels of the condition and its presentation. There are children at:

- Level 1 "requiring support".
- Level 2 "requiring substantial support".
- Level 3 "requiring very substantial support".

These ratings pertain to social communication skills deficits, restricted and repetitive behaviours and an overall rating. They have become embedded in the degree of financial support allocated through the various support schemes and school systems in some countries, although this nexus was not originally intended.

Autism spectrum disorder in ICD-11 now incorporates both childhood autism and Asperger's syndrome from the ICD-10 under a single category characterised by social communication deficits and restricted, repetitive and inflexible patterns of behaviour, interests or activities. Guidelines for autism spectrum disorder have also been updated to reflect the current research. Qualifiers are provided for the extent of impairment in intellectual functioning and functional language abilities.

Autism spectrum disorder is the focus of intense research and study, but neurological and genetic research into causation have not been definitive. MRI scans and volumetric studies have suggested that although there is no difference in brain size at birth, children with autism spectrum disorder may experience an increased rate of head growth from early infancy, particularly in the cerebral cortex, cerebellum and limbic system. However, no relationships have been found between brain volume and measures of autism symptom severity. Atypical "cell packing" has been noted in the cerebellum, whilst possible early frontal lobe dysfunction and anomalies in the limbic system have also been speculated.

Previous "non-scientific" theories, such as the early pronouncements from the psychodynamic movement of the 1960s, included the notion that autism was the result of attachment and bonding difficulties early in life, giving rise to the pejorative term "refrigerator mothers". This hypothesis has largely been confined to history but was played out on film in the incongruous 1960s Elvis Presley movie "Change of Habit", where a young autistic girl, mistreated and neglected, is described as being "trapped behind a wall of hate".

Autism spectrum disorder is sometimes referred to as a "neurobiological" disorder, some research implicating increases in blood serotonin but reduced dopamine activity. These findings are far from definitive and may simply relate to "chicken and egg" theories of causation. Autism spectrum disorder is also known to have increased heritability risks. Genetic factors would appear to substantially increase a family's susceptibility to autism spectrum disorder, but the search for specific genes or chromosomes implicated in incident rates has thus far proved elusive.

Molecular genetic studies have to date been unable to isolate specific DNA sequences responsible for a genetic component to autism spectrum disorder. "Interest" has been expressed in a number of chromosomes, but a complex multifactorial interaction is seen more likely to be involved. Several genetic syndromes are known to present with autistic-like behaviours, and studying the specific genes associated with these syndromes may provide some further insights into any genetic causative factors of autism spectrum disorder. Ongoing research also explores the possible association between external agents such as medications, alcohol, tobacco, food additives and other chemicals and the susceptibility of genes to variations and mutations possibly implicated in autism spectrum disorder, but no definitive findings have as yet been reported.

Two alarming statistics have consistently stood out in the profile of autism spectrum disorder. Firstly, autism spectrum disorder is far more likely to occur in boys than in girls. In severe autism spectrum disorder, the gender ratio is often quoted as being four boys to each girl diagnosed. In mild autism spectrum disorder (particularly when DSM-IV criteria for Asperger's disorder was applied), this ratio was 10 boys to each girl, although considerable anecdotal evidence and debate continues as to whether girls are in fact "under-diagnosed" with mild autism spectrum disorder. This is thought to reflect the subtle differences in symptomatology between males and females, particularly early in the developmental cycle, whereby girls may present with better social interaction, communication, symbolic play and "masking" skills than boys, and similarly less stereotypic behaviours than boys.

Another disturbing element of autism spectrum disorder, particularly in its more severe manifestation, is the high incidence of seizure disorders. Epilepsy is reported in approximately 25% of such children, and most concerningly, many of the convulsive episodes encountered do not necessarily result in clear evidence of epilepsy as tested by EEG (electroencephalograph) methods. Reference is also made to the phenomenon of "silent seizing", whereby there would appear to be episodes of staring and absence but not associated with discernible epileptic activity.

External causation factors of autism spectrum disorder have been proffered in recent decades, notably by Dr Andrew Wakefield who claimed "scientific proof" of a direct causative link between MMR vaccinations (measles, mumps, rubella) and autism spectrum disorder. Described as "the scientific scam of the century" and disproven through many follow-up research projects, they led to Doctor Wakefield being disbarred from practising medicine.

Similarly, simple medical treatments and "cures" for autism spectrum disorder, for example the use of various complementary medicines such as DMG, secretin and melatonin, have proved inconclusive, with limited evidence supporting their use in autism spectrum disorder, and concerns about possible detrimental side effects.

A third areas of high interest to researchers is the incidence of "comorbid" conditions associated with autism spectrum disorder. High levels of anxiety are consistently noted and are hypothesised to be the cause of some stereotypic and maladaptive behaviours. Attentional difficulties are also common, as can be obsessive and compulsive traits and oppositional behaviours. There is also evidence of increased rates of mental illness amongst people with autism spectrum disorder, and this is also true of other neurodevelopmental disorders.

Many eminent scholars, practitioners and researchers have tried to explain the breadth and variety of the "Autism Spectrum", and its relationship with other neurodevelopmental and behavioural conditions. The noted Swedish researcher Professor Christopher Gillberg introduced the acronym "ESSENCE" ("Early Symptomatic Syndromes Eliciting Neurodevelopmental Clinical Examinations") in 2010. This refers to any number of neurodevelopmental/neuropsychiatric disorders that can present in early childhood, including

- Attention deficit hyperactivity disorder.
- Autism spectrum disorder.
- Developmental coordination disorder.
- Intellectual disability.
- Tourette syndrome.
- Early onset bipolar disorder.

- Behavioural phenotype syndromes.
- Neurological and seizure disorders.
- Pervasive demand avoidance syndrome.

These are usually "comorbid" with each other and difficult to distinguish between early in the developmental cycle. They may share genes, environmental risk factors and clinical symptoms. "Overlap" can occur between symptoms and diagnoses. It is stressed that "ESSENCE" is not a diagnosis in itself, but a means of alerting clinicians and researchers to the variety and interplay of symptoms demonstrated by children.

Increased knowledge and awareness of autism spectrum disorder has had the positive effect of arousing interest in specific treatment programmes and methodologies, particularly when these are applied early in the developmental cycle and as soon as possible after initial diagnosis. "Early intervention" programmes with differing theoretical and philosophical underpinnings have proliferated, including

- Precision teaching programmes such as TEACCH.
- Highly structured behavioural interventions such as Applied Behavioral Analysis.
- Relational-based social and emotional interventions.
- Structured play-based programmes such as "Floortime".
- Developmentally based curricula including "early start" programmes such as the "Denver" model.
- Pharmacological treatments.
- Specific therapeutic programmes such as Speech Pathology and Occupational Therapy.

It has proven difficult to clearly establish through empirical research whether such interventions produce consistent or sustained benefit. This may reflect a number of possible factors:

- The brevity of some early intervention programmes.
- The disparity between quantitative and qualitative outcomes of research and measurement methods.
- The perhaps subject and subtle nature of "progress" itself.

Many programmes in fact combine elements of some or all of the above treatment approaches or "integrative" models. Given the breadth and complexity of the "Autism Spectrum", it is perhaps not surprising to find that there is no simple answer to the question of the "best" treatment method.

Attention deficit/hyperactivity disorder (F90)

Perhaps one of the most controversial childhood diagnostic conditions, attention deficit/hyperactivity disorder is defined through a consistent pattern of inattention and/or hyperactivity-impulsivity as manifested in:

- Inattention.
- Hyperactivity and impulsivity.
- Onset before 12 years of age.
- Presence of symptomatology in two or more setting (e.g. home, school, work).

ADHD is described as beginning in childhood. Several symptoms need to be present before 12 years of age, and a precise age of onset is not described or specified, because "symptoms are hard to distinguish from highly variable normative behaviours before age 4 years", and because retrospective diagnosis to such an early age would often be difficult. Thus, ADHD cannot be diagnosed unless there was clear symptomatology prior to age 12 years.

A diagnosis of attention deficit hyperactivity disorder requires that symptomatology must be present and observable in at least two settings, for example school and home, which creates the need to have reliable sources of information across settings. It is therefore most often identified during the early school years. DSM-5-TR quotes incidence rates of approximately 7% worldwide but with considerable variation across nations. Prevalence is described as being higher in "special" populations such as out-of-home care, correctional settings and across children already diagnosed with other neurodevelopmental disorders or genetic disorders.

No clear biological or genetic marker has been found for attention deficit hyperactivity disorder. It is described as a "risk factor" for suicidal ideation and behaviour in young children, and there are other "functional" consequences such as reduced academic performance, peer relationship difficulties, accidental injury and poor self-application.

Treatment of attention deficit hyperactivity disorder usually occurs through a combination of specific drugs such as stimulant or non-stimulant medications, and behavioural management and support processes, and anecdotal evidence suggests that the latter methodologies tend to be more effective when medications are in use. Medications are frequently the main treatment modality, but these are not recommended for very young children unless absolutely necessary for the safety and wellbeing of the child and family, for example when their behavioural symptoms are sufficiently challenging as to render educational and therapeutic programme ineffective, or when a child's impulsive behaviours include absconding, dangerous climbing and jumping, or unsafe object use.

Formal diagnosis is often delayed until six years of age, or completion of at least one year's formal education, allowing more accurate observation of attentional difficulties in the structured setting of school. DSM-5-TR specifies a number of subtypes of attentional disorders:

- F90.2 Combined Presentation (with both inattention and hyperactivity).
- F90.0 Predominantly Inattentive Presentation.
- F90.1 Predominantly Hyperactive/Impulsive Presentation.

Also codified are:

- F90.8 Other Specified Attention-Deficit/Hyperactivity Disorder.
- F90.9 Unspecified Attention-Deficit/Hyperactivity Disorder, when children do not meet the full criteria for Attention Deficit/Hyperactivity Disorder, or when there is insufficient information for the practitioner to make a more specific diagnosis.

Controversy regarding this diagnostic category stems from three factors:

- The disputation or disbelief from many sources that attentional deficit-based conditions are in fact neurological disorders. Opinion is still abroad that the behaviours associated with ADHD are simply a manifestation of inappropriate behavioural management and parenting.

- The emphasis upon medications, either stimulants or non-stimulants. Considerable clinical and ethical probity needs to be applied to the use or recommendation of such medications. As psychologists have no training in medical or pharmacological interventions and no prescribing rights, assessment of ADHD in its various forms should be conducted as far as possible through a "team" approach with experienced paediatricians.
- The differing responses of government and non-government agencies and service providers to the support of young children with ADHD. In many jurisdictions, children with diagnoses of ADHD are not regarded as meeting eligibility criteria for support funding or programme inclusion.

As with other behaviourally based diagnostic categories, assessment and diagnosis of ADHD is best achieved through direct observation, preferably across different settings such as home and school, as well as a clinician's office. Assessment questionnaire and checklist-based assessment tools for ADHD include:

- BRIEF2 (Behavior Rating Inventory of Executive Function).
- Conners 4th Edition.
- Achenbach System of Empirically Based Assessment-Attention Problems Scale.
- Child Behaviour Checklist DSM Oriented ADHD subscale.
- Strengths and Difficulties Questionnaires (Hyperactive Subscale).

As with autism spectrum disorder, attention deficit hyperactivity disorder cannot be diagnosed by response to questionnaires and checklists alone. It is the combination of information and evidence derived from these, plus direct observations and information from other informed sources, that guide a psychologist in his or her clinical practice and decision-making.

Attention deficit hyperactivity disorder is viewed predominantly as a "frontal" disorder through deficits in executive function. Neurological studies suggest a number of diffuse or "soft" abnormalities in the neurology of children with ADHD, implicating reduced size of cerebellum, and anomalies in the prefrontal cortex. Research is ongoing.

Developmental coordination disorder F82

This diagnostic category has been present in successive editions of DSM as well as ICD. In ICD-11, it is referred to as developmental motor coordination disorder (Code 6A04). It is under the general heading of "motor disorders" in DSM-5-TR and refers to delayed acquisition and execution of coordinated motor skills, manifested in clumsiness, slowness and inaccuracy of performance. These delays and difficulties must "persistently interfere with activities of daily living", and other conditions such as intellectual disability or neurological conditions such as cerebral palsy must be excluded. It can be difficult to accurately differentiate this diagnosis from aspects of global developmental delay.

Stereotypic movement disorder F98.4

This is characterised by:

- Repetitive, seemingly driven and apparently purposeless motor behaviour.
- Subsequent interference in social or academic functioning, possibly resulting in self-injury.

What is a neurodevelopmental disorder? 35

In ICD-11, this is coded as "Stereotypic Movement Disorder, Unspecified" (Code 6A06.Z). Stereotypic movement disorder must be differentiated from neurodevelopmental conditions such as autism spectrum disorder, or medical or genetic conditions. There are some genetic disorders which are characterised by specific patterns of movement. These are generally described as being behavioural "phenotypes" as opposed to "stereotypies", where certain movement patterns are intrinsic to the genetic condition. An example of this is Smith-Magenis Syndrome with its characteristic "self-hug" behaviour.

Tic disorders

Tourette's Disorder 307.23.
Persistent (Chronic) Motor or Vocal Tic Disorder 307.22.
Provisional Tic Disorder 307.21.
Other Specified Tic Disorder 307.20.
Unspecified Tic Disorder 307.20.

Tic disorders generally develop between four and six years of age. Their frequency and severity vary considerably over time. In young children, they are generally "transient". They can be associated with conditions such as attention deficit/hyperactivity disorder and obsessive-compulsive disorder, and are best assessed, diagnosed and treated by specific specialist services such as Tic disorders clinics attached to major children's hospitals.

Other specified neurodevelopmental disorders F88

Again, new to DSM-5-TR, this category

> applies to presentations in which symptoms characteristic of a neurodevelopmental disorder that cause impairment in social, occupational or other important areas of functioning predominate, but do not meet the full criteria for any of the disorders in the neurodevelopmental disorders diagnostic class.

An example given in DSM-5-TR is neurodevelopmental disorder associated with prenatal alcohol exposure, which is known more widely as foetal alcohol spectrum disorder.

Unspecified neurodevelopmental disorder F89

This category mirrors the above, but adds that it is to be used when a clinician chooses not to specify the reason that criteria for other neurodevelopmental disorders are not met when there is insufficient information to make a more specific diagnosis.

Pervasive demand avoidance syndrome (not classified by DSM-5-TR or ICD-11)

Not all "behavioural conditions" make their way into DSM or ICD but still attract considerable interest, research and discussion. DSM 5 marked two important changes in format for the Diagnostic and Statistical Manual. Firstly, the change from Roman Numeral iteration (DSM IV) to simple numeric type (DSM 5) implied that new or revised versions of the Manual may come about more quickly and easily than previously.

The second was the inclusion of "Conditions for Further Study", for example "Persistent Complex Bereavement Disorder" and "Internet Gaming Disorder". There are perhaps as many behavioural presentations as there are children, and DSM-5-TR and ICD-11 represent the best scientific efforts to confirm the existence and nature of these through research and debate. One example of a possible future neurodevelopmental disorder for inclusion is pervasive demand avoidance syndrome (PDA).

First described by Professor Elizabeth Newson (Child Development Unit, Nottingham Hospital) in the 1980s, the term generally referred to children who were "puzzling" in presentation, not "classically Autistic" and often likely to attract the DSM-IV diagnosis pervasive developmental disorder (not otherwise specified). They were often seen as "too sociable, too imaginative and too comfortable in role play" to meet diagnostic criteria for autistic-type conditions but were challenging none the less.

The central difficulty relates to their avoidance of and resistance to demands and requests, ranging from explicit instructions to subtle hints.

Children described with PDA tend to have high levels of anxiety and a need to "control" situations. Their avoidance is often described as "compulsive and obsessive". These behaviours are "pathological". However, with their higher levels of sociability, they can often be charming and creative in their avoidance strategies, for example through negotiating, manipulating or distracting. Research into PDA suggests the following:

Children with PDA in comparison to those with autism spectrum disorder are less likely to:

- Have caused anxiety to parents before 10 months of age.
- Show stereotypic motor mannerisms.
- Show (or have shown) echolalia or pronoun reversal.
- Show speech anomalies in pragmatics.
- Show (or have shown) stereotypic toe walking.
- Show compulsive adherence to routines.

Children with PDA when compared to autism spectrum disorder are more likely to:

- Resist demands obsessively (100%).
- Be socially manipulative (100% by age 5 years).
- Show normal eye contact.
- Show excessive lability in mood and impulsivity.
- Show social imitation skills (including gestures and personal style).
- Show role play (more extended and complete than mere imitation).
- Show other types of symbolic play.

Early research into pervasive demand avoidance has shown no gender preference, in stark contrast to autism spectrum disorder. Research also indicates that PDA can be differentiated from other diagnostic categories such as oppositional defiant disorder, attention deficit hyperactivity disorder (including attention deficit disorder) and attachment disorders. Also noted from the research of Phil Christie (Director of Children's Services, Elizabeth Newsom Centre, Nottingham) are the following:

- Children with PDA appear to be more "passive" in the first 12 months of life. It is prognosticated that this leads to greater efforts on the part of parents to adapt to their child's behaviour in these early months, to the point where they are unprepared for later behavioural challenges.

- Although better social skills are described in children with PDA, it is also suggested that their social overtures and responses are superficial, unsubtle and lacking depth. Children with PDA are suggested to lack "social identity".
- As well as problems with lability and a need to "control", children with PDA are described as having delayed language skills, possibly as a direct consequence of their early history of passivity.
- There is some suggestion of a neurodevelopmental component to PDA through developmental markers such as delayed or absent crawling (greater than 50%), clumsiness and awkward movements.

Pervasive demand avoidance (PDA) does not appear in either DSM-5-TR or ICD-11, but research continues into the possibility of greater recognition of this behavioural cluster, particularly in the context of Gilberg's "ESSENCE" theory. It will be remembered that "Semantic-Pragmatic Disorder" was similarly not included in DSM-IV as a diagnostic category, but "Social (Pragmatic) Communication Disorder" made its way into DSM 5. This is the very nature of research and debate, particularly for constellations of behaviour lacking "hard" neurological or physical markers.

Bibliography

Abbott, R., and Burkitt, E. (2023), "Genetics and Neurodevelopmental Disorders", In Abbott, R. and Burkitt, E. (Eds.), Child Development and the Brain from Embryo to Adolescence, Bristol University Press.

Al-Beltagi, M. (2023), "Pre-autism: What a Paediatrician Should Know about Early Diagnosis of Autism", World Journal of Clinical Pediatrics, 12(5), pp 273–294.

American Psychiatric Association (1980), Diagnostic and Statistical Manual III, American Psychiatric Association.

American Psychiatric Association (1987), Diagnostic and Statistical Manual III-R, American Psychiatric Association.

American Psychiatric Association (1994), Diagnostic and Statistical Manual-IV TR, American Psychiatric Association.

American Psychiatric Association (2013), Diagnostic and Statistical Manual 5, American Psychiatric Association.

American Psychiatric Association (2022), Diagnostic and Statistical Manual 5 TR, American Psychiatric Association.

Ashok, A. H., Baugh, J., and Yeragani, V. (2012), "Paul Eugen Bleuler and the Origin of the Term Schizophrenia", Indian Journal of Psychiatry, 54(1), pp 95–96.

Asperger, H. (1944), "Die Autistischen Psychpathen in Kindersalter", Archiv Fur Psychiatrie und Nervenkrankheiten, 117, pp 76–136.

Attwood, A. (2006), Asperger's and Girls, Future Horizons.

Attwood, A. (2008), The Complete Guide to Asperger's Syndrome, Jessica Kingsley Publications.

Baron-Cohen, S. (2008), Autism and Asperger's Syndrome: The Facts, Oxford University Press.

Baron-Cohen, S. (2018), "The Truth about Hans Asperger's Nazi Collusion", Nature, 557(7705), 305–306.

Bishop, D. V. M. (1989), "Autism, Asperger's Syndrome and Semantic Pragmatic Disorder: Where are the Boundaries?", British Journal of Disorders of Communication, 24(2), pp 107–121.

Blume, H. (1998), "Neurodiversity: On the Neurological Underpinnings of Geekdom", The Atlantic, https://www.theatlantic.com/magazine/archive/1998/09/neurodiversity/305909/

Christie, P., Duncan, M., Fidler, R., and Healy, Z. (2011), Understanding Pathological Avoidance Syndrome in Children, Jessica Kingsley Publishers.

Courchesne, E., Carper, R., and Askhoomoff, N. (2003), "Evidence of Brain Overgrowth in the First Year of Life in Autism", The Journal of the American Medical Association, 290(3), pp 337–344.

de Villiers, J. (2023), "Aetiology of Neurodevelopmental Disorders", In McCarthy, J. M., Alexander, R. T., and Chaplin, E. (Eds.), Forensic Aspects of Neurodevelopmental Disorders: A Clinician's Guide, Cambridge University Press.
Deer, B. (2020), The Doctor Who Fooled The World: Andrew Wakefield's War on Vaccines, Scribe Publications.
Di Filippis, M. (2018), "The Use of Complementary Alternative Medicine in Children and Adolescents with Autism Spectrum Disorders", Psychopharmacol Bulletin, 48(1), pp 40–63.
Gillberg, C. (2010), "The ESSENCE in Child Psychiatry: Early Symptomatic Syndromes Eliciting Neurodevelopmental Clinical Examinations", Research in Developmental Disabilities, 31(6), pp 1543–1551.
Haines, C. (2012), Silently Seizing: Common, Unrecognised and Frequently Missed Seizures and their Potentially Damaging Impact on Individuals with Autism Spectrum Disorders, AAPC Publishing.
Horwitz, A. (2015), "DSM-I and DSM-II", In Cautin, R. L. and Lilienfeld, S. O. (Eds.), The Encyclopedia of Clinical Psychology, Wiley.
Howlin, P. A., Charman, T., and Ghaziuddin, M. (2011), The SAGE Handbook of Developmental Disorders, SAGE Publications.
Joseph, L., Soorya, L. V., and Thurm, A. (2023), Autism Spectrum Disorder, Hogrefe.
Kanner, L. (1943), "Autistic Disturbances of Affective Contact", Nervous Child, 2, pp 217–250.
Krishnaswami, S., McPheeters, M. L., and Veenstra-VanderWeele, J. (2011), "A Systematic Review of Secretin for Children With Autism Spectrum Disorders", Pediatrics, 127(5), e1322–e1325.
Lord, C., Rutter, M., DiLavore, P., Risi, S., Gotham, K., Bishop, S., Luyster, R., and Guthrie, W. (2012), Autism Diagnostic Observation Schedule (2nd Edition), Manual, Western Psychological Services.
McGlade, A., Whittingham, K., Barfoot, J., Taylor, L., and Boyd, R. N. (2023), "Efficacy of Very Early Interventions on Neurodevelopmental Outcomes for Infants and Toddlers at Increased Likelihood of or Diagnosed with Autism: A Systematic Review and Meta-Analysis", Autism Research, 16, pp 1–16.
MGM (1953), "Time Bomb" movie.
Moriyama, I. M., Loy, R. M., Robb-Smith, A. H. T., Rosenberg, H., and Hoyert, D. L. (2011), History of the Statistical Classification of Diseases and Causes of Death, Centers for Disease Control, Center for Health Statistics.
Muhle, R., Tretacoste, S. V., and Rapin, I. (2004), "The Genetics of Autism", Pediatrics, 113, pp 472–486.
Muir, J. (2006), "The Neurobiology of Autism", The Clinician: Child & Adolescent Mental Health Service Statewide Network (CAMHSNET), Volume 3 Acceptance and the Autistic Disorders.
Nicoll, N. (2006), "What is Autism Spectrum Disorder?", The Clinician: Child & Adolescent Mental Health Service Statewide Network (CAMHSNET), Volume 3 Acceptance and the Autistic Disorders.
Njotto, L. L., Simin, J., Fornes, R., Odsbu, I., Musssche, I., Callans, S., Engstrand, L., Bruyndonckx, R., and Brusselaers, N. (2023), "Maternal and Early-Life Exposure to Antibiotics and the Risk of Autism and Attention Deficit Hyperactivity Disorder in Childhood: A Swedish Population-Based Cohort Study", Drug Safety, 46(5), pp 467–478.
O'Reilly, B., and Wicks, K. (2013), The Australian Autism Handbook, Jane Curry Publishing.
PDA Society, United Kingdom, "Pathological Demand Avoidance Syndrome-A Reference Booklet for Clinicians", www.pdasociety.org.au
Reed, G. M., et al. (2019), "Innovations and Changes in the ICD-11 Classification of Mental, Behavioural and Neurodevelopmental Disorders", World Psychiatry, 18(1) pp 3–19.
Rubinsztein, J. S. (2019), "Asperger's Children: The Origins of Autism in Nazi Vienna by Edith Sheffer", The British Journal of Psychiatry (Review), 214(3).
Sanua, V. D. (1990), "Leo Kanner (1894–1981): The Man and the Scientist", Child Psychiatry & Human Development, 21(1), pp 3 23.
Singer, J. (2016), Neurodiversity: The Birth of an Idea, Kindle.
Universal Pictures (1969), "Change of Habit", movie.
Urwin, R. (2006), "The Genetics of Autism", The Clinician: Child & Adolescent Mental Health Service Statewide Network (CAMHSNET), Volume 3 Acceptance and the Autistic Disorders.
Waterhouse, L., Wing, L., Spitzer, R., and Siegel, B. (1992), "Pervasive Developmental Disorders: From DSM III to DSM III-R", Journal of Autism and Developmental Disorders, 22, pp 525–549.

Weaving, L. S., Ellaway, C. J., Gecz, J., and Christodoulou, J. (2005), "Rett Syndrome: Clinical Review and Genetic Update", Journal of Medical Genetics, 42, pp 1–7.
Wing, L. (1997), "A History of Ideas on Autism", Autism, 1(1), pp 13–23.
World Health Organisation (1993), "The ICD-10 Classification of Mental and Behavioural Disorders: Diagnostic Criteria for Research", World Health Organisation.
World Health Organisation (2015), "International Statistical Classification of Diseases and Related Health Problems Volume 1", World Health Organisation.
Yankowitz, L. D., et al. (2020), "Evidence against the 'Normalization' Prediction of the Early Brain Overgrowth Hypothesis of Autism", Molecular Autism, 11(51), pp 1–17.
Zehetner, A. A. (2011), "Psychopharmacology: The Use of Medication to Treat Challenging Behaviours in Children and Adolescents" In Dossetor, D., White, D., and Whatson, L. (Eds.), Mental Health of Children and Adolescents with Intellectual and Developmental Disabilities, IP Communications.

3 Genetic and chromosomal disorders

The science of human genetics, whether applied to general human development or to the specifics of disability, behaviour, health and well-being, is relatively young in historical terms, but progressing at an exponential rate, delving ever deeper into the basic building blocks of life and changing forever the way in which we conceptualise who we are. It is analogous to our understanding of the cosmos through successive generations of exploration techniques such as the Hubble Space Telescope and now the James Webb Space Telescope; we can now observe and study in their minutiae processes and materials that have always existed but which were hitherto invisible to humanity (Table 3.1).

Psychologists are not trained medical practitioners or geneticists. However, if they are working in the field of neurodevelopmental disorders in young children, they will need at least a working knowledge of basic genetic concepts as they apply to developmental disorders with confirmed genetic causation or association. Indeed, psychological associations and societies around the world stipulate that psychologists involved in the domain of neurodevelopmental disorders need to maintain as current an understanding of the role of genetics in neurodevelopmental disorders as possible.

Table 3.1 Timeline of genetic discoveries: National Human Genome Research Institute

1859	Darwin; "On The Origin Of Species"
1865	Mendel; Heredity "transmitted in units"
1869	Miescher; DNA isolated
1879	Flemming; discovery of mitosis (cell replication)
1902	Garrod; discovery of first "genetic mutation"
1909	Johannsen; "genes", "genotypes" and "phenotypes"
1911	Morgan; chromosomes carry genes
1941	Beadle and Tatum; genes direct formation of enzymes
1944	Avery, McLeod and McCarty; DNA transforms cell properties
1953	Watson, Crick and Wilkins; the Double Helix
1955	Tjio; confirms there are 46 chromosomes
1959	Lejeune; Trisomy 21 (Down Syndrome)
1961	Guthrie; introduces genetic tests for newborns
1966	Nirenberg et al; the 4-letter genetic code
1975	Sanger, Maxam and Gilbert; rapid DNA sequencing
1983	Huntington's Disease first genetic defect mapped (chromosome 4)
1987	First comprehensive genetic "map"
1990	Human Genome Project commenced
1999	Chromosome 22 the first chromosome "mapped"
2003	Human Genome Mapping Complete

DOI: 10.4324/9781003565338-5

Psychologists will not be directly involved per se in the diagnosis of these conditions but may be called upon to undertake developmental or intellectual assessments, to assist with behavioural management programmes, and to clarify the degree of impact caused by genetic conditions. For example, there may be circumstances where funding support agencies will not simply accept a diagnosed genetic condition unless specific evidence is provided regarding the impact of this condition upon developmental milestones, intelligence and adaptive behaviour or daily living skills.

Another, perhaps more important reason for psychological engagement with children with specific genetic conditions is that they can present with behavioural challenges which are sometimes highly specific to the condition. This is called a "behavioural phenotype". An educated grounding in these concepts is therefore necessary, including the types of specific genetic and chromosomal disorders, the specific disabling impacts, behavioural challenges and appropriate support strategies.

Phenotypes

A phenotype is defined as a constellation of symptoms related to a specific cause, for example a genetic mutation or anomaly. Phenotypes can relate to physical characteristics such as facial appearance, medical and physical conditions, and behavioural and emotional traits. There are many examples of phenotypes in genetic abnormalities, and it is unusual for a genetic condition to be referred to as a "spectrum" disorder, due to the more limited range of symptoms found in genetic syndromes. Examples include the distinctive facial features associated with Down syndrome and velocardiofacial syndrome, the physical movement patterns and behavioural presentations associated with Smith-Magenis syndrome, the obsessive eating found in Prader-Willi syndrome, the "elfin-like" appearance and reported "musicality" associated with Williams syndrome, and the disturbed sleeping patterns associated with Angelman syndrome. These will be explored in more detail in a later chapter.

Chromosomes and genes: Basic facts

Our bodies are made up of millions of cells. Each cell contains a complete copy of a person's genetic plan or blueprint. The genetic material is packaged into long strands that are made up of DNA (deoxyribonucleic acid) and are called chromosomes. In humans, all the cells, except the egg or sperm cells, contain 46 chromosomes, made up of 23 pairs, one from each parent. In each cell, females have 44 autosomes (the non-sex chromosomes) and two copies of the X chromosome (XX), whilst males have 44 autosomes (the non-sex chromosomes) and an X and a Y chromosome (XY).

These pairs are usually identical in content, except of course in the male of the species who has an X chromosome and a Y chromosome (Figure 3.1):

A chromosome is like a string of beads. Each bead represents a gene, and each chromosome contains thousands of genes, all comprised of the chemical called DNA. The information contained in genes is in the form of a chemical "genetic code". It is estimated that there are between 50,000 and 100,000 genes in every cell of the body. There are approximately 8,300,000 possible combinations of chromosomes and that makes for an almost infinite number of genetic combinations. In the overwhelming majority of live births, this process of coding works perfectly, giving us our unique genetic "brand"- appearance, personality, temperament, even skill sets. But not even nature is perfect,

42 *Diagnosing Young Children with Neurodevelopmental Disorders*

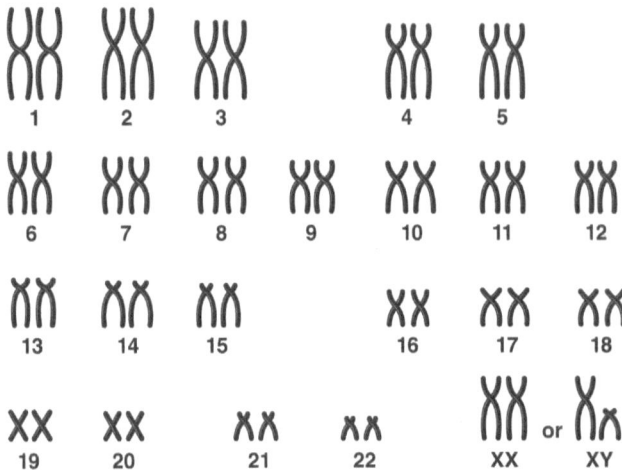

Figure 3.1 The normal sequence of chromosomes

and sometimes errors occur in the process of formulating, coding and copying genes and chromosomes.

A genetic disorder is considered "rare" if it occurs in 1 in every 2,000 live births or less. On that statistical basis, there are currently more than 7,000 genetic disorders, which can affect every facet of a person's development: Health, growth, metabolism, intellect, behaviour, emotionality and psychological and psychiatric well-being. This number is increasing all the time as the science of genetic assessment and diagnosis progresses. It is not that these more recently discovered disorders and syndromes are necessarily "new". It is more that the genetic basis for many disorders and symptoms could not previously be confirmed. Some of these genetic and chromosomal anomalies are extremely relevant to early childhood development, and are summarised below, and later expanded upon. They can be grouped into four broad categories:

- Extra chromosomes, or even a missing chromosome.
- "Translocation" of chromosomes.
- Microdeletions or microduplications within chromosomes.
- Individual genetic mutations.

Examples of these four broad categories are given below:

Extra chromosomes, for example "trisomy"

A trisomy occurs when there are three copies of a chromosome instead of two. The best-known example of a trisomy is Down syndrome (Trisomy 21), where there are three copies of chromosome 21. Others include Patau syndrome (Trisomy 13), Klinefelter syndrome (XXY) and XXX syndrome. There are also conditions where there are more than three copies of chromosomes, for example XXXY syndrome, 48XXYY syndrome and XXXXX Syndrome, but these are exceedingly rare. And there exists at least one example of a "missing chromosome" syndrome, Turner syndrome (XO syndrome) (Figure 3.2).

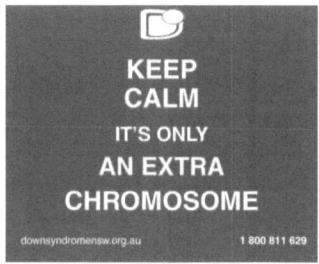

Figure 3.2 Down Syndrome Association of NSW fridge magnet

Translocation disorders

A translocation disorder refers to a circumstance where data from one chromosome is overlaid or imprinted onto another chromosome. These are rare. For example, part of chromosome 21 can overlay other chromosomes, often chromosome 14, causing a variant of Down syndrome.

Microdeletion and microduplication disorders

Microdeletion syndromes occur when some genetic material is missing from a copy of a chromosome. This error occurs soon after the original 23 chromosomes divide into pairs (except for the X chromosome for males), and synchronisation of the genetic data takes place. The genetic data which is "deleted" is measured in megabase pairs, and most deletions involve one megabase pair or less.

The most commonly occurring microdeletion syndrome is velocardiofacial syndrome (vcfs, or 22q11.2 syndrome), referring to the fact that the deletion occurs on the "long arm" (q) of chromosome 22, at a highly specific site numbered 11.2. This type of codifying is consistent in all microdeletion and microduplication syndromes. Other well-known microdeletion syndromes include Cri du Chat syndrome (Deletion 5p Syndrome), Smith-Magenis syndrome (17p11.2 Syndrome) and Prader-Willi syndrome (15q11-q13).

Microduplication syndromes, as the name would imply, are caused by a repetition of genetic material in a particular chromosome. Again, the size of a duplication is measured in megabase pairs. Examples of microduplication disorders include Duplication 3q Syndrome (Hirschhorn syndrome), Duplication 9p syndrome and Duplication 15q syndrome. Such is the advance of genetic science that "sub-micro" deletions and duplications can even be detected.

Genetic mutations

When a gene or a coded "message" is changed in some way, a different "message" is given to the body cells. Such a change is called a "mutation". When a mutation occurs, it is permanent and can be passed down through the generations of a family. These are often referred to as "point mutations". There are many such mutations; in fact, advances in genetic assessment techniques are discovering an ever-increasing number of such mutations. It is not necessarily that the number or frequency of mutations are increasing, rather that the accuracy and scope of assessment procedures is improving over successive generations of genetic science.

Examples of mutations as they apply to young children who may require assessment include Rett syndrome and Marfan syndrome.

Mutations may emanate from various causes, including exposure to certain chemicals or environmental antagonists, or simple "coding errors", which might occur during cell division. Mutations can, but not necessarily will, be passed on through successive generations, if the mutations are contained in the egg or sperm cells. Spontaneous mutations often occur "de novo", when neither parent has been a "carrier" of the mutation. When mutations are passed on, it is by a complex "mathematical" process, depending upon which parent is the "carrier" of the mutated gene. Reference is again made to the advances in genetic testing and analysis, to the point where there is growing interest in "pre-mutations" and their impact upon human development.

Multifactorial inheritance

Multifactorial Inheritance refers to the pattern of inheritance, through generations of a family, of disorders and characteristics which are due to an interaction of genetic and environmental factors. Although these conditions tend to "run in families", the patterns are less predictable than for disorders which are due to changes or mutations in a single gene. Some examples of multifactorial inheritance include:

- Birth defects such as spina bifida.
- Cancer.
- Cardiovascular conditions.
- Mental illness.
- Neurodevelopmental disorders such as autism spectrum disorder.

Autism spectrum disorder is a good example of multifactorial inheritance. For example, when mild autism spectrum disorder was described as "Asperger's Disorder" during the 1990s, Professor Simon Baron-Cohen was instrumental in highlighting the heritability factors associated with the condition, even going so far as to emphasise the correlation between Asperger's disorder and parental occupation.

Condition arising from environmental agents

Medical texts also refer to disorders known to be directly associated with environmental agents, for example fetal alcohol spectrum disorder. Most developed countries have specialist diagnostic clinics for possible fetal alcohol spectrum disorder. Other such conditions include fetal Dilantin syndrome and fetal Valproate syndrome (both being agents within anticonvulsant medications), and fetal warfarin syndrome (a drug often necessary to prevent blood clotting following major surgery such as heart transplants).

In the 1980s and 1990s, the United States endured a period of heavy usage of "Crack Cocaine" (PCE), and many so-called "crack babies" were born during this time. However, no specific disorders or conditions have been found to result for people whose mothers' used cocaine while pregnant. Studies focusing on children under six years of age have not shown any direct, long-term effects of prenatal cocaine exposure on language, growth or development as measured by test scores; however, PCE is still thought to be associated with premature birth, birth defects, attention deficit hyperactivity disorder and other conditions. The effects of cocaine on a foetus are thought to be similar to those of tobacco but less severe than those of alcohol.

That neurodevelopmental conditions could be associated with chemical exposure was dramatically illustrated during the prevalence of "Pink Disease" (infantile acrodynia) in the first half of the twentieth century. This disease was mainly attributed to the use of teething balms and powders containing mercurous chloride with young children. Symptoms were in some respects similar to those of autism spectrum disorder and included

- Irritability.
- Neurosis.
- Photophobia (light sensitivity).
- Hyperhidrosis (excessive sweating).
- Hypotonia (low muscle tone).
- Ataxia (lack of coordination).
- Digestive problems, (including weight loss, appetite loss, vomiting and constipation).
- Anaemia.
- Excessive salivation.
- Respiratory problems.
- Lethargy.
- "Extreme misery".
- Loss of speech.
- Loosening of teeth.
- Swollen extremities.
- Marked reddening of the extremities, particularly the hands and feet, hence the reference to "pink".

Incidence rates for Pink disease were reported as 1 in 500 children during the disease's peak, and once the causal link between the disease and mercury chloride (calomel) was established and the offending chemical removed in 1954, Pink disease virtually ceased to exist, although support groups still function for older sufferers of the disease.

Some concluding notes on genetic disorders

Firstly, the individual names of genetic disorders can be confusing but easily explained. Some are simply named after the medical specialist most closely associated with the discovery, conceptualisation and understanding of a condition, for example Down syndrome is named after Professor John Langdon Down. There are many such examples. Some are named after more than one specialist, for example Smith-Magenis syndrome (Doctors Anne Smith and Ellen Magenis). Others bear the names of hospitals or research institutions, such as "Floating-Harbor Syndrome", an amalgam of Boston Floating and Harbor General, California. Some are simply labelled according to the deletion or duplication site (for example 18q duplication), or the specific symptoms associated with the condition (velocardiofacial syndrome or vcfs). Others are essentially anagrams of symptoms, for example SHORT Syndrome, referring to Short Stature, Hyperextensibility of joints, Ocular depression, Rieger anomaly and teething delay.

The second point to appreciate is that the study of genetics is still a relatively "young" specialty but rapidly developing. It is a most exciting time to be involved in genetics, particularly since the human genome project. An important offshoot of this recency is

46 *Diagnosing Young Children with Neurodevelopmental Disorders*

that many of the physicians, scientists and geneticists whose names have been attached to disorders, are still alive and practising. They attend international conferences to discuss their research and findings and are generally amenable to discussing their work with others as colleagues.

Genetic testing is generally "ordered up" by paediatricians who may be concerned about the presentation of a young child they may be treating. Many genetic disorders present with distinctive facial and/or physical characteristics which stand them apart from the normal population. This is often a paediatrician's first reference point to consider further exploration. Such characteristics are frequently described as "dysmorphic". Doctors frequently consult textbooks such as "Recognizable Patterns of Human Malformation", which includes photographs as well as diagnostic criteria, descriptions of characteristics, aetiology and prognosis, and important on-line updates of research into syndromes.

In more recent years, paediatricians and geneticists have had increasing access to on-line matching systems such as "Face-Match", which provide additional speed and accuracy of diagnostic confirmation or suspicion. Genetic testing is conducted using either FISH tests (fluorescence in-situ hybridisation) or CGH array (comparative genomic hybridisation). Results are reported back to parents and to referring doctors, and if results are positive, families are offered post-assessment genetic counselling (Figure 3.3).

Genetic syndromes with specific behavioural phenotypes can also be associated with an increased risk of other neurodevelopmental disorders such as autism spectrum disorder, and with such "co-morbidity", the autistic-type symptoms will sometimes present in an atypical manner, perhaps being "reflected" through the particular phenotypic "lens" of the condition. This is often referred to as "symptom shadowing" or "symptom overshadowing".

Smith-Magenis syndrome, for example, presents with phenotypic hand movements, which may be interpreted (or misinterpreted) as "stereotypies". They can also present with an overriding resistance to and anxiety at "change", and a lack of empathic skills which can "mirror" the "theory of mind" deficits associated with autism spectrum disorder.

The last and most important consideration to address is the distress that simply reading about the sheer volume of genetic disorders, and the complexity of the difficulties

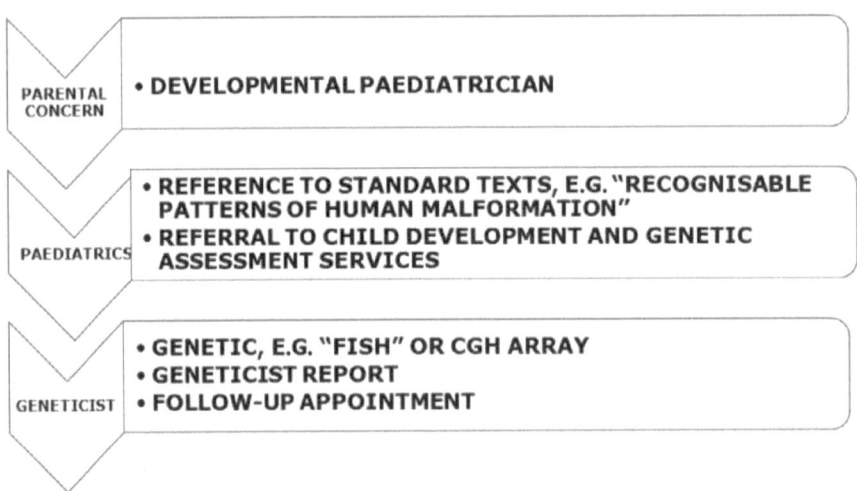

Figure 3.3 The path to genetic assessment

caused, needs to be put into perspective. Genetic anomalies and disorders of this nature consume a great many chapters and pages in textbooks and medical dictionaries and are couched in highly technical medical terminology. The textbooks are often illustrated with graphic photographic material and contain frightening figures and statistics about the severity of disabilities, medical complications and mortality rates.

With "new" genetic disorders being reported more and more frequently, another question remains – are these in fact "new" genetic mutations or simply those which were already extant but unable to be seen and examined? Recent studies using the most contemporary assessment and diagnostic techniques have revealed a slew of previously unlabelled genetic mutations causing significant developmental interruption to young children.

What needs to be remembered however is that most of the described conditions are in fact extremely rare, to the point where "incidence rates" cannot necessarily be estimated. In studies of childhood intellectual disability, it has been estimated that only 25% of children diagnosed with an intellectual disability can be found to have an underlying causative genetic disorder. This means that in approximately three quarters of cases, no specific causation can be attributed.

If there is a possible "downside" to the rapid progression of genetic assessment techniques, it is this. Science is detecting more and more genetic and chromosomal anomalies, including "sub-microdeletions", "sub-microduplications" and pre-mutations". But it is not at all certain in many of these instances whether there are any negative implications arising from these anomalies. Good, well-constructed research into genetic disorders requires adequate sample sizes and traditional peer-reviewed studies. This is not possible when it is known that there are only a few children in a country presenting with a particular anomaly.

Parents are therefore often placed in an invidious situation where they are informed that something appears to be "wrong" with their child's genetic makeup, but no information can be given as to what this anomaly actually means. Research indicates that parents derive their most useful information from support groups, allied health professionals and other parents.

Parents have described the impact of a lack of knowledge about their child's specific disorder. Uncertainty and confusion, feelings of isolation, fears for the future, mental health issues and frustration can permeate their emotional reactions, particularly when specific chromosome disorders have no associated "label", let alone possible ramifications and long-term prognosis.

In our "age of information", social media and "connectability", families are increasingly bombarded by information, some of which is useful and some not. Many find great comfort in making on-line contact with families in similar situations where they can "compare notes" through social media about rare genetic disorders. Specialists can also participate in these on-line forums, sharing their expertise with a far wider audience than previously possible.

The ever-increasing knowledge of genetic disorders means also that standard genetic textbooks are increasingly hard-pressed to update their published editions to keep pace with new discoveries, and it is suggested that psychologists interested in this vital domain of knowledge seek access to on-line sources of information such as the International Behavioural and Neural Genetics Society's, "Genes, Brains and Behavior" (GBB), "app", providing updated information and research articles on a regular basis.

The next chapter offers a representative sample of genetic and chromosomal disorders in more detail. Preference has been given to a representative range of Trisomy conditions, microdeletion and microduplication disorders, genetic mutations, and one disorder caused by environmental factors such as substance abuse. Hopefully these descriptions will introduce and explain the concepts and principles which relate to genetic and chromosomal disorders in general.

Bibliography

Baron-Cohen, S. (2008), Autism and Asperger's Syndrome: The Facts, Oxford University Press.
Chandler, L. S., and Lane, S. J. (2014), Children with Prenatal Drug Exposure, Routledge.
Dally, A. (1997), "The Rise and Fall of Pink Disease", Social History of Medicine, 10(2), pp 291–304.
Fisch, G. (Ed.) (2003), Genetics and Genomics of Neurobehavioural Disorders, Humana Press.
Genetic Alliance; The New York-Mid-Atlantic Consortium for Genetic and Newborn Screening Services (2009), Understanding Genetics: A New York-Mid-Atlantic Guide for Patients and Health Care Professionals, Genetic Alliance.
Gilmore, L. (2018), "Supporting Families of Children with Rare and Unique Chromosome Disorders", Research and Practice in Intellectual and Developmental Disabilities, 5(1), pp 8–16.
Hagerman, R. I., Protic, D., Rajaratnam, A., Salcedo-Arellano, M. J., Aydin, E. Y., and Schneider, A. (2018), "Fragile-X Associated Neuropsychiatric Disorders", Frontiers in Psychiatry, 9, pp 1–9.
Hong, D., et al. (2021), "Genetic Syndromes Screening by Facial Recognition Technology: VGG-16 Screening Model Construction and Evaluation", Orphanet Journal of Rare Diseases, 16, 344.
International Behavioural and Neural Genetics (on-line app), "Genes, Brains and Behaviour", https://www.ibngs.org/.
Jones, K. L., Jones, M. C., and Del Campo, M. (2021), Smith's Recognizable Patterns of Human Malformation (8th Edition), Saunders/Elsevier.
Kerrie, S., and Austin, D. W. (2011), "Ancestry of Pink Disease (Infantile Acrodynia) Identified as a Risk Factor for Autism Spectrum Disorders", Journal of Toxicological and Environmental Health, 74(18), pp 1185–1194.
Magalini, S. I., and Magalini, S. C. (1997), Dictionary of Medical Syndromes, Lippincott-Raven Publishers.
Milani, D., Ronzoni, L., and Esposito, S. (2015), "Genetic Advances in Intellectual Disability", Journal of Pediatric Genetics, 4(3), pp 125–127.
National Human Genome Research Institute, https://www.genome.gov/.
Paige Harden, K. (2022), The Genetic Lottery: Why DNA Matters for Social Equality, Princeton University Press.
Selikowitz, M. (2008), Down Syndrome, Oxford University Press.
Society for the Study of Behavioural Phenotypes (SSBP), Information Sheets, https://ssbp.org.uk/.
Weaving, L. S., Ellaway, C. J., Gecz, J., and Christodoulou, J. (2005), "Rett Syndrome: Clinical Review and Genetic Update", Journal of Medical Genetics, 42, pp 1–7.
Wright, C. F., et al. (2023), "Genomic Diagnosis of Rare Pediatric Disease in the United Kingdom and Ireland", The New England Journal of Medicine, 388, pp 1–12.

4 Selected genetic and chromosomal disorders

This section details a selection from the plethora of genetic and chromosomal disorders now known to medical science, particularly if they are known to be associated with developmental, cognitive, behavioural, psychological or psychiatric disorders. Many of these syndromes and disorders are also associated with other medical complications, some of which are summarised in Table 4.1 to provide an insight into the number and complexity of issues faced by the parents and families of children with these genetic and chromosomal disorders.

Disorders with extra or missing chromosomes

Down syndrome

First described separately by Doctors John Langdon Down and Eduard Seguin in 1866 from physical and behavioural presentation, Down syndrome has presumably always existed. Artistic representations of people with Down syndrome, often beatific in nature, appeared in churches in Germany as early as 1505. Initially, the causative factors of

Table 4.1 Comorbidity with various genetic disorders

Medical condition	Syndrome/Disorder
CARDIO	22q11.2, Downs, Marfans, Turner, Williams, Wolf-Hirschhorn
HEARING	Down, Turner, Wolf-Hirschhorn
DISEASE	Down, Kleinfelter, Turner, Wolf-Hirschhorn, 15q
EPILEPSY	Down, 22q11.2, Rett, Wolf-Hirschhorn, Phelan-McDermid, 15q
JOINTS/MUSCLES	Down, Marfan, Kleinfelter, Smith-Magenis, Williams, Pitt-Hopkins, Phelan-McDermid, Retts, Wolf-Hirschhorn, 15q
PREMATURE DEATH	Hirschsprung, Turner, Down
GENERAL HEALTH	Williams, Prader-Willi, Turner
DEVEL. REGRESSION	Retts
INTELLECTUAL DELAY	Almost universal, ranging mild to severe
AUTISM SPECTRUM DISORDER	22q11.2, Fragile X, 15q
ADHD	Turner, 22q11.2, Williams, 15q, NF1
LEARNING DIFFICULTY	Kleinfelter, 22q11.2, Turner, Williams, NF1
SOCIAL INTERACTION DIFFICULTY	22q11.2, Turner, Fragile X, Williams, 15q
NEUROLOGY/BRAIN DISORDERS	Smith-Magenis, Wolf-Hirschhorn, 22q11.2

DOI: 10.4324/9781003565338-6

50 *Diagnosing Young Children with Neurodevelopmental Disorders*

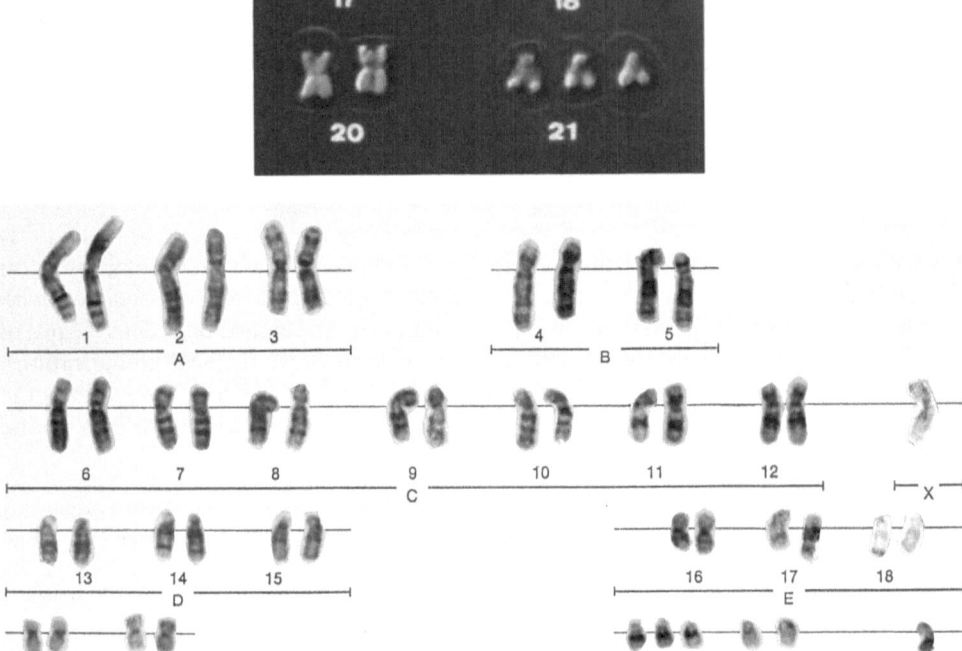

Figure 4.1 Clear evidence of Trisomy 21

Down syndrome were not understood, but unfortunately Down described it as "a reversion to a primitive Mongolian ethnic stock", and the term "Mongolism" was applied for many years. It was not until 1959 that Lejeune and his colleagues confirmed the presence of an extra chromosome 21 as causative (Figure 4.1).

Down syndrome is one of the most common genetic disorders and is the most frequently occurring chromosomal disorder. The incidence rate is approximately 1 in every 700 births, but with a significantly higher risk of occurrence when mothers are aged 35 and above (Table 4.2).

Table 4.2 Incidence by maternal age of Down syndrome

Maternal age	Incidence of Down syndrome
20 YEARS	1 IN 2,000
25 YEARS	1 IN 1,200
30 YEARS	1 IN 900
35 YEARS	1 IN 350
40 YEARS	1 IN 100
45 YEARS	1 IN 30

Mathematical distortion of these figures stems from the fact that in most developed countries, women aged 35 or above constitute only a small proportion of total pregnancies, so it cannot be extrapolated that the majority of babies with Down syndrome are born to older mothers. In fact, 20% of children with Down syndrome are born to mothers aged 25 years or less. There are in fact three different types of Down syndrome:

- **Trisomy 21**, when every cell in the human body possesses an extra Chromosome 21. Trisomy 21 reflects 95% of individuals with Down syndrome.
- **Translocation**, whereby a part of Chromosome 21 attaches itself to another chromosome, frequently chromosome 14. These equate to 4% of people with Down syndrome.
- **Mosaicism or Mosaic Down Syndrome**, whereby only some cells have the extra chromosome 21, therefore analogous to a "mosaic". It is generally described that individuals with Mosaicism present with milder physical features and higher intellectual skills. Mosaicism occurs in approximately 1% of cases.

Babies and toddlers with Down syndrome progress through their developmental milestones at a slower rate than non-affected children. If one considers standardised developmental assessments and age equivalent scores, it is not unusual for young children with Down syndrome to be functioning in the moderate range of developmental delay, acquiring standard milestones at approximately 50% the expected rate.

In other words, a 4-year-old child with Down syndrome would be expected to be attaining developmental age equivalent results of approximately 2 years. As they grow older, children with Down syndrome will likewise tend to be assessed with moderate intellectual disabilities on standardised measures of intelligence. Naturally, variations can occur, with some children and individuals functioning in the mild range of delay, but others more severely delayed.

Approximately 5–10% of children with Down syndrome will also present with autism spectrum disorder, although making such comorbid diagnoses is challenging, as it can be difficult to delineate "true" signs of autism spectrum disorder from behaviours related to their intellectual disability. Approximately 1% of boys with Down syndrome have comorbid diagnoses of Klinefelter syndrome, whereby there is an additional X chromosome.

Individuals with Down syndrome are likely to experience a number of physical and mental health issues more frequently than non-affected individuals, including

- Upper respiratory tract infections.
- Glue ear.
- Visual difficulties caused by either short or long-sightedness, squints, nystagmus, cataracts and Keratoconus (an unusually shaped cornea).
- Hypermobility of joints and low muscle tone.
- A condition known as atlantoaxial instability, whereby there is increased mobility in the atlantoaxial joint in the neck.
- Congenital or acquired hypothyroidism.
- Hirschsprung disease occasioning constipation and toileting difficulties.
- Leukaemia.

Individuals with Down syndrome can also present more often with a range of cardiac disorders, mainly different types of septal defects. Later in life, they are inclined to experience higher rates of Alzheimer's disease. They are also more vulnerable to late-onset seizure disorders – by 50 years of age, approximately 10% of people with Down syndrome will have experienced a seizure. Although children with Down syndrome generally present with less externalised behavioural difficulties than other children, there is research suggesting that as adults, people with Down syndrome can experience more mood, anxiety and other psychiatric difficulties than the normal population. The knowledge base for prevalence of mental health difficulties in people with disabilities is expanding, but is still inadequate.

Klinefelter syndrome (47XXY syndrome)

Klinefelter syndrome (47XXY syndrome), results from two or more X chromosomes in males. The syndrome was named in 1942 after American endocrinologist Harry Klinefelter, who worked with Fuller Albright and E. C. Reifenstein at Massachusetts General Hospital in Boston. Primary features are infertility and small poorly functioning testicles. Symptoms may also include weaker muscles, greater height, poor coordination, less body hair, breast growth and less interest in sex. Intelligence is usually normal, however, reading difficulties and speech problems are more common.

Symptoms are typically more severe if three or more X chromosomes are present, for example 48XXXY syndrome or 49XXXXY syndrome. Klinefelter syndrome occurs randomly. The extra X chromosome comes from the father and mother nearly equally. Older mothers may have a slightly increased risk of a child with the syndrome, but the condition is not typically inherited from one's parents. Klinefelter syndrome is one of the most common chromosomal disorders, occurring in 1 to 2: 1000 live male births.

As babies and children, XXY males may have weaker muscles and reduced strength. As they grow older, they tend to become taller than average. They may have less muscle control and coordination than other boys of their age. During puberty, the physical traits of the syndrome become more evident, because these boys do not produce as much testosterone as other boys. They have less muscular bodies, less facial and body hair, and broader hips. As teens, XXY males may develop breast tissue and also have weaker bones and a lower energy level than other males. By adulthood, XXY males look similar to males without the condition, although they are often taller. About 10% of XXY males have gynecomastia (enlarged breast tissue) noticeable enough that they may choose to have cosmetic surgery. Affected males are often infertile, or may have reduced fertility.

XXY males are also more likely than other men to have health problems, such as autoimmune disorders, breast cancer, venous thromboembolic disease and osteoporosis. In contrast to these potentially increased risks, rare X-linked recessive conditions are thought to occur less frequently in XXY males than in normal XY males, since these conditions are transmitted by genes on the X chromosome, and people with two X chromosomes are typically only carriers rather than affected by these X-linked recessive conditions.

Some degree of language, learning or reading impairment may be present, and neuropsychological testing often reveals deficits in executive function. Also, delays in motor development may occur. XXY males may sit up, crawl and walk later than other infants. They may also struggle in school, both academically and with sports.

48XXYY or 48XXXY syndromes occur in 1:18,000–50,000 male births. The incidence of 49XXXXY syndrome is 1: 85,000–1:100,000 male births, making these variations extremely rare. Additional chromosomal material can contribute to cardiac, neurological, orthopaedic and other anomalies. Mosaicism 47XXY/46XX syndromes with clinical features suggestive of Klinefelter Syndrome are very rare.

Turner syndrome (45 x OR 45XO syndrome)

Turner syndrome, also known 45X, or 45X0, is a genetic condition in which a female is partly or completely missing an X chromosome. Henry Turner first described the condition in 1938, and in 1964 it was determined to be due to a chromosomal abnormality. Symptoms vary. Often, a short and webbed neck, low-set ears, low hairline at the back of the neck, short stature, and swollen hands and feet, are seen at birth. Typically, affected girls develop menstrual periods and breasts only with hormone treatment, and are unable to have children without reproductive technology. Heart defects, diabetes and low thyroid hormone occur more frequently.

Most people with Turner syndrome have normal intelligence but may have difficulty with spatial visualisation skills and mathematics. Vision and hearing problems occur more often. Turner syndrome occurs in between 1:2,000 and 1:5,000 females. Ninety-nine percent of Turner syndrome conceptions are thought to end in miscarriage or stillbirth, and as many as 15% of all spontaneous abortions have the 45X karyotype. Generally, people with Turner syndrome have a shorter life expectancy, mostly due to heart problems and diabetes.

Turner syndrome is not usually inherited. In most cases, it is a sporadic event, and the risk of recurrence is not increased for subsequent pregnancies. Turner syndrome manifests itself differently case by case, with no two individuals sharing the same features. While most of the physical findings are harmless, significant medical problems can be associated with the syndrome, including:

- Physical features such as short stature, broad chest, low-set ears and obesity, and characteristic facial features.
- Reproductive difficulties and sterility, and absence of menstrual periods.
- A range of cardiac abnormalities.
- "Horseshoe" kidney.
- Visual impairments.
- Ear infections and hearing loss.
- Attention deficit hyperactivity disorder.
- Non-verbal learning disability, particularly in maths and spatial relations.
- Thyroid disorders such as hypothyroidism.
- Increased risk of Type 1 and Type 2 diabetes.
- Social interaction difficulties, and psychological symptoms of depression, possibly related to age at diagnosis and increased substance use.

Microdeletion syndromes

Velocardiofacial syndrome (22q11.2 syndrome)

Velocardiofacial syndrome is the most frequently occurring microdeletion syndrome and is described as a "model for understanding microdeletion disorders" due to its prevalence, specific phenotype and the amount of research relevance it holds for other conditions and to genetic disorders in general. The earliest descriptions of the disorder date from the 1950s by Sedla-kova in Czechoslovakia, based more on specific symptoms than aetiology, and the label "velocardiofacial syndrome" was formally constructed in 1978 by Robert J. Shprintzen, (Upstate Medical University Syracuse USA). Originally labelled therefore as Shprintzen Syndrome, it was renamed velocardiofacial syndrome (VCFS) or 22q11.2 Syndrome at the behest of Professor Shprintzen.

54 Diagnosing Young Children with Neurodevelopmental Disorders

"Velocardiofacial Syndrome" refers to the three primary areas of impact of the syndrome:

- Velo (From the Latin "Velum"): Structural abnormalities of the palate, often requiring complex surgery, and structural problems of the pharynx, again requiring complex surgery. Cleft palates, including asymmetrical cleft palates, are common.
- Cardio: Heart abnormalities, again often requiring early surgical intervention, which is generally successful.
- Facial: The tendency for the syndrome to present with similar facial characteristics.

Velocardiofacial syndrome is currently estimated to occur in 1:2,000 to 1:4,000 live births. Approximately 20 years ago, incidence rates were often reported as 1:16,000, but these statistics have been revised over the last two decades, reflecting the progress made in specific genetic assessment techniques rather than any increase in incidence of occurrence.

Velocardiofacial syndrome is caused oxymoronically by a large microdeletion of approximately 6 megabase pairs on chromosome 22 at q11.2. It is equally prevalent in males and females. The disorder can be inherited or can occur de novo.

As well as the three labels (Shprintzen syndrome, 22q11.2 syndrome and velocardiofacial syndrome), a specific variant of the disorder – DiGeorge Sequence – shares the same microdeletion site but with additional symptomatology, including hypothyroidism and hypoplastic immune system (Figures 4.2 and 4.3).

The specific defects associated with velocardiofacial syndrome are detailed below:

VELO:

- Cleft palate.
- Velo-pharyngeal incompetence.
- Eating and swallowing difficulties.
- Hypernasality.

CARDIO:

- VSD (ventrical septal defect).
- Tetralogy of Fallot.

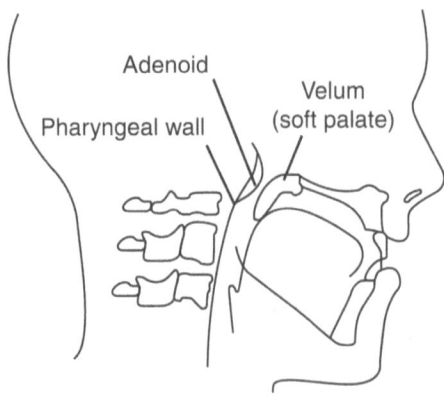

Figure 4.2 Schematic diagram of velocardiofacial syndrome

Selected genetic and chromosomal disorders 55

Ventrical Septal Defect = a hole between 2 bottom chambers LV and RV.
Tetralogy of Fallot = pulmonary stenosis, right ventricular hypertrophy (thickening), overriding aorta and ventrical septum defect.
Truncus Arteriosis = only 1 large vessel leaving heart, not 2.
Patent Ductus Arteriosis = an open connection allowing oxygenated blood from high pressure aorta back into low pressure pulmonary artery which has de-oxygenated blood.
Interrupted Aortic Arch often occurs with ventricular septal defect.
Tricuspid Artresia = failure of tricuspid valve to develop.

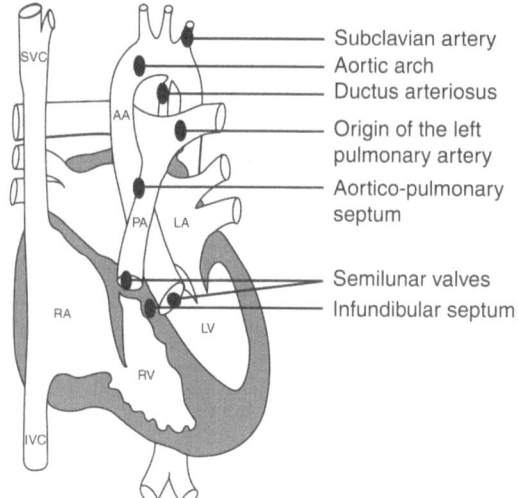

Figure 4.3 Cardiac anomalies in 22q11.2 syndrome

- Truncus arteriosis.
- Patent ductus arteriosus.
- Interrupted aortic arch.
- Tricuspid artresia.

FACIAL:

- Characteristic facial features including:

  - elongated face.
  - almond-shaped eyes.
  - wide nose.
  - small ears.

In addition, up to 170 other health issues can occur, including:

- eye problems.
- middle-ear infections (otitis media).
- hypoparathyroidism.
- immune system problems.
- weak muscles.
- curvature of the spine (scoliosis).
- leg pains and cramps.

Velocardiofacial syndrome is an intensively researched condition in relation to neurological and psychological difficulties and anomalies, including:

- Low IQ scores, with a mean of approximately 70 often reported.
- Spatial reasoning difficulties.

Table 4.3 Rates of psychiatric disorder in studies of vcfs

Shprintzen et al. 1992	*Chronic paranoid schizophrenia 10%*
Pulver et al. 1994	Schizophrenia or schizoaffective disorder 29%
Papolos et al. 1996	Bipolar I Disorder 30%
	Bipolar II Disorder 30–47%
	Schizoaffective disorder 20%
	Psychosis 40%
Murphy et al. 1999	Psychosis 30%
	Schizoaffective Disorder 26%
	Bipolar Disorder 2%
	Major depressive disorder 12%
	Psychosis not otherwise specified 2%
Provenzani et al. 2022	1:10 people with 22q11.2 deletion experience psychosis
Leader et al (2023)	45% of sample presented with diagnosed psychotic disorders
Wallen, Gillberg et al. (2023)	43% of adults with major depressive episodes

- Significant learning difficulties, particularly in relation to mathematics.
- Attentional difficulties.
- Epilepsy.
- Increased rates of autism spectrum disorder.
- Increased rates of anxiety.
- Social interaction difficulties.

Perhaps the most alarming statistic of all is that in adolescence and adulthood, people with vcfs have a significantly increased incidence of mental health disorders, with particular concern about prodromal behaviours, psychotic symptoms, depressive illnesses and chronic anxiety. Table 4.3 summarises the consistency of research findings over a number of decades and illustrates the possible importance of this syndrome in understanding the genetic mechanisms potentially involved in the causation of schizophrenia and other mental health disorders:

This frequency of psychosis is complex and the subject of intense research. Specific genes associated with the microdeletion site are thought to play a role in the regulation of dopamine. Research is also focusing upon structural and "architectural" abnormalities of the brain, including decreased overall brain volume due to diminution of grey matter, enlargement of the frontal lobe, decrease in tissue volume in the left parietal lobe and decrease in right cerebellar tissue volume.

The possible "downstream" implications of these anomalies are becoming clearer over time. Individuals with 22q11.2 syndrome appear to have atypical patterns of visual exploration, particularly when attempting to recognise and interpret facial expressions of emotionality in others. They are also more likely to experience increased social anxiety and present with poorer social skills than the general population. This confluence of symptoms and findings has been described as indicative of a "homogeneous" subtype of schizophrenia, suggestive of the "overshadowing" of symptoms which is known to occur with some genetic disorders.

The "community" of parents of children with vcfs, along with researchers and practitioners, constitute a strong, coherent presence, including the Velocardiofacial Syndrome Education Foundation, which is active in community and research-based education through conferences, publications and media awareness campaigns.

Smith-Magenis syndrome

Originally described by Doctors Anne Smith and R. Ellen Magenis in 1982, and with clear delineation of symptoms by 1986, Smith-Magenis syndrome is a microdeletion at chromosome 17p11.2. Approximately 25 genes are located in that region, including RA11 which is thought to be responsible for most of the syndrome's characteristic features:

- Prominent facial features, short hands and fingers, and reduced range of movement at the elbows.
- Early failure to thrive.
- Cardiac defects, renal anomalies, brain anomalies, eye abnormalities, hearing loss and spinal scoliosis.
- Severe sleep disturbances caused by "phase shift" in circadian rhythms, with melatonin produced during the day rather than at night. This is a feature unique to Smith-Magenis syndrome.

Individuals with Smith-Magenis syndrome tend to present with moderately delayed intellectual skills and delayed language skills. They often present with a hoarse voice, and a high threshold to pain. They have an increased incidence rate of autistic-type features, particularly reduced empathy, repetitive questioning, insistence on sameness and a restricted range of activities. They are frequently extremely anxious. They also present with a stereotypic "self-hug" movement. The most concerning features of Smith-Magenis syndrome relate to maladaptive behaviours (Table 4.4).

Smith-Magenis syndrome is rare. It occurs in 1:25,000 to 1:50,000 live births, equally distributed by gender. It is felt that the condition may be under-diagnosed due to the more subtle presentation of phenotypic symptoms in early childhood. As with velocardiofacial syndrome, there is a strong linkage and partnership between parents and professionals in the ongoing research into and management of Smith-Magenis syndrome.

Williams syndrome (Williams-Beurens syndrome)

First described in 1961 by J.C.P. Williams and colleagues, Williams syndrome is caused by a microdeletion at chromosome 7q11.23, encompassing a region of some 17 genes, and is estimated to have an incidence rate of 1:20,000 live births. Most people with

Table 4.4 Behavioural symptoms in Smith-Magenis syndrome

Difficulty or characteristic	Prevalence
Sleep disturbance	65–100%
Impulsivity	80% or higher
Hyperactivity	Over 80%
Autistic traits	70–93%
Self-hugging	"Highly characteristic"
Physical aggression	Generally over 70%
Destructive behaviour	81%
Self-injury	Over 70%
Intellectual disability	Over 75%

Williams syndrome share a wide range of physical, social and cognitive characteristics, which may occur to a greater or lesser degree:

- Distinctive facial features: Long upper lip, small chin, "generous" lips, chubby face, upturned nose and flattened nose bridge. Some may have a squint.
- Weight and growth problems: The newborn may have a low birth weight and gain weight slowly. Adults are usually shorter than average.
- Feeding difficulties: Including swallowing difficulties and excessively slow eating.
- Hyperacusis: Extreme sensitivity to sound, including a significant startle response to normal sounds.
- Dental problems: Including smaller than normal teeth, oddly shaped teeth, widely spaced teeth and a misaligned bite.
- Cardiovascular defects: Common heart problems include narrowed aorta (aortic stenosis) and narrowed pulmonary artery (pulmonary stenosis).
- Hypercalcaemia: Higher than normal levels of calcium in the blood.
- Colic: It is thought that the colic or irritability frequently experienced by babies with Williams syndrome may be caused by hypercalcaemia.
- Hernias: Including groin and umbilical (belly button) hernias.
- Kidney problems: Including variations in shape and function.
- Muscle and joint problems: Including poor muscle tone, weak muscles, overly loose joints, muscle contractures and poor physical coordination.
- Speech delays: Receptive language delays are more frequent than expressive language difficulties.

Intellectual and personality traits may include developmental delays, intellectual disabilities and below average IQ, learning difficulties, poor spatial skills and attention deficit hyperactivity disorder (ADHD). People with Williams syndrome are often "overly sociable", with no fear of strangers nor social interaction. They are often musical. As with other genetic disorders, people with Williams syndrome can have comorbid diagnoses of autism spectrum disorder, but as with other genetic disorders, caution must be applied to differentiating between phenotypic behaviours associated with Williams syndrome and the behavioural traits commonly associated with autism spectrum disorder.

Prader-Willi syndrome

Prader-Willi syndrome is more complex in aetiology than some other microdeletion syndromes. After its initial description as "polysarcia" by John Langdon Down in the 1860s, symptoms were further detailed by endocrinologists Doctors Prader, Labhart and Willi in the 1950s, but it was not for some time that a small deletion was noted on chromosome 15 for some individual cases. By the 1980s, it was confirmed that Prader-Willi syndrome was caused by "the lack of expression of maternally imprinted/paternally expressed genes" in the region 15q11-15q13. This is now referred to as the Prader-Willi syndrome critical region (PWSCR). The two mechanisms causing Prader-Willi syndrome are:

- A deletion of chromosome 15 of paternal origin.
- The inheritance of two maternally derived (but not paternally derived) chromosome 15's.

Selected genetic and chromosomal disorders 59

This phenomenon is known as "maternal uniparental disomy", and this factor is extremely complex. Interested readers may wish to pursue this information further through reference to specific texts on genetics, but essentially it means that other syndromes such as Angelman's syndrome can be associated with the same deletion point.

Prader-Willi syndrome ranges in incidence from 1:22,000 to 1:25,000. It has a developmental phenotype characterised by:

- Significant hypotonia at birth and failure to thrive during infancy.
- Overeating, developmental delay and/or intellectual disability and short stature during childhood.
- Obesity and psychiatric issues during adulthood.

It is the obsessive craving for and seeking of food which marks the most general understanding of Prader-Willi syndrome as a phenotypic disorder. Intellectual skills are described as variable and possibly indicative of two different subtypes of the syndrome. Autistic-type features are also reported as variable, again suggestive of subtypes. There is generally a strong need for routine, and sleep disorders and difficulties with body temperature regulation are also described. Subtype variations are also described in relation to later mental health issues such as psychosis and depression.

Charles Dickens described in "Pickwick Papers" a "fat and red-faced boy in a state of somnolency", as "young dropsy", "young opium eater" and "boa constrictor", in a possible early reference to someone with Prader-Willi syndrome.

Wolf-Hirschhorn syndrome

Wolf-Hirschhorn syndrome is a rare microdeletion syndrome occurring in approximately 1:50,000 live births, the deletion occurring at chromosome 4p. Its characteristic symptoms are:

- Severe growth restriction.
- Microcephaly.
- Hydrocephalus.
- Corpus callosum agenesis.
- Severe general learning disability.
- Severe comprehension and speech delays.
- Seizures.
- Ataxic gait.
- Hypotonia muscle hypertrophy.
- Microcephaly.
- A distinct "Greek warrior helmet" face.
- Contracture of hands, wrists and feet.
- Poor development of secondary sexual characteristics.
- Closure defects such as cleft lip or palate, coloboma of the eye, cardiac septal defects.
- Hypoplasia of the kidneys and genital tract.
- Hernias.
- Immunodeficiency.

Children with Wolf-Hirschhorn syndrome often pass away prior to birth or in the first year of life. Approximately one-third die within the first two years of life, generally of heart defects, aspiration pneumonia, other severe infection or from seizures.

Microduplication syndromes

Microduplication syndromes tend to occur less frequently than microdeletion syndromes, but advances in genetic assessment techniques are bringing more to light. They can be very rare and incidence rates not always reported. There can be a consequent dearth of research information about micro-duplication syndromes. A number of microduplication syndromes are listed below:

Duplication 3q syndrome: Falek and colleagues originally described this syndrome in 1966, but it was initially confused with Brachmann-de Lange Syndrome. It was Hirschorn and others who confirmed the duplication on chromosome 3q21 in 1973. This syndrome features growth deficiency, intellectual disability with brain abnormalities including seizures, characteristic facial appearance, cardiac defects, chest deformities and hernias.

Duplication 9 syndrome (Trisomy 9p syndrome): This was first identified by Rethore and colleagues in 1970, and features growth deficiency, severe intellectual disability, microcephaly and other dysmorphic physical characteristics. It is a very rare disorder.

Duplication 10p syndrome: The duplication point described by Yunis and Sanchez in 1974 is 10q25, and the syndrome is characterised by moderate to severe intellectual disability, and characteristic facial and physical features. Heart and renal malformations are common, and many children with the syndrome are reported to die in the first year of life.

Duplication 15q syndrome: From Prader-Willi syndrome, it was noted that there was a possibility of a duplication on chromosome 15q. 15q microduplication syndrome, described by Fujimoto and colleagues, is rare, and the cause is hypothesised to arise from "unbalanced translocations". Severe to profound intellectual disability is described, as are a range of dysmorphic physical characteristics. Congenital heart defects are reported to be the primary cause of death.

Genetic mutations

Fragile x syndrome

This is the single most identifiable inherited cause of intellectual disability and also the most commonly occurring single-gene mutation leading to diagnoses of autism spectrum disorder (Figure 4.4). The mutation occurs on the X chromosome at Xq27.3 and is described as "dynamic" because the underlying cause of the mutation can increase over generations. First described by Martin and Bell in 1943, and then by Lubs in 1969 and Sutherland (1977), the genetic mutation was not confirmed by DNA testing until 1991 by Oberle. Research is ongoing into causation, characteristics and heritability. Incidence rates vary according to whether individuals who are effectively not impacted by the genetic mutation are included in studies, but the prevalence rate is generally reported as 1:3,600. Males are generally more affected that females, particularly in terms of intellectual disability.

The core features of Fragile X syndrome vary from mild intellectual and emotional difficulties to severe intellectual disability and autism spectrum disorder, but with most functioning in the mild to moderate range of intellectual disability and with language skills in advance of spatial and mathematical skills. Speech and language skills are colourfully

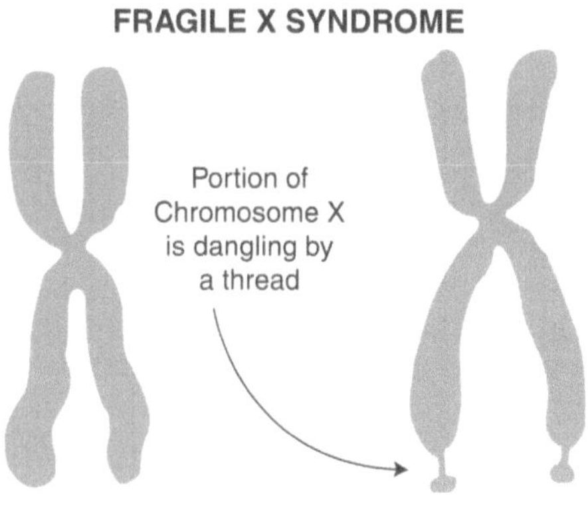

FRAGILE X SYNDROME

Figure 4.4 Schematic representation of Fragile X syndrome

described as featuring "jocular litanic phraseology", and repetitive, perseverative and echolalic features as well. Social interaction difficulties are common, often described with high social anxiety and aversion of eye gaze. Sensory sensitivities are not uncommon, as are stereotypic and maladaptive behaviours such as hand-biting, hand flapping, body rocking, running and pacing.

The rate of diagnosis of autism spectrum disorder in Fragile X is high, but as in other genetic conditions, the autistic-type presentation is not necessarily consistent. For example, studies have demonstrated that the "Theory of Mind" difficulties associated with autism spectrum disorder are more likely to be associated with short-term memory deficits in individuals with Fragile X syndrome.

Attentional difficulties are common in Fragile X syndrome but are exacerbated by the high levels of anxiety experienced by individuals with Fragile X syndrome. The level of symptomatology in Fragile X syndrome is also demonstrated to vary considerably dependent upon the severity of intellectual disability.

Individuals with Fragile X syndrome are often prone to illness early in life, particularly reflux and ear infections, and visual issues. Over time, there is longitudinal evidence of declining IQ scores, but this may be an artefact of intelligence testing per se as research does not indicate declining mental age scores over time. Fragile X syndrome is inherited, but the mechanism for this and the various permutations depend upon a number of genetic factors, including which parent carries either the "pre-mutation" or the "full mutation". Texts such as "Understanding Fragile X Syndrome" (Carvajal and Aldridge) provide excellent guides to this process.

Rett syndrome

The German neurologist Andreas Rett described, and filmed, characteristic behaviours and appearance of a group of affected girls in 1966. Research since then has confirmed the aetiology, characteristic phenotype and incidence rate of what is now known as Rett syndrome. It is a genetic mutation leading to a severely degenerative trajectory of skills and predominantly affects girls. The genetic mutation has been specified as X-linked, occurring at Xq28, affecting the "binding protein" MECP2. It occurs in approximately 1:10,000 females, and although it is known to occur in males, that incidence rate has not been possible to calculate due to its rarity of occurrence.

Rett syndrome was at one stage regarded as part of the broad spectrum of autistic disorders and included in DSM IV-TR as such, but the confirmation of the genetic mutation in 1999 was factored into the subsequent release of DSM 5 in 2013 where Rett syndrome was no longer seen as a component of autism spectrum disorder. The developmental trajectory of Rett syndrome is summarised below:

- Apparently normal gestation and birth history.
- Physical appearance and head circumference normal at birth.
- Subsequent head growth falling below expected norms.
- Sub-optimal developmental progress.
- Disturbance in spontaneous movements, noted at approximately 3 months.
- Diminution of language and hand use skills approaching 2 years of age.
- Stereotyped hand movements such as twisting, patting, face or hair rubbing.
- Initial hypotonia changes to hypertonia and dystonia.
- Inability to walk, or presence of dyspraxic gait.
- Irregular breathing patterns, including breath-holding, forced expiration and non-epileptic vacant spells.
- Scoliosis.
- Constipation.
- Reduction in height over time.
- Epilepsy, with incidence rates over 75% reported.
- Physical movement regression can result in many women with Rett syndrome being confined to wheelchairs as they grow older.

Assessing intellectual skills in individuals with Rett syndrome, particularly post-regression, is made extremely complex by the lack of speech and language and the loss of hand function, but it is estimated that most individuals with the disorder have severe intellectual disabilities. Again, there is strong parent and professional liaison for Rett syndrome, for example national Rett syndrome associations partnering with various research organisations to monitor the prevalence of the disorder, to coordinate research and to make recommendations regarding support and service provision.

Tuberous sclerosis

Tuberous sclerosis is a rare genetic disease that causes benign tumours to grow in the brain and several areas of the body, including the spinal cord, nerves, eyes, lung, heart, kidneys and skin. It is caused by mutations in either the *TSC1* or the *TSC2* gene, and occurs in approximately 1:5,00 to 1:10,000 births. The term "tuberous sclerosis" refers to characteristic "tuber" or potato-like nodules in the brain, which are affected by calcium over time and become hard or sclerotic. It is a lifelong condition with a highly variable prognosis, depending upon the severity of symptoms. Some sufferers can lead relatively independent lives, but others can be severely affected. Common neurological symptoms include:

- Brain tumours.
- Seizures.
- Developmental delay and intellectual disability, ranging from mild to severe.
- Behavioural and emotional difficulties such as aggression, attention deficit hyperactivity disorder, obsessive-compulsive disorder, and repetitive, destructive and even self-harm behaviours.

Selected genetic and chromosomal disorders 63

- Autism spectrum disorder is a frequent comorbid diagnosis.
- Skin abnormalities.
- Kidney problems.
- Lung lesions.

Awareness of some of the symptoms of tuberous sclerosis was as early as 1835, but it was Doctor Désiré-Magloire Bourneville who first reported and categorised tuberous sclerosis in 1880 in a young patient with seizures, hemiplegia, renal tumours and "mental sub-normality".

Neurofibromatosis type 1 (NF1)

Neurofibromatosis type 1 (NF1) is a genetic mutation on the NF1 gene that causes tumours to grow along nerves. These tumours are usually benign but may cause a range of symptoms, including:

- Birthmarks known as café au lait spots: light or dark brown patches that can occur anywhere on the body.
- Soft, non-cancerous tumours on or under the skin (neurofibromas).
- Clusters of freckles in unusual places such as the armpits, groin and under the breasts.
- Problems with the bones, eyes and nervous system.

Children with NF1 are usually of average intelligence but can experience specific learning difficulties and comorbid conditions such as attention deficit hyperactivity disorder and autism spectrum disorder. Behavioural difficulties can also occur, particularly in relation to disinhibition. NF1 occurs in approximately 1: 3,000 children.

Pitt-Hopkins syndrome

This is not only a rare genetic disorder caused by a mutation on chromosome 18q21.2, but also includes significant amounts of deleted genetic material. Early interest and research into this syndrome is accredited to Doctors David Pitt and Ian Hopkins at the Royal Children's Hospital in Melbourne in 1978. Features of the syndrome include severe developmental delay and intellectual disability, characteristic facial features, epilepsy in approximately 40% of cases, and "overbreathing" whilst awake. Stereotypic movements of the hands and sometimes the head from side to side are common, possibly occurring in over 80% of such children. More specifically, there are repeated hand-to-mouth movements, hand clapping, flapping, wringing, swaying or lateral movements. These may have a communicative function. Aggression, anxiety, disruptiveness and sleep disturbances are occasionally reported. A major feature of Pitt-Hopkins syndrome is the breathing abnormality, characterised by paroxysms of hyperventilation followed by breath-holding until cyanosis, but only whilst the child is awake.

Turnpenny-Fry syndrome

Turnpenny-Fry syndrome is an exceptionally rare genetic disorder and a graphic example of the advances in genetic assessment techniques. Professor Peter Turnpenny is Consultant Clinical Geneticist and Honorary Clinical Professor, University of Exeter Medical School, and Doctor Andrew Fry is Clinical Senior Lecturer in Genetics at The Institute of Medical Genetics, University Hospital of Wales.

Turnpenny-Fry syndrome is caused by a mutation on the PCGF2 gene and is characterised by differing degrees of intellectual disability, developmental delay, distinctive facial dysmorphism and skeletal abnormalities. At the time of writing, fewer than 20 cases of this disorder have been reported world-wide. Cardiac and hearing difficulties have been reported in relation to this syndrome, as have behavioural challenges such as possible autism spectrum disorder and attention deficit hyperactivity disorder, but with so few reported cases of the disorder, it is not possible to make generalised statements about comorbidities.

Disorders caused by environmental agents

Fetal alcohol spectrum disorder (FASD)

Of all the "substance abuse" related disorders which occur in early pregnancy, maternal alcohol use is regarded has the "earliest, most debilitating, and longest-lasting effect on the foetus". Ironically, alcohol is not an illicit substance. It is legal, freely available, advertised and socially accepted, and governments of all persuasions profit from its popularity and availability through taxes and excises. The French Paediatrician Doctor Paul Lemoine initially recognised the association between maternal alcohol consumption and foetal damage in 1968. He noted similar dysmorphic features amongst a cohort of infants whose mothers had taken alcohol during pregnancy. The condition was named "Fetal Alcohol Syndrome" in 1973 by the University of Washington, based on three specific components:

- Dysmorphic facial features.
- Growth delay.
- Central nervous system effects.

The term fetal alcohol spectrum disorder (FASD) was broadly adopted in 2015. The core diagnostic criteria for FASD needs a clear and substantiated history of maternal alcohol consumption, and the amount and timing of consumption are vital. The "classic" features of FASD include:

- Dysmorphic facial features.
- Growth retardation.
- Central nervous system deficits.
- Possible intellectual disability, with verbal IQ often better than non-verbal scores.
- Poor working memory skills.
- Difficulties with "cause-effect" reasoning.
- Learning difficulties and difficulties with abstract thinking.
- Problems of executive function and attention deficit hyperactivity disorder.
- Behavioural problems related to hypersensitivity, hyposensitivity or sensory stimulation.
- Defiant behaviours.
- Social communication and cognition deficits.
- Emotional difficulties.

In addition, FASD has been associated with a range of visual, hearing, dental, cardiac, renal and skeletal conditions. The impact of alcohol on the developing foetus varies by trimester. In the first trimester, alcohol can cause damage to the brain and other organs, and may be seen through smaller head size, small wide-set eyes, a thin upper lip and

Table 4.5 Diagnostic criteria for fetal alcohol spectrum disorder

Fetal alcohol spectrum disorder (FASD)

Diagnostic criteria	Diagnostic categories	
	FASD with 3 sentinel facial features	FASD with < 3 sentinel facial features
Prenatal alcohol exposure	Confirmed or unknown	Confirmed
Neurodevelopmental domains Brain structure/Neurology Motor skills Cognition Language Academic achievement Memory Attention Executive function, including impulse control and hyperactivity Affect regulation Adaptive behaviour, social skills or Social Communication	Severe impairment in at least three neurodevelopmental domains	Severe impairment in at least three neurodevelopmental domains
Sentinel facial features Short palpebral fissure Smooth philtrum Thin upper lip	Presence of 3 sentinel facial features	Presence of 0, 1 or 2 sentinel facial features

other birth defects. The child may experience early growth difficulties. Alcohol during the second and third trimester may not cause immediately obvious signs, but damage to the brain can later be manifest in learning and behavioural problems such as poor attention and memory, impulsiveness and difficulties with "cause-and-effect" reasoning. Long-term impacts may include social and employment issues, reduced life expectancy and a higher risk of substance abuse and suicide.

Assessment and diagnosis of FASD is a complex and specialised multidisciplinary process, and with few specialist assessment clinics, it is therefore under-recognised and undiagnosed. It is described as a "hidden harm". Two sub categories are defined: FASD with three sentinel facial features and FASD with less than three sentinel facial features (Table 4.5).

Any assessment of FASD must include a thorough case history and documentation of birth defects, adverse pre-and post-natal exposures (including alcohol) and known medical conditions, including genetic or other syndromes, and full growth history. The current guidelines and recommendation surrounding FASD are in the process of review, with a predicted release date for these revisions in 2025. One recommendation is that the precise wording and format of the guidelines should be more closely aligned to those of DSM-5-TR.

Incidence rates for FASD vary considerably across the globe for a host of socio-economic and cultural reasons, but it is possible to single out specific "population" groups of concern where incidence rates significantly higher and risk factors are more complex:

- "Aboriginal" populations.
- Incarcerated populations.
- Children in care.

Table 4.6 Incidence of fetal alcohol spectrum disorder by geographic zone

Incidence rates of FASD per 1,000 population by geographic region

Geographic region	Lowest reported	Highest reported
Global Average	7.7	14.6
Africa	7.8	14.8
The Americas	8.8	16.6
Eastern Mediterranean	0.1	0.2
Europe	19.8	37.4
South-East Asia	1.4	2.7
Western Pacific	6.7	12.7

Countries and regions where the incidence of FASD exceeds 1% of population are at particular risk, and in one study of 187 nations, 76 countries were found to be in that risk demographic. In these countries, it was extrapolated that the risk of FASD was in fact higher than the risk of some common birth defects such as Down syndrome and Spina Bifida in developed countries such as the United States. Incidence rates vary significantly from study to study, survey to survey, but not the general trend (Table 4.6).

Bibliography

Australian Guide to the Diagnosis of Fetal Alcohol Syndrome Disorder (FASD) (2020), Telethon KIDS Institute, and University of Sydney.

Baker-Gomez, S. (2004), Missing Genetic Pieces-Strategies for Living With VCFS, Desert Pearl Publishing.

Bassett, A. S., and Chow, E. W. C. (2008), "Schizophrenia and 22q11.2 Deletion Syndrome", Current Psychiatry Reports, 10(2), pp 148–157.

Campbell, L. E., Corliss, C., Duijff, S., Green, A., and Roche, L. (2024), "Psychological Interventions for Individuals with 22q11.2 Deletion Syndrome: A Systematic Review", Advances in Neurodevelopmental Disorders, 8(4), pp 511–523.

Carvajal, I. F., and Aldridge, D. (2011), Understanding Fragile X Syndrome: A Guide for Families and Professionals, Jessica Kingsley Publishers.

Cassidy, S. B., and Driscoll, D. J. (2009), "Prader-Willi Syndrome", European Journal of Human Genetics, 17(1), pp 3–13.

Dubourg, L., Kojovic, N., Eliez, S., Shaer, M., and Schneider, M. (2023), "Visual Processing of Complex Social Scenes in 22q11.2 Deletion Syndrome: Relevance for Negative Symptoms", Psychiatry Research, 321(7), 115074.

Duijff, S. N., Klaasen, P. W., Swanenburg de Veye, H. F., Beemer, F. A., Sinnema, G., and Vorstman, A. S. (2018), "Cognitive Development in Children with 22q11.2 Deletion Syndrome", The British Journal of Psychiatry, 200(6), pp 462–468.

Fisch, G. (Ed.) (2003), Genetics and Genomics of Neurobehavioural Disorders, Humana Press.

Ge, R., et al. (2023), "Source-Based Morphometry Reveals Structural Brain Abnormalities in 22q11.2 Syndrome", Human Brain Mapping, 45(1), pp 1–15.

Genetic Alliance; The New York-Mid-Atlantic Consortium for Genetic and Newborn Screening Services (2009), Understanding Genetics: A New York-Mid-Atlantic Guide for Patients and Health Care Professionals, Genetic Alliance.

Goodspeed, K., et al. (2018), "Pitt-Hopkins Syndrome: A Review of Current Literature, Clinical Approach, and 23 Patient Case Series", Journal of Child Neurology, 33(3), pp 233–244.

Hemmings, C., and Bouras, K. (2016), Psychiatric and Behavioural Disorders in Intellectual Disability (3rd Edition), Cambridge University Press.

Howlin, P. A., Charman, T., and Ghaziuddin, M. (2011), The SAGE Handbook of Developmental Disorders, SAGE Publications.

Jones, K. L., Jones, M. C., and Del Campo, M. (2021), Smith's Recognizable Patterns of Human Malformation (8th Edition), Saunders/Elsevier.

Kobrynski, L. J., and Sullivan, K. E. (2007), "Velocardiofacial Syndrome, DiGeorge Syndrome: The Chromosome 22q11.2 Deletion Syndromes", The Lancet, 370, pp 1443–1452.

Kwiatkowski, D. J., Whittemore, V. H., and Thiele, E. A. (Eds.) (2010), Tuberous Sclerosis Complex: Genes, Clinical Features and Therapeutics, Wiley-Blackwell.

Lange, S., et al. (2017), "Global Prevalence of Fetal Alcohol Spectrum Disorder Among Children and Youth: A Systematic Review and Meta-analysis", JAMA Pediatrics, 171(10), pp 948–956.

Leader, G., Curtin., A., Shprintzen, R., Whelan, S., Coyne, R., and Mannian, A. (2023), "Adaptive Living Skills, Sleep Problems, and Mental Health Disorders in Adults with 22q11.2 Deletion Syndrome", Research in Developmental Disorders, 136, p. 104491.

Murphy, K. C., et al. (1999), "High Rates of Schizophrenia in Adults with Velocardio-Facial Syndrome", Archives of General Psychiatry, 56, pp 940–945.

Murphy, K. C., and Scambler, P. J. (2005), "Velo-Cardio-Facial Syndrome-A Model for Understanding Microdeletion Disorders", Cambridge University Press.

Papolos, D. F., et al. (1996), "Bipolar Spectrum Disorders in Patients Diagnosed with Velo-Cardio-Facial Syndrome: Does a Hemizygous Deletion of Chromosome 22q11 Result in Bipolar Affective Disorder?", American Journal of Psychiatry, 153, pp 1541–1547.

Peippo, M., and Ignatius, J. (2011), "Pitt-Hopkins Syndrome", Molecular Syndromology, 211(20), pp 171–180.

Popova, S., et al. (2023), "Fetal Alcohol Spectrum Disorders", Nature Reviews Disease Primers, 9(11), pp 1–21.

Popova, V., Lange, S., Gmel, G., and Rehm, J. (2017), "Estimation of National, Regional, and Global Prevalence of Alcohol use During Pregnancy and Fetal Alcohol Syndrome: A Systematic Review and Meta-analysis", The Lancet Global Health, 5, pp e290–e299.

Provenzani, U., et al. (2022), "Prevalence and Incidence of Psychotic Disorders in 22q11.2 Deletion Syndrome: A Meta-analysis", International Review of Psychiatry, 34(7-8), pp 676–688.

Pulver, A. E., et al. (1994). "Psychotic Illness in Patients Diagnosed with Velocardio-Facial Syndrome and their Relatives", The Journal of Nervous and Mental Disease, 82, pp 476–478.

Sanders, A. F. P., Hobbs, D. A., Knaus, T. A., and Beaton, E. A. (2022), "Structural Connectivity and Emotional Recognition in Children and Adolescents with Chromosome 22q11.2 Deletion Syndrome", Journal of Developmental Disorders, 53(10), pp 4021–4034.

Schaefer, G. B., Kleimola, C. K., Stenson, C., and Daley, S. E. (1996), Wolf-Hirschhorn Syndrome: A Guidebook for Families, Munroe-Meyer Institute for Genetics and Rehabilitation.

Selikowitz, M. (2008), Down Syndrome, Oxford University Press.

Semel, E., and Rosner, S. R. (2003), Understanding Williams Syndrome: Behavioural Patterns and Interventions, Cambridge University Press.

Shprintzen, R. J., et al. (1992), "Late-onset Psychosis in the Velocardio-Facial Syndrome", American Journal of Medical Genetics, 42, pp 141–142.

Smercornish, S., and Schmitt, J. E. (2024), "Neuroanatomical Correlates of Cognitive Dysfunction in 22q.11.2 Deletion Syndrome", Genes (Basel), 15(4), 440, https://doi.org/10.3390/genes15040440

Smith, A. C. M., Boyd, K. E., Brennan, C., et al. (2002), "Smith-Magenis Syndrome", In: Adam MP, Feldman J, Mirzaa GM, et al., editors. GeneReviews® 13(2), pp 1–17. https://www.ncbi.nlm.nih.gov/books/NBK1310/

Turnpenny, P. D., et al. (2018), "Missense Mutations of the Pro65 Residue of PCGF2 Cause a Recognizable Syndrome Associated with Craniofacial, Neurological, Cardiovascular, and Skeletal Features", American Journal of Human Genetics, 103, pp 786–793.

Upadhyaya, M., and Cooper, D. N. (Eds.) (2012), Neurofibromatosis Type 1, Molecular and Cellular Biology, Springer Publications.

United Nations Trade and Development (2024), "UN List of Least Developed Countries", https://unctad.org/.

Wallen, L., Gillberg, C., Fernell, E., Gillberg, C., and Billstedt, E. (2023), "Neurodevelopmental and Other Psychiatric Disorders in 22q11.2 Deletion Syndrome from Childhood to Adult Age: Prospective Longitudinal Study of 100 Individuals", American Journal of Medical Genetics, 193(20), https://doi.org/10.1002/ajmg.c.32052

5 Population demographics

Is it possible to calculate accurately how many children worldwide may have diagnoses of neurodevelopmental disorders, how many may be eligible for such diagnoses but unaccounted for, how evenly or unevenly these numbers are distributed around the globe, and how do these demographics relate to the characteristics of different countries and regions? Terminology varies, such as "Third World" countries, "under-developed" nations, "low-to-middle income" countries (LMIC's) and "Less developed countries" (LMCs), and reference is made to several surveys which are on the public record, particularly through agencies such as the United Nations, UNICEF and the OECD.

In September 2015, all 193 member states of the United Nations agreed to adopt 17 sustainable development goals (SDGs) as a means to end extreme poverty, reduce inequality and injustice and protect the planet by the years 2030. From this came the "Global Burden of Disease, Injuries, and Risk Factors Study" in 2016, which reported the following statistics:

Worldwide, there were estimated to be approximately 53 million children with neurodevelopmental disorders and disabilities, approximately 50 million of whom were in low- or middle-income countries. This represents 8.4% of children.

At least 250 million children under the age of 5 years, across the 195 countries surveyed, were described as experiencing "suboptimal developmental outcomes". One interpretation of the complex data set involved suggested that even a figure of 350 million children may be an underestimate. The highest rates of occurrence were on the subcontinent and in sub-Saharan Africa.

The survey studies concluded that the global burden of developmental disabilities had not significantly improved since 1990, suggesting that inadequate global attention was being paid to the developmental potential of children who survived childhood as a result of "child survival programs", particularly in sub-Saharan Africa and south Asia. The survey also confirmed the nexus between relative advantage and disadvantage as a factor of socio-demographic conditions in individual countries and regions, and not surprisingly the higher the socio-economic index (SDI), the lower the proportion of children with disabilities, chronic health conditions and sub-optimal developmental outcomes (Figure 5.1).

Similarly, the 2019 World Health Organization and the United Nations Children's Fund (UNICEF) Study, published in 2023, reported that approximately 317 million children and adolescents worldwide experienced health conditions, which contributed towards having a neurodevelopmental disorder. The five most prevalent medical conditions contributing to developmental disabilities were hearing loss, intellectual disability, attention deficit hyperactivity disorder, cerebral palsy and vision loss.

DOI: 10.4324/9781003565338-7

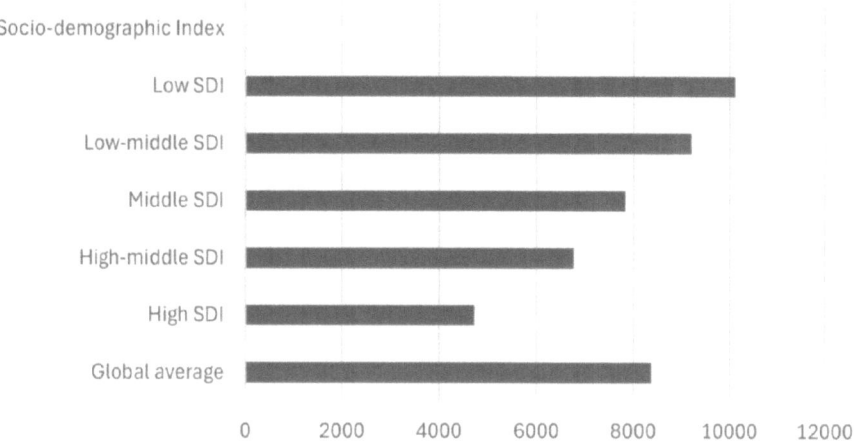

Figure 5.1 Incidence of childhood disability per 100,000 population as measured by the socio-demographic index (SDI)

The UNICEF study further reported that there were approximately 80 million children in the 3–4 years age range experiencing low cognitive, social and/or emotional development, and that one in 10 children had a moderate to severe functional difficulty.

It is not just on the sub-continent or in sub-Saharan Africa that such disproportionate statistics are reported. Indigenous Australian children, living in urban, rural and remote areas, are described as having an increased risk of adverse neurodevelopmental outcomes, including being at risk for a range of specific childhood neurodevelopmental disorders such as cerebral palsy, foetal alcohol spectrum disorder and autism spectrum disorder. Indigenous Australian children are reportedly 30% more likely to have a physical disability and are at a higher risk of developmental and intellectual difficulties compared with non-Indigenous children. The prevalence of neurodevelopmental disorders in some remote communities in Australia is reported to be as high as 30% of the paediatric population.

There are many reasons for this extreme imbalance of developmental outcomes in young children from low, middle-income and "developing" countries, and geographic regions. Some of the factors contributing to this imbalance relate to socio-economic factors, which in turn have "downstream" impacts on basic health, diet, education, access to diagnostic, medical, therapeutic and financial support, for example:

- Inadequate dietary intake.
- Untreated underlying health difficulties.
- Lack of community knowledge and awareness of neurodevelopmental disorders, their symptoms and causative factors.
- Reluctance to approach medical and other support services for a variety of reasons, including community attitudes and possible stigma, financial hardship preventing or restricting travel, logistical difficulties in transport and access.

- Attitudes and suspicions about specialist medical services, for example an adherence to specific beliefs or a mistrust in external sources of information and support.
- A lack of specialist medical services such as paediatricians, and a lack of knowledge of the cause, nature and prevalence of neurodevelopmental disorders.

To help account for these imbalances, the United Nations and its internal agencies conduct surveys to determine which countries are at greatest economic, social, medical and welfare disadvantage. The most recent publication by the United Nations Trade and Development Index of "Least Developed Countries" (LCDs) lists 45 countries which meet that description. The index is formulated on the basis of the following criteria:

- Income.
- Health and education.
- Economic vulnerability.
- Environmental vulnerability.

In its 2024 assessment, the overwhelming proportion of countries deemed to be "less developed" were in sub-Saharan Africa. Others were distributed in South-East Asia, South America and the South Pacific. There are of course pockets of poverty and less than optimal development in other parts of the world, for example in the remote outback desert regions of Australia, but the discrepancy between sub-Saharan Africa and the rest of the world is obviously a great concern from a humanitarian standpoint, but also from an epidemiological stance (Figure 5.2).

If the prevalence of neurodevelopmental disorders in both the sub-continent, sub-Saharan Africa and other remote areas of the globe, are indeed under representations, then global incidence estimates for various neurodevelopmental disorders are also brought into question. This in turn can affect the motivation and sense of urgency, which should follow on from these statistics to pay more attention to the strategies needed to begin correcting this imbalance.

The statistics surrounding the prevalence of autism spectrum disorder dramatically illustrate the complex nexus between socio-economic conditions, cultural beliefs and attitudes, diagnostic and reporting standard, service access:

- Various studies estimate that approximately 95% of autistic individuals live in low-middle income countries, with an increasing prevalence attributed to improved diagnostic testing and an increasing number of children surviving their first 5 years. But the prevalence of autism spectrum disorder may still be an under estimation. Globally, it is estimated that only 1% of autism spectrum disorder emanates from sub-Saharan Africa, and the absence of data from large-scale epidemiological studies compromise the incidence rates.
- An additional challenge to the accurate understanding of autism spectrum disorder prevalence rates in sub-Saharan Africa is the lack of assessment and diagnostic tools that are sensitive to local variations, including cultural interpretations of disability in sub-Saharan Africa. Adaptation of such tests can be impeded because of complex copyright laws and the costs involved in adaptions for local conditions.

Is there a simple solution to the depth and severity of the problems faces in developing countries such as sub-Saharan Africa? The UNICEF Global Report outlines the

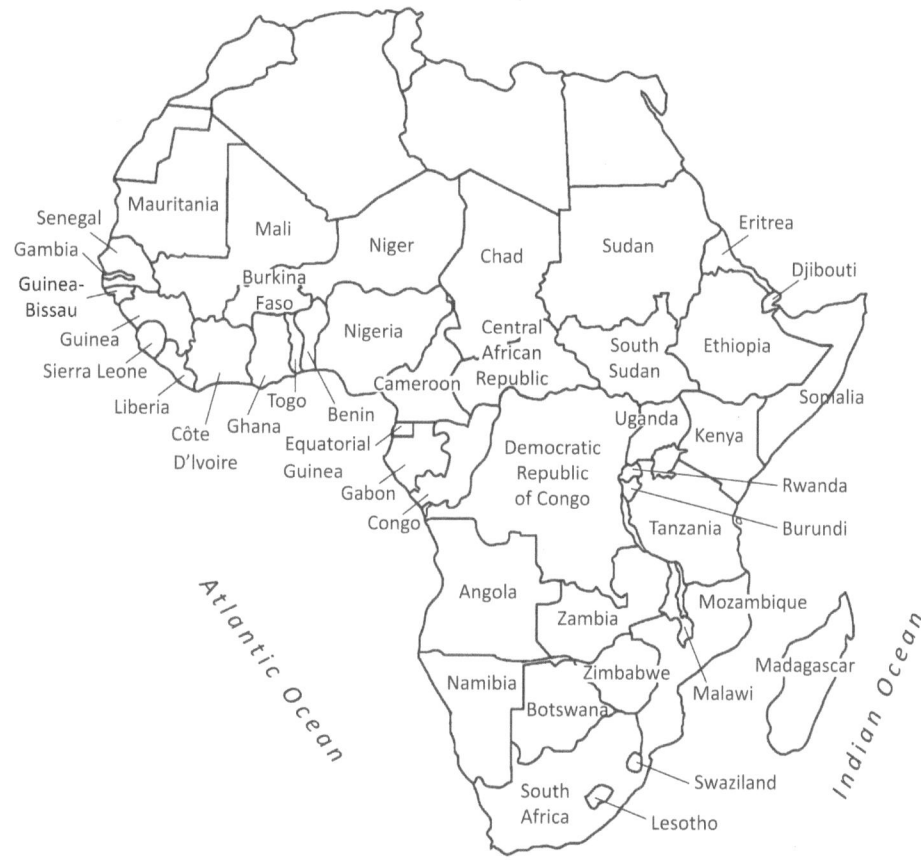

Figure 5.2 Sub-Saharan "less developed" countries

actions needed for "A Way Forward" to address the many socio-economic, political, cultural and geographic barriers to meaningful progress. A number of "Action Areas" are listed:

1 Strengthening coordination and accountability mechanisms to improve outcomes for children and young people with developmental disabilities and their families.
2 Deepening commitment at all levels.
3 Creating opportunities for young people with developmental disabilities and their families to participate in advocacy, leadership, policy, programming and monitoring.
4 Addressing the social determinants of health, well-being and participation of children with developmental disabilities in policies, programmes and financing.
5 Strengthening multisectoral policymaking to address inequities in healthcare and optimise development and health trajectories.
6 Strengthening services throughout the life-course in line with a twin-track approach to inclusive and people-centred evidence-based care.
7 Ensuring that caregivers and children with developmental disabilities have access to information and support.

8 Removing barriers to participation in society, address stigmatisation and discrimination, and foster environments that enable meaningful inclusion of children with developmental disabilities and their families in all spheres of life.
9 Strengthening health information systems, monitoring of programmes and services, and research for data-driven decisions and accountability.
10 Developing inclusive plans and protocols for health emergency preparedness and response.

There is obviously a great deal to be done.

Bibliography

Bolajoko, O., et al. (2024), "Early Childhood Development Strategy For The World's Children With Disabilities", Frontiers in Public Health, 12, pp 1–12.

De, P., and Chattopadhyay, N. (2019), "Effects of Malnutrition on Child Development: Evidence from a Backward District of India", Clinical Epidemiology and Global Health, 7, pp 439–445.

Gonete, A. T., Alemu, T. G., Mekonnen, E. G., and Takele, W. W. (2021), "Malnutrition and Contributing Factors among Newborns Delivered at the University of Gondar Hospital, Northwest Ethiopia: A Cross-Sectional Study", British Journal of Medicine Open, 11, pp 1–10.

UNICEF (2023), Global Report (2019), "A World Ready to Learn: Prioritizing Quality Early Childhood Education", UNICEF, www.unicef.org.

UNICEF, (2023), Global Report on Children with Disabilities: From the Margin to the Mainstream, UNICEF, www.unicef.org (undated).

United Nations Trade and Development (2024), "UN List of Least Developed Countries", UNICEF, www.unicef.org.

Part II
Why do we assess and diagnose neurodevelopmental disorders?

Why do we assess young children? This section explores the technical, bureaucratic and systemic functions of developmental assessments: eligibility for support funding and programmes, entry into preschools and schools, and accuracy of information about a child's diagnosis, strengths, weaknesses and immediate needs.

But of paramount importance is the consideration of parental needs. What emotions, anxieties, fears and doubts do families bring to the assessment context? How does this affect the manner in which neurodevelopmental assessments are conducted?

6 Why do we assess young children?

What is an "assessment", particularly as it pertains to young children? Is it an informal appraisal through guided or informal observations and interactions of what they can do? Is it a medical examination conducted in a surgery or a clinic? Is it an interview with parents, caregivers, therapists and teachers to consider possible programmes of assistance, therapy and intervention? Is it a process of aligning behaviours and symptoms to an objectified diagnostic criterion? Does it involve trying to satisfy external criteria for access to support, for example a level of intelligence or developmental competence? It is of course all of these functions and a lot more.

Psychologists engage in the assessment and diagnostic process with young children in many different contexts. Sometimes a child may be referred to them because a diagnosis of a particular condition (e.g. a genetic disorder such as Down syndrome) has already been made, but additional information is required about the impact of the particular syndrome or disorder upon a child's level of ability. Sometimes referrals are made to psychologists because there is no obvious evidence of any specific disorder or syndrome, but there are concerns about a child's apparent developmental progress or behavioural presentation. This scenario can occur, for example, when there are concerns about possible autism spectrum disorder or developmental delay. Sometimes assessments and diagnoses are required for "systemic" reasons, for example eligibility for funding or programme support such as early intervention services. At other times, assessment may be necessary to assist in clarifying a child's needs to assist teachers and therapists in establishing goals and priorities for intervention.

But the overriding purposes for assessing young children are to help allay the fears and concerns of the parents, and to assist them in appropriate planning and decision-making. Psychologists help to clarify whether parental concerns about behaviours, skills and progress are justified, and to support them in deciding which actions to take to remediate delays. Sometimes the role of psychologists is to direct families to further assessment services, including medical assessments, assessment of hearing and vision, speech pathology or occupational therapy assessments. The role of psychologists can also extend to helping families predict and prepare for future needs and eventualities, and to inform them about future options for assistance, therapy, education and "life-planning."

Psychologists also assess young children to help families understand their role in the development of their young children, to advocate for them if necessary in the complex maze of bureaucratic "eligibility requirements" and to be "on hand" to support families when they experience anxiety, frustration and concern about their child's progress, their own ability to help.

Psychologists are well-placed to fulfil these many and varied professional roles, through their training, experience and professional orientation within the "helping professions". Many have "systemic experience" with government departments and non-government agencies involved in supporting young children and their families. Psychologists are skilled at clinical interviews, report and submission writing, providing accurate and sympathetic feedback, and understanding the roles of other professions.

Governments throughout the developed world have a significant history of providing support services for children with various chronic health conditions, disabilities and disorders. More recently in historic terms, governments have recognised the need to support access to early intervention and therapeutic programmes such as specialised preschools and treatment programmes, early enrolment into special schools and the recognition that some children are best supported in special school contexts, but others more appropriately helped in mainstream schools or special classes within these. There is also increasing government recognition of the rights of parents to broader choices in service choices for their child.

For example, government funding programmes have been established throughout the developed world both to ease the financial burdens families have to face in order to access therapy and intervention services of their choosing, and to recognise the additional stresses placed upon parents' shoulders through the extra hours required to spend with their child, caring for basic needs, foregoing employment opportunities to be "at home" more often, purchasing equipment and attending training programmes.

There are of course differences across countries, states, territories, local councils and counties, boroughs and districts, for "entry criteria" to such programmes and service delivery models, but common elements include the need for medical practitioners, psychologists and other professionals to assess and confirm specific diagnoses and clarify their impact upon a child's functionality. There is therefore a premium upon the skills of psychologists engaged in early childhood assessments to provide the following:

- Appropriate assessment procedures.
- Accuracy of diagnostic terminology and criteria.
- Informative and accurate report-writing.
- Proactive advocacy where necessary for and with families.

To fulfil these various roles effectively, psychologists working with young children and their families also need to have experience and skill in areas such as:

- Collating background referral information from families and other sources.
- Conducting appropriate triage or prioritisation in maintaining referral waiting lists.
- Liaising with other professionals such as medical practitioners, therapists, preschools and schools and other psychologists.
- Staying abreast of research and practice in assessment and diagnosis of young children, and psychological and medical advances in child development.
- Keeping "up to date" with political and bureaucratic policies and procedures regarding eligibility criteria and service provision.

Many of these skills are learned "on the job" depending upon a psychologist's career path and employment context; indeed, there is a rich history of young "early career"

Why do we assess young children? 77

psychologists being "paired" with more experienced practitioners from whom to learn. Other skills, areas of knowledge and expertise can come through additional study and training born out of a psychologist's interest in particular frames of reference, through conferences, workshops, seminars and webinars. Whichever the "avenue", psychologists should never cease to learn and develop new knowledge and skills as child development itself is never static.

There is however a clear distinction between the "developed world" and the "developing world". In the former, there are assessment and diagnostic services, trained paediatricians, geneticists and psychologists with in-depth knowledge of neurodevelopmental delays and disorders, financial and material assistance for families seeking help, and specific intervention and educational facilities and programmes available to remediate developmental delays and disorders and to maximise the potential of young children.

These assumptions cannot be made of the "developing" countries such as Sub-Saharan Africa or the sub-continent, where there can be paucity of resources and knowledge, services and expertise in matters paediatric and developmental. In a later chapter, the impact of this "disadvantage" will be detailed in relation to prevalence rates of neurodevelopmental disorders, through factors of causation, assessment and diagnosis, and service provision.

How do parents perceive and experience assessments?

In 1983, a remarkable example of "focus group" research was undertaken in Australia, and the results published and distributed as a booklet throughout assessment and diagnostic centres and clinics. Titled "To Parents of Children with Disabilities, from Parents of Children with Disabilities", the publication allowed the parents of children with disabilities free reign to talk openly and honestly about their experiences, and describe the information and knowledge they would like to share with other parents to help them better prepare for the "journey" ahead. There were seven chapters in this booklet:

- "Finding out": The initial discovery that a family has a child with a disabling condition.
- "The earlier the better": Descriptions and explorations of early intervention services.
- "The professionals": How families can make the most of their involvements with the various professionals they will meet.
- "Getting together": Finding ways for parents and families to support each other.
- "Family matters": Exploring the dynamics in a family which includes a child with a disability.
- "What about education": Selecting appropriate schools and educational programmes.
- "When I'm 64": Planning for the future.

The stories told are honest and heart-felt, sometimes positive and sometimes not. There were tales of appreciation of the services and information afforded to families by various disability support agencies, assessment centres, hospitals and clinics, but also stories of dismay and confusion at the perceived treatment of their concerns, fears and needs. Perhaps "things have changed" in terms of awareness of early childhood disability since the publication's times, but revisiting this "view of the past" is important and revelatory because of the insights and experiences of families traversing the assessment and diagnosis process for their child. Upon "finding out" that their child had a disability, one family commented:

> The future was just an unknown void; all our hopes and plans were dashed to pieces. We had no idea what was in store for us. We had no prior experience with children with disabilities, or their families. We desperately needed some solid base, some information on which to rebuild our shattered future. I was devastated and numb. People said that everything would work out fine, but I thought: "How would you know, it's not happening to you?" Now, one year later, we seem to have got it all together again. We feel that life is okay-different, but okay. I never thought it would happen, but it did.

Of her experience of an initial medical assessment for her young child, another mother wrote:

> I was sitting in the doctor's waiting room, a feeling of panic mounting steadily inside me. I knew there was something wrong with my son-he was almost one year old and just not developing properly. I felt I couldn't stand it anymore-I wasn't coping. It took great effort to hold back my tears. The doctor showed me into his room. 'How are you today?' he enquired. 'I'm fine thanks Doctor', I replied." Later, she added: "As a parent of a child with a disability, I have found that the emotional trauma I have gone through has been largely ignored.

From another interview:

> I felt a desperate need to have a "label", probably in case there was a cure. I went from service to service, but no one said anything different. After a while I realised it didn't matter and it is more important to find some practical help for my child.

Although published some decades ago, the stories told by parents then are as relevant now as they were at the time. The emotional responses to receiving unwelcome news about one's young child are timeless and universal, even if the manner in which "emotionality" is expressed may vary from country to country, culture to culture, ethnicity to ethnicity. DSM-5-TR recognises this phenomenon of different expressions of shock, anger, confusion, disbelief, depression and fear through its description of "Cultural idiom of Distress", and one has only to watch the world news to observe the range of emotional responses to tragedy joyous occasions, success, loss and the like. Emotionality can range from hysteria to "stiff upper lip", rage and violence to simmering discontent, introversion to externalised displays of emotionality, unbridled joy to polite applause.

Do these parental responses reflect the experiences of all parents of young children as they enter, probably for the first time, the process of "assessment"? Parental reactions to the "assessment process", the acceptance or dismissal of diagnostic information, and indeed parental perceptions of their child's abilities, behaviours and levels of performance, can be influenced by such factors as their pre-assessment knowledge of, and exposure to, disabling conditions. For example, parents who had little foreknowledge of developmental delays and disorders tended to experience more shock and denial than did parents who had more pre-assessment understanding.

In one study, three groups of parents were identified:

- Those who were knowledgeable and "inquisitive".
- Those with less initial knowledge but already felt that "something was wrong" (the "passionate" group).
- Those who were "experienced" with the assessment and diagnostic process, disability services and terminology.

The "inquisitive" group were described as being less accepting of categorical diagnoses, whilst the "passionate" group were more inclined to accept a diagnosis to speedily learn what to do to support their child and find appropriate services. The third group, comprising parents who were requesting review or follow-up assessments, was seen as having acquired considerable knowledge over time and experience about their child's disability, and tended to perceive assessment as a means of ratifying their decisions and affirm their current knowledge.

Other avenues of research suggest that formal developmental assessments, as distinct from questionnaire-based assessments, serve two important functions in helping parental perceptions of their children. One line of study suggests that watching another adult interact with their child, manage their behaviours and elicit skills and achievements not otherwise known to them, was capable of changing parental expectations of their children, and of clarifying their understanding of their child's levels of abilities.

Of course, these categories may be over-generalisations, and the proliferation of knowledge brought about through electronic and social media has meant that every parent can pre-read and even attempt to "self-diagnose" disorders, but the implications of these different parental groupings are important for the manner in which assessments are conducted, from initial referral to meeting with parents and child, establishing rapport, conducting an assessment, formulating an appropriate diagnosis, and providing feedback through meetings and written reports. For instance:

- Why has a family come to you for assessment? Is it because they have been specifically referred or as sometimes occurs, "strongly urged" by other professionals, friends or family members?
- Are they seeking confirmation of previous assessment outcomes?
- Are they seeking specific diagnostic "labelling" because this may be required for service, school or funding eligibility?
- Is it always necessary to conduct a formal assessment at a first meeting, or is it best to meet with families first, and listen and discuss whilst they put forward their feelings, experiences and points of view?
- Is it best to assess a young child in your office or rooms, or to observe the child in a more naturalistic environment such as a preschool?
- How can a psychologist best support a family in the period immediately after an assessment has been conducted and a diagnosis made?
  - Do some families need time to be alone and do their best to understand and assimilate the news they have been given?
  - Are there families who immediately want to "move forward" with support and management options for their children, becoming instantly "action-orientated"?
  - Do some parents need to address their own emotional responses first before focussing upon their child's future?

- Are there families who become clinically orientated and seek further opinions of the veracity of a diagnosis made?
- Do some parents become depressed and less than able to make immediate decisions and plans?

An awareness on the part of psychologists of their family's immediate needs is therefore important and how they should clinically assist, but it is also true some of these decisions are not always in the hands of psychologists to make. There may be logistic or employment conditions and strictures placed upon practitioners which predetermine what will occur. But at the heart of any involvement with a family of a young child is the need to understand their experiences, opinions, expectations and needs and as far as possible accommodate these factors in the workplace. It is even more paramount to understand the emotional state of families and the impact that this can have upon the manner in which psychologists approach developmental assessments. Parents may in fact not even "be ready" for engagement in assessment and diagnosis, but may feel that they have no choice but to attend.

Psychologists worldwide, regardless of their clinical focus, must be appropriately trained, qualified and registered with an appropriate professional body or association, and these "guilds" serve to provide ethical and professional guidelines and parameters for appropriate psychological practice in whichever field of psychology one may choose to engage in. In relation to psychologists engaging in disability-oriented work, psychological societies universally set standards and expectations, competencies and standards to facilitate "best practice" clinical involvement. The Australian Psychological Society in 2009, for example, published an in-house article entitled "Psychology and Disability", and a number of issues were canvassed around assessment and diagnosis, advocacy and family support:

- Although the "nature" of disabling conditions had not necessarily changed, there had been significant shifts in the various classification systems for various conditions, with a direct impact upon the levels of support required and attainable. This emphasised the need for current diagnostic knowledge.
- Changes and developments in diagnostic categorisation had driven the need for new assessment tools with increased focus upon the levels of support needed, as opposed to "deficits, incapacities or disabilities". Knowledge of new and updated assessment tools was therefore needed.
- Assessment tools for measurements of "adaptive behaviour" skills were noted in their importance and relevance to service planning and provision, behavioural support and community involvement, where previously levels of intelligence through psychometric testing were sufficient criteria for diagnosis of (for example) intellectual disability.
- The importance of developments in the field of genetics, particularly related to behavioural phenotypes, was stressed.
- Psychologists were seen as having a critically important role in making evidence-based decisions and judgements about diagnoses, therapeutic support programmes, family support initiatives, school enrolment practices, and even government policy, emphasising the need for up-to-date knowledge and awareness of scientific method as it applied to various treatment options.
- The emergence of multi-disciplinary employment opportunities for psychologists through trans-disciplinary practice was seen as vital: "It would be a bold Psychologist indeed who believe they could go it alone".

- The forging of close working relationships with colleagues in paediatrics, psychiatry, nursing, speech pathology, occupational therapy, social work and other professions was highlighted. It was also suggested that an understanding of such professional practices needed to be nourished in undergraduate and postgraduate university programmes.
- Within these expanding roles for psychologists, extra responsibilities were noted, including the need for psychologists to "moderate" their communication and expectations to meet the needs of other professionals and staff members, and to use "plain language" and a brevity of detail in reports.

The American Psychological Association's (APA) Code of Ethics includes a list of principles for psychologists engaging with individuals with disabilities. They include the need to:

- *Learn about various disability paradigms, models and their implications for services, including relevant Federal and state laws and legislations.*
- *Examine one's beliefs and emotional reactions towards disabilities, and increase one's knowledge and skills through training, supervision, education and consultation. Also, understand the experiences of people with disabilities and recognise social and cultural diversity in the lives of people with disabilities.*
- *Recognise that families of individuals with disabilities have both strengths and challenges, including their being at an increased risk of abuse.*
- *Provide a "barrier-free" physical and communication environment for clients with disabilities, including the use of appropriate language and respectful behaviour. Also learn about the opportunities and challenges presented by assistive technologies.*
- *Apply the most psychometrically appropriate assessment approaches for clients with disabilities and determine whether accommodations in assessments are appropriate to yield a valid test score. Also appropriately balance quantitative, qualitative and ecological perspectives, in interpreting assessment data of clients who have disabilities.*
- *Recognise the wide range of individual responses to disability when developing and implementing psychological interventions, and keep clients' perspectives paramount when advocating for client self-determination, integration, choice and least restrictive alternatives.*
- *Recognise and address health promotion issues for individuals with disabilities.*

Similarly, the British Psychological Society Code of Conduct details broad beliefs and statements regarding respect, competence, responsibility and integrity, and specific guidelines are provided for "delivering psychological services for young people with neurodevelopmental difficulties and their families". This document reiterates that:

Psychological approaches are key to understanding the difficulties of children with neurodevelopmental conditions. They are based on a detailed assessment to develop a formulation of the child's difficulties. A psychological approach that considers behaviour in its wider context (e.g. social, cultural, gender, class and race) is important, as some children who appear on first assessment to have neurodevelopmental difficulties may, in fact, have attachment difficulties. A diagnosis may form part of a formulation. This can be a contentious area: Some families and young people do not want a diagnosis, whereas others ask for one so that the child can access other services, particularly in a school context.

The British Psychological Society described psychological assessments in the following terms, with specific considerations of the following:

- The ongoing process of assessment, rather than it being a "one-off" event.
- The need to review diagnoses over time as a child's developmental status may change.
- The professionals involved in assessment will typically include:
  - A paediatrician or child psychiatrist.
  - An applied psychologist, whether clinical, educational or neuropsychologist.
  - A speech and language therapist.
  - An occupational therapist skilled in sensory assessment.
- Assessment will include several different modalities, including:
  - A clinical interview and developmental history through a structured discussion with parents.
  - Observations of the child in various settings, such as school and in social situations with other children.
  - Information gathered from other sources, such as questionnaires.
- These methods allow for the following factors to be assessed:
  - Mental health and behaviour.
  - Communication abilities.
  - Cognition or intellectual ability.
  - Neuropsychological functioning.
  - Achievement and adaptive functioning.
  - The recognition that: "A good assessment recognises that beliefs about the cause and course of neurodevelopmental difficulties are influenced by culture, and the reaction to diagnostic labels will also differ across cultures".

Educational and developmental psychologists, clinical psychologists and generalist psychologists the world over have long been engaged in the assessment and diagnosis of disabling conditions in young children, often in the context of multi-disciplinary or trans-disciplinary teams and agencies. They can practise their psychological services in a range of settings:

- Child development units within public children's hospitals or health services.
- Specialist facilities within such hospitals, for example Neonatal Intensive Care Units, Child Development Units and Departments of Psychological Medicine.
- Community health centres, and specialist assessment and diagnostic teams attached to these.
- Private paediatric and child development centres, perhaps specialising in particular disorders such as autism spectrum disorder.
- Private early intervention programmes.
- Private practice/sole trader clinics or private multi-disciplinary teams.

These different settings and employment contexts may be viewed differently by families, particularly when they are unfamiliar with child development difficulties and service provision. The psychologists working in these contexts may bring differing levels of training and experience to their professional roles.

They may have the luxury of being closely supervised, mentored and monitored in the exercise of their roles, or they may by necessity or isolation be thrown onto their own resources, initiative and intuition to "learn on the run".

And it is into this sometimes dynamic, sometimes confusing, professional environment that parents come for assistance, when they are perhaps at their most vulnerable. They may be young and inexperienced as parents, scared, angry, confused, shocked or combinations of these conflicting emotions. They may bring with them specific cultural, ethnic and religious beliefs and attitudes, practices and understandings, which may be to a degree contradictory to the values, beliefs and understandings of the assessment and diagnostic service, its personnel and its "charter".

The assessment and diagnostic process is therefore dynamic, and at the heart of its dynamism is the fundamental tenet that parents and their children are there for assistance, advice, guidance, reassurance, direction and as much "certainty" as can be given.

Bibliography

American Psychological Association (2022), "Guidelines for Assessment of and Intervention with Persons with Disabilities", www.apa.org.

Arnold, S. (2009), "Supports, Empowerment and Self-Direction: The Emerging Paradigm in the Disability Sector", InPsych, the Bulletin of the Australian Psychological Society, 33(6), pp 16–17.

Australian Psychological Society (2018), "Australian Psychological Society Code of Ethics", www.psychology.org.au.

British Psychological Society Code of Ethics and Conduct (2021), www.bps.org.uk.

British Psychological Society Division of Clinical Psychology, "Delivering Psychological Services for Children and Young People with Neurodevelopmental Difficulties and their Families", www.bps.org.uk.

Diemann, P., and Kasten-Koller, U. (2011), "Maternal Evaluations of Young Childrens' Developmental Status", Psychological Tests and Assessment Modelling, 53, pp 214–227.

Ellis, J., and Whaite, A. (1983), To Parents of Children with Disabilities, from Parents of Children with Disabilities, Social Evaluation and Research Ltd.

McVilly, K. R. (2009) "What do Psychologists Need to Know about People with Disability?", InPsych, the Bulletin of the Australian Psychological Society, 33(6), p 13.

Shahat, A. R. S., and Greco, G. (2021), "The Economic Costs of Childhood Disability: A Literature Review", International Journal of Environmental Research and Public Health, 18, pp 1–25.

7 Parental experience of assessment and diagnosis

The birth and parenting of a child: Love and labour. Unbridled joy and excitement, sometimes tempered by anxiety and anticipation. Pride, expectations, laughter, fear, frustration, exhaustion, exaltation. So many mixed emotions and sensations surround the birth of a child and the impacts that this event has upon the lives of parents. But what happens if something goes wrong? What happens if these emotions are clouded by fear, apprehension, bad news, confusing or ill-informed comments made by others, or the underlying power of one's own intuition as a parent that things are not as they should be with their newborn?

Perhaps a child is born with an easily recognisable disorder or a chronic health condition, and at the very moment when joy and excitement should surround a family, shock, fear and confusion intrude and dominate. Or a child may not exhibit any obvious difficulties, but parents gradually come to suspect that something is wrong or concerning. They seek advice from a variety of sources: Community health professionals, doctors, other parents, including of course their own. Each of these attempts to reassure and to clarify, but unintentionally may further confuse and add to the nagging suspicions. A family may be led down a long and tortuous road of appointments, tests, assessments and opinions, often couched in terminology which is foreign and incomprehensible.

What do these experiences do for a family? Why would it be so important to consider the emotional states of families of young children negotiating diagnostic assessment to the best of their ability the path through this maze? Why would they seek to endure the frantic round of referrals, appointments, assessments, meetings and reports, while simultaneously endeavouring to manage their emotions and thoughts, their busy work and family lives, and their own fears and expectations?

Parents rarely come totally "equipped" for parenthood. There is no simple "User's Manual" or universal method for "success". They do their best, and they learn. They rarely have pre-understanding of disabling conditions or chronic health problems, unless of course through other family members or friends. But their emotional reactions to the turbulent events which unfold need to be understood by reference to classic psychological theories as they occur within the complex world of disability.

Emotional responses such as "complex grief"

Psychologists will of course be familiar with the classic stages of grief espoused by Elizabeth Kubler-Ross in 1969, originally 5 in number but gradually extended to at least 7:

- Shock and disbelief.
- Denial.

- Guilt.
- Anger and bargaining.
- Depression and reflection.
- Reconstruction.
- Acceptance.

This model generally applied to the loss of a loved one, through death, separation or removal, but the question was often posed: How do these stages and this process relate to "loss" when the object of the "loss" and subsequent grief is forever present? In 2004, the Author had the privilege to contribute to a book, "Lessons from my Child" (in Australia and Japan, but "A different Kind of Perfect" in the United States). This derived from a simple invitation to parents of children with various disabling and health conditions to "tell their stories", unedited but as far as possible aligned to the seven classic stages of grief and loss. The book commences with the following conundrum:

> Grief comes to every single one of us at some stage of our lives. It is one of the few emotional states that all societies acknowledge through ritual and ceremony-a Christian funeral or Hindu cremation are first and foremost socially instituted ways of allowing people to express their sorrow. But how does grief manifest itself when nobody has died? This is the dilemma that faces parents of children with disabilities.

Although grief is technically defined as a personal and emotional reaction to a significant loss, most commonly the death of a loved one, it can also stem from the loss of dreams, ideas, hopes and expectations – the loss of what "might have been". It is this sense of loss that drives the grieving process in parents of children with disabilities or disorders, coupled by the fact that the source of the loss and grief is there every single day to reignite the sense of loss.

No two people will experience and express grief in exactly the same way, and there is no "right" way to feel or behave whilst mourning. More importantly, people do not necessarily pass through the various stages of grief in a sequential manner-they may ebb and flow, wax and wane in terms of their reactions to significant loss. They may even experience multiple "stages" of grief simultaneously, and such feelings and reactions can be triggered by any number of circumstances.

In 1962, Olshansky suggested the theory of "chronic sorrow" as it applied to the families of children with disabilities, whereby they may never truly achieve real "acceptance" of their child's disability, but remain in a state of constant flux, at times appearing content with their lives, but at other times returning to fully-fledged grief for a time, for example at times coinciding with significant transitions or anniversaries such as a child's birthday, or his/her first day at school. But although grief is not experienced as a series of discrete stages, it is worthwhile exploring these theoretical "stages" as they pertain to the life of real families with children who have disorders or disabilities.

Shock

> I was devastated and numb. People said that everything would work out fine, but I thought: How would you know? It's not happening to you.

> I knew that we were being told a good deal about our child's condition, but I was just so numb that I really didn't hear or remember. I ended up writing down questions as they came to mind so that I could bring them up at the next opportunity.

Shock is often characterised by sensations of numbness or disbelief. Some people report a sense of "paralysis" and of being "disconnected" from the reality of one's situation. But when a family has a young child to care for and raise, an immediate reality tends to take over-one must keep functioning in order to care for a child.

When the shock emanates from news such as confirmation of a diagnosis of a disorder or disability, this reality is again immediately "in-play". One must function. There are appointments and assessments to keep, therapy sessions to attend, needs to be met. This "busyness" may have the effect of delaying and interrupting the grieving process-a parent may offer such thoughts as "I don't have time to grieve", and the impact of such deferment of feeling may not occur until much later. There may be delayed grief, and responses not unlike those associated with trauma.

Disbelief

> I didn't want to see my baby. I just cried and cried. I didn't want to look at my baby, touch or hold my baby. I didn't want to talk to anyone. I just wanted to be on my own and I cried and cried.

> I knew there was something wrong with him, but no one seemed to be able to help. I tried so hard to love him as I saw my friends love their children. I sat with him in my arms and cried. I thought that it may be possible for his skin to absorb my tears as they dropped onto him and that he would feel my love in them.

Disbelief is simply that. "I do not believe this is happening". "I do not believe what I am being told". "They must be wrong!" "How would they know, and how can they be so certain?" This can particularly be the experience when a young child with no obvious physical signs of "difference" or disorder is diagnosed. Families often, and quite rightly, "disbelieve", and are entitled to question information given them. A common occurrence in coming to terms with a possible disability or disorder diagnosis is that such a diagnosis may not occur in one single event or consultation. A child may (for example) have been assessed by a community nurse, a general practitioner, a paediatrician, a geneticist, a speech pathologist or a psychologist, before a diagnosis of a disorder (e.g. autism spectrum disorder) is confirmed. There is a "drip-feed" process occurring whereby each individual practitioner adds to the gradual realisation that something really is "wrong" with one's child. This may in some cases mitigate the sense of shock, but not the sense of loss.

The pain of not knowing was greater than the pain of knowing.

Denial

> I freely admit that when my son was very young, I held off making contact with other parents for as long as possible. That would have meant admitting to myself the one thing that I was desperately trying to shut out-that my child was different.

"**Denial**" is a most logical and understandable response to an unpleasant and unwanted event. It is as though the mind automatically engages in a protective "retreat" – "this is not happening!" It is an attempt to introduce distance between our experience and ourselves. It is akin to a pain reliever, and those in denial are perhaps yelling "this is not what I want!"

It is often associated with an "end of expectations", the realisation that a family's expectations and hopes for their young child may not eventuate. Denial can be transient or sustained, perhaps as a function of the expectations parents held for their child.

Denial is a natural part of the grieving process even though it at times presents a degree of "inconvenience" for practitioners wishing to support and assist families. It is a means by which parents can express their sense of loss and disappointment, anger and sadness. People in denial are sometimes considered as "obstructionist", but this is not true. Parents can manifest denial as a means of trying to deal with loss, when their inherent belief systems would otherwise dictate that "awful things happen to other people but not to me". People shield themselves from the possibility that they may have to deal with loss, tragedy or unwanted outcomes, but are not prepared when difficult circumstances do arise.

Denial has a protective function-it "buys time" to blunt the initial shock and to search for the necessary strength and courage to deal with a crisis for which one is not ready to confront.

Guilt

> Everyone told us that it wasn't our fault. That's all very well, but we chose to have the child, we conceived our child and brought our child into the world. It's hard not to feel guilty.
>
> I felt that because my child was different, I must be different or have some fault. I must have made some awful mistake.

"Guilt" is often associated with denial: A parent may ask, "What did I do wrong?" "Is it my fault?" Sometimes no amount of rational explanation about "causation" can assuage these feelings until parents are more able to take such information on-board. There are also cultural factors and imperatives associated with feelings of guilt, and these will be discussed later in this chapter.

Guilt associated with a disabled child can be expressed in a number of ways. One is by "telling a story" that explains how parents may feel "responsible" for their child's disability. Their stories can often be persuasive. Another way of manifesting guilt is through the "belief" that the child's disability may be a form of punishment for past actions. Guilt can also be expressed through the belief that because "good things happen to good people", it must follow that "bad things happen to bad people". Parents may feel that they must be "bad people" because they have a child with a disability, and this can be accompanied by feelings of shame and guilt.

An important consideration needs to be made for families who have children diagnosed with specific genetic disorders, particularly if they are in fact heritable. The level of guilt experienced by families in these situations can be palpable – "I DID pass on this disorder!"

Anger and bargaining

> Why did this have to happen to the child I wanted too much?
>
> Nothing worse could have happened to me. I found the best way to deal with my emotions and with my child was to push them from my mind, reject them totally. It was an enormous blow to my self-esteem. I realise now that I considered the birth

of my other children as a boost to my self-image. This time I felt somehow, imperfect and inadequate, and unattractive. I just didn't want to know.

"Anger and bargaining". Anger is a most powerful, automatic and basic human response. It is akin to "fight vs flight". Anger primarily arises from anxiety when people feel overwhelmed and powerless. It can temporarily calm our anxieties and restore a semblance of control. Anger is also ingrained in our psychological sense of fairness: "This is not fair! I did not cause this and I did not deserve this!" "I will do whatever it takes to change this!"

People deal with anger in different ways. Some "vent" physically and verbally, some turn the anger inwards and experience bitterness. Some harness and channel their anger into purposeful action, such as establishing support groups or lobbying for enhanced service provision for children with disabling conditions. This notion of "displacement" is very important to understand and accept, particularly if as a professional one has been the apparent "target" of such anger: You are not actually the target of this anger. You were simply "in the firing line" and in the wrong place at the wrong time.

Bargaining arises from anger. In its simplest terms, it is manifest in intentions to "do whatever it takes" to redress a situation; "I'll do anything to resurrect my marriage". "I'll avoid repeating the mistakes at work if I can only have a second chance". This is much more difficult in the context of disability, but is often manifest in parents seeking out the best "treatment options" for their child:

> My dream is to invent a pill which will magically cure my daughter, and when I have done it I will cure her and not share it with anybody else.

This is perfectly reasonable and understandable, but can sometimes be misguided. Take for example, a family who over-commit themselves financially to engage their child in a treatment methodology which is expensive and not necessarily proven to be effective. Families need and deserve current and accurate information about intervention strategies and modalities, therapeutic concepts, educational options and other vital decisions relating to their children.

Psychologists may not always agree with such decisions, but it needs to be asked: Are families also entitled to the "dignity of failure?" If the answer is "yes", then part of the psychologist's role with families is to accept such choices and decisions, but also to be ready to support families when what they wanted to attempt or to achieve does not come to fruition.

Depression

> At one time dying seemed to be the only way of halting the pain. I think it was a form of self-protection.

> It was two years before one of us acknowledged something was wrong. As we'd sensed it for some time but not expressed it, it was almost a relief to be told. However, emotionally, those 2 years were the most harrowing I've ever experienced. Some time after being told I became really depressed.

Depression is clinically defined as a prolonged feeling of intense sadness, often accompanied by associated feelings of worthlessness, inadequacy and lethargy. Again, they are understandable reactions to grief and loss, disappointment and frustration – they are reactions to specific incidents that have been difficult to come to terms with. Generally, these symptoms pass with time and resolution. They are inherent in "reactive depression".

This needs to be clearly distinguished from clinical depression, which is a more chronic state of being, and less likely to be resolved without specific interventions such as therapeutic programmes and/or medication. Families of children with disorders or disabilities, if they do experience depression, are again faced with the difficulty of unresolved grief. Whereas sadness and depression in the context of (for example) the death of a loved one can resolve over time, parents of children with disabilities are in constant daily reminder of the source of their sadness.

Also, they are generally extremely busy and "time poor", and have "no time to heal". They must remain "functional", they might say they are not "super parents" but simply "work harder". In fact, there is research to suggest that therapeutic outcomes for children with disabilities are less optimal if one or both parents are experiencing ongoing depression. Depression is also described as being an opportunity for reflection, sometimes defined as "pining":

> Without warning I would find myself thinking about my baby and his problems and what might have been. I would always try to shut it out because I felt so guilty thinking such a 'wicked' thought.

Acceptance

> Sometimes I think that I've finally accepted my child's disability, then something small happens and I burst into floods of tears. I wonder if it is something you never really accept. There's always a scar on your heart.

"Reconstruction" and "Acceptance" are generally considered to mark the "end" of the grieving process if an "ending" is in fact possible. The term "closure" has in recent decades become an overused cliché – it is extremely debatable whether grieving as a process has a tangible endpoint.

Parents of children with disabilities often refer to "moments of clarity" when they as far as possible come to terms with the past, the present and the future for themselves and their children. There is a "letting go" of previous hopes and expectations and an understanding that "it is what it is". Some parents who have written about their "journey" through the grieving process refer to acceptance as the "end of the chapter" but not the end of the story, as there are always new challenges, experiences, highs and lows to go through.

In recent years, Kubler-Ross and David Kessler have talked of "Finding Meaning" as an additional stage in the grief process, that death or loss has to have an inherent meaning or that one can "channel" the feelings of loss and despair into some form of purposeful action or response: Relatives of murder victims devote time, intellect and energy to the pursuit of justice not just for their lost relative or child, but for the betterment of society in general; parents of children with disabilities politicise the plight of their child and activate and lobby for better services for those similarly affected; there are searches for cures and treatments for others to use, financial commitments made to support charities and other worthy causes. These means of "operationalising" one's despair, grief and sorrow can serve as a means of harnessing and redirecting the immense emotional energy generated and expended through grief.

On the other hand, there is considerable debate as to whether a stage-based model of grief, such as those espoused by Kubler-Ross and Kessler, can readily apply to the emotional responses of families to the diagnosis in their children of disabilities or chronic medical conditions. Grief and mourning are not necessarily pathological responses to the perceived "loss" of the "idealised child" and are not necessarily universal or inevitable reactions to such circumstances. A literal interpretation of the "stage model" of grief and loss might presume that parents would progress in their own way through denial, anger, bargaining and depression before reaching an acceptance of their child's disability, but current research suggests alternate propositions.

One hypothesis introduces the notion of "positive illusions", which suggests that in certain circumstances people experiencing crisis achieved better outcomes when they maintained what some professionals may have perceived as "unrealistic expectations". There is also the theory that families could be viewed as "adapting and evolving when supported". What may occur is sometimes defined as "cognitive adaptation" as a way parental awareness of and response to disability can progress over time. This is inherent in the theory of "positive psychology", which presumes that parents have the innate capacity to overcome significant unexpected events, and over time can experience increased understanding regarding their role, resulting in further personal growth and development.

"Cognitive Coping" may be defined as thinking about specific situations, such as the diagnosis of a child with a developmental disorder, in ways that may enhance one's sense of well-being. This may include (for example) attributing to such an experience the realisation that one's child will remain a source of happiness and love, that parents will learn "life lessons", feel pride in achievements, develop new strengths and provide different means of reaching fulfilment. In so doing, individuals may feel they have gained "control" over difficult emotions and situations, find new "meaning" in their lives and move "beyond chronic sorrow", even though there will always be "reminders" – unexpected events that might rekindle deeply held emotions (Figure 7.1).

And it is not just the parents of children with disabling conditions who must work through the emotional journey, which can become such a significant part of their role of parents. The siblings of children with disabilities, whether younger or older, also have their own reactions to their roles, expectations, responsibilities and experiences within a family with a disability focus. Research has highlighted the challenges faced by siblings. Anger, confusion, depression, jealousy, anxiety, and even guilt, can be part of their "journey", as they come to terms with the changed expectations, responsibilities, relationships and understandings of "family life", as well as joy and pride in the achievements of their sisters and brothers. It is not uncommon for psychologists to organise and offer such services as "siblings groups" and workshops, to enable siblings to come together, share their experiences, vent their emotions, frustrations, joys and fears about their disabled siblings.

The role of culture, faith, spiritualist and ethnicity in the grieving process: "spirituality and faith"

We live in a most rich and diverse world, with multiple belief and value systems, customs, mores and practices. There is increased migration between nations, sometimes for economic reasons and sometimes political, for seeking greater opportunity or fleeing

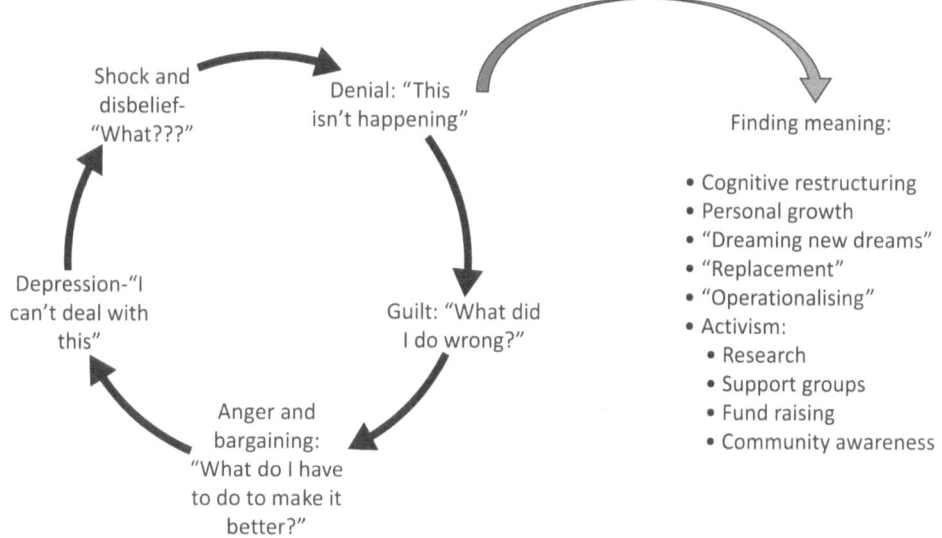

Figure 7.1 The cycle of grief

oppression, war and violence. The world is becoming more of a "melting pot", and this brings both riches and challenges. In some countries, this increased diversity is celebrated, in others reviled and rejected. This diversity can apply to all realm of life and society, including childhood disability. The role of individual faiths, beliefs and societal factors may therefore play an important role in helping individual families to understand and accept news of a childhood disability, and to work through the grieving process and the uncertain course of the "journey", which lies ahead for themselves and their child.

It is not possible for psychologists to fully understand the multitudinous belief systems in our world, but it is implicit in the role to not preclude an acceptance of beliefs and practices beyond one's immediate understanding as these apply to their clients.

Indeed, the relevant national psychological societies and associations would suggest that such understandings are obligatory for Psychologists. The first General Principle of the Australian Psychological Society's Code of Ethics emphasises that Psychologists should:

> have a high regard for the diversity and uniqueness of people and their right to linguistically and culturally appropriate services.

DSM-5-TR states that disorders are not defined in a vacuum, but in relation to cultural, social and familial norms and values. Culture is "transmitted, revised, and recreated" within families, and "thresholds of tolerance for specific symptoms or behaviours differ across cultures, social settings and families". Therefore, clinical judgement that specific behaviours or symptoms of disorder requiring diagnosis and support depend at least to a degree on the cultural norms inherent to the belief systems, traditions and practices of the family or social system within which they occur. "Cultural" factors may contribute to either "stigma" or "support" for disabling conditions. They may influence coping strategies and resilience, but may also influence acceptance or rejection of a specific diagnosis and subsequent recommendations for treatments or therapies.

DSM-5-TR lists three concepts which may provide a framework for better understanding of the cultural complexities of assessment, diagnosis, treatment and follow-up:

Cultural syndrome: A cluster of symptoms found within certain cultures, communities or groups, but not necessarily recognised as an "illness" within that culture, even when clearly regarded as such by others external to the culture.
Cultural idiom of distress: A way of talking about suffering amongst individuals of a particular cultural group. This may imply "shared concepts" of pathology, and ways of describing, expressing the feelings of distress. An "idiom of distress" may not be associated with any particular symptoms or diagnoses. One need only to watch TV or on-line news broadcasts of floods, earthquakes, war and other devastations to appreciate the different expressions of grief, loss, pain and anger.
Cultural explanation or perceived cause: "A label, attribution, or feature of an explanatory model that provides a culturally conceived aetiology or cause for symptoms, illnesses or distress".

August bodies such as the United Nations, the OECD and UNICEF have listed many examples of the differing beliefs of, knowledge about, attitudes towards and reactions to, the diagnosis of disabling conditions in young children. Some of these examples are very explicit and perhaps pejorative and do not necessarily reflect the beliefs held by all members of individual societies. They are generalisations and should be regarded as such. For example:

- In Sub-Saharan Africa, common beliefs about the causes of childhood disability may include sin or promiscuity of the mother, an ancestral curse or demonic possession.
- In some South Asian cultures, a girl may be expected to be like her mother, and a boy similar to his father. If this does not occur, it can be interpreted as a "disturbance of the natural order". Or a family may perceive a child with disability as being taken over by 'djinn' or spirits, as a "changeling".

In China and other South-East Asian communities, the strong traditional links to Buddhist and Confucian principles can be reflected through attitudes towards disability. There is a high value on family hierarchy based on age, gender and generational status. "Harmony" in family and society is maintained by self-restraint and collectivism, with everyone acting in accordance with their hierarchical status. Maintaining "face" means that "shameful" family affairs cannot be disclosed to outsiders.

People in "collective" cultures may hold stigmatising attitudes towards people who "deviate from the norm", for example those with disabling conditions. There may be less tolerance towards "diversity" than in more pluralistic cultures. Parents in collective cultures may be concerned about possible stigma arising from a family member perceived as "different".

It is not the intention of this publication to overgeneralise or accredit these different responses to particular societies, faiths or religions, but it is instructive for psychologists to be aware of some of the varied dynamics which may be associated with childhood disability so they may better understand the needs of client families. Take the possible different understandings of "causation":

- In some cultures and language groups, there may be no equivalent words or terms for "disability", "developmental delay" or "Autism Spectrum Disorder".
- The causation of a disability may in some cultures be attributable to "payback", retribution or previous parental sins, defects of character or parental promiscuity.

- There may be beliefs around the influence of "spirits" or "devils", and that a child's condition is contrary to the natural order of the world. A child with a disability may be seen as a "bad omen" for the community.
- Even if a disability is recognised by a family, they may be reluctant to accept it due to "the web of social meanings" that may push them to resist the diagnosis. For example, there may be material consequences such as limited marital prospects.
- One parent may fear rejection from the other, even to the abandonment of one parent.

There can also be societal conflict about the appropriateness of support and treatment for a child with a disabling condition:

- Support for a child with a disability frequently focuses upon helping a child towards increasing levels of independence, but independence may not be highly valued in some social milieus.
- There may be misgivings about medical, educational or psychological "treatment" of neurodevelopmental disorders, but a belief and trust in "traditional" medicines and practices, such as witchcraft or traditional "healers".

Logistical issues such as access to and availability of services can also influence acceptance of disability in developing countries:

- There can be a paucity of suitably qualified medical specialists, therapists and teachers, and a lack of expert knowledge, services support programmes. Even where services may exist, there is not necessarily universal trust in these resources.
- Access to services which may be "remote" may simply not be affordable or able to be factored into the daily lives of individual families.
- Access to services may involve financial costs beyond the reach of individual families.
- The differentiation between "medical" conditions, delayed development and mental health concerns may not be well understood.

Faith and spirituality, strong beliefs and customs, can also play a positive role in accepting diagnoses and engaging in remediations and therapies, educational programmes and community support. Families with strong religious and spiritual beliefs, family and societal ties may find the resilience and determination to accept and master difficult situations easier because of their beliefs. They may be more inclined to "positively reframe" the difficulties they are facing. In some cultures, the presence of a disability may be viewed as "God's Will" and another test or challenge for a family to tackle. Some societies may view the plight of a young child with a disability as a "communal responsibility", where everyone has a useful role in the support of its members.

Psychologists involved in assessing young children therefore need to be aware of the emotional and psychological "journeys" that their families have commenced and are to continue. Psychologists also need to be aware of, sympathetic to, and cognisant of, the cultural, spiritual and linguistic framework within which a disability has occurred. Parents who come to psychologists for assessment services will do so both because they want to and because they must. The motivations behind these needs and wants may vary greatly however, and it cannot be taken for granted that there is a single simple "agenda" for referral and assessment.

Psychologists must therefore be extremely mindful of the competing and confusing emotions that may impact upon a family's engagement and participation in the assessment process. They need to be flexible in their practices and routines, ready to listen and respond to the needs, doubts and fears of families, and even to abandon formalised assessment procedures either temporarily or completely if circumstances dictate this course of action.

They may, for example, need to allow for the presence of family members or friends to act as advocates, interpreters, emotional supports and corroborating witnesses. Psychologists need to allow time for discussion and feedback, questions and answers, agreement or rejection of diagnostic pronouncements and proposed courses of action. Families act in the best interests of their young children, and also in their own best interests in a protective sense, but not in emotional or cultural vacuums.

The process of reacting to and dealing with childhood disability is complex indeed, and reference is sometimes made to "complex" or "unresolved" grief, but this notion has not yet achieved full acceptance. DSM 5 listed a number of "conditions for further study", one of which was persistent complex bereavement disorder, but the subsequent DSM-5-TR describes "Prolonged Bereavement Disorder" (F43.8), which is demarcated by:

> the death of a loved one, at least 12 months ago, of a person who was close to the bereaved individual (for children and adolescents, at least 6 months ago).

Thus, "complex grief" occurs in the context of "loss" through death, and the bereavement is further defined by duration. No reference is made to the complex process of grieving for the "loss" of the child a family may have felt they had expected and deserved, the experiences they had anticipated, instead supplanted by feelings, responsibilities, complications and adversities that were not envisaged.

Although the process of psychological assessment and diagnosis is in many respects "linear" and "systematic", it cannot be assumed that the process of absorbing complex information, bad or confronting news, unfamiliar terminology, and statements of belief contrary to those of a particular family, ethnicity or cultural belief system, will similarly be predictable or straightforward. There must be patience, consideration and support of any individual family's needs, hopes, expectations, beliefs and misgivings. It is indeed "complex".

Bibliography

Adams, S. N. (2024), "The Unmasking of Autism in South Africa and Nigeria", Neuropsychiatric Disease and Treatment, 20, pp 947–955.

Affleck, G., Tennen, H., and Gershman, K. (1985), "Cognitive Adaptations to High-Risk Infants: The Search for Mastery, Meaning, and Protection from Future Harm", American Journal of Mental Deficiency, 89(6), pp 653–656.

Allred, K., and Hancock, C. (2012), "On Death and Disability: Reframing Educators' Perceptions of Parental Response to Disability", Disabilities Study Quarterly, 32(4).

American Psychiatric Association (2013), Diagnostic and Statistical Manual 5, American Psychiatric Association.

American Psychiatric Association (2022), Diagnostic and Statistical Manual 5 TR, American Psychiatric Association.

American Psychological Association (2022), "Guidelines for Assessment of and Intervention with Persons with Disabilities", www.apa.org.

Australian Psychological Society (2018), "Australian Psychological Society Code of Ethics".

Bayat, M. (2007), "Evidence of Resilience in Families of Children with Autism", Journal of Intellectual Disability Research, 51, pp 702–714.

Dowling, C., Nicoll, N., and Thomas, B. (2004), Lessons from my Child, Finch Publishing.

Dunst, C. J., and Trivette, C. M. (2009), "Capacity-Building Family-Systems Intervention Practices", Journal of Family Social Work, 12(2), pp 119–143.
Ellis, J., and Whaite, A. (1983), To Parents of Children with Disabilities, from Parents of Children with Disabilities, Social Evaluation and Research Ltd.
Ferguson, P. M. (2002), "A Place in the Family: An Historical Interpretation of Research on Parental Reactions to Having a Child with a Disability", Journal of Special Education, 36(3), pp 124–147.
Franz, L., Chambers, N., von Isenberg, M., and de Vries, P. J. (2017), "Autism Spectrum Disorder in Sub-Saharan Africa: A Comprehensive Scoping Review", Autism Research, 10(5) pp 2–42.
Grinker, R. R., and Cho, K. (2013), "Border Children: Interpreting Autism Spectrum Disorder in South Korea", Ethos, 41(1), pp 46–74.
Gupta, A., and Singhal, N. (2004), "Positive Perceptions in Parents of Children with Disabilities", Asia Pacific Disability Rehabilitation Journal, 15(1), pp 21–33.
Harrison A. J., Bradshaw L. P., Naqvi N. C., Paff M. L., and Campbell J. M. (2017), "Development and Psychometric Evaluation of the Autism Stigma and Knowledge Questionnaire (ASK-Q)", Journal of Autism and Developmental Disorders, 47, pp 3281–3295.
Harrison, A. J., Naqvi, N. C., Smit, A. K., Kumar, P. N., Muhammad, N. A., Saade, S., Yu, L., Cappe, E., Low, H. M., Chan, S.-J., and de Bildt, A. (2023), "Assessing Autism Knowledge across the Global Landscape Using the ASK-Q", Journal of Autism and Developmental Disorders, 54, pp 1897–1911.
Harrison, A. J., Paff, M. L., and Kaff, M. S. (2019), "Examining the Psychometric Properties of the Autism Stigma and Knowledge Questionnaire (ASK-Q) in Multiple Contexts", Research in Autism Spectrum Disorders, 57, pp 28–34.
Hus, Y., and Segal, O. (2021), "Challenges Surrounding the Diagnosis of Autism in Children", Neuropsychiatric Disease and Treatment, 17, pp 3509–3529.
Kessler, D. (2019), Finding Meaning: The Sixth Stage of Grief, Simon and Schuster.
Klein, S., and Schive, K. (2001). You will Dream New Dreams: Inspiring Personal Stories by Parents of Children With Disabilities, Kensington Book Publishing.
Kubler-Ross, E., and Kessler, D. (2014), On Grief and Grieving, Scribner.
Lynch, P., et al. (2023), "Experiences of Identifying Pre-school Children with Disabilities in Resource Limited Settings-An Account from Malawi, Pakistan and Uganda", Disability and Society, 39(8) pp 1–21.
Moses, K. (2003), The Impact of Childhood Disability: The Parent's Struggle, CdLS (Cornelia De Lange Syndrome) Foundation Newsletter.
Olshansky, S. (1962), "Chronic Sorrow: The Response to having a Mentally Defective Child", Families in Society: The Journal of Contemporary Social Services, 43, pp 191–193.
Otufat-Shamsi, S. (2015), "Developmental Disabilities in Children Across Different Cultures", World Forgotten Children Foundation Newsletter, 9(2).
Paget, A., Mallefwa, M., Chinguo, D., Mahebere-Chirambo, C., and Gladstone, M. (2016), "'It Means you are Grounded'-Caregivers' Perspectives on the Rehabilitation of Children with Neurodisability in Malawi", Disability and Rehabilitation, 38(3), pp 223–234.
PSP Learning Hub (2021), "Children with Disability -Culture and Identity". https://psplearninghub.com.au/
Rochefort, M., Paradis, A., Rivard, M., and Dewar, M. (2023), "Siblings of Individuals with Intellectual Disabilities or Autism: A Scoping Review using Trauma Theory", Journal of Child and Family Studies, 32(11), pp 1–19.
Taylor, S. E., Kemeny, M. E., Reed, G. M., Bower, J. E., and Gruenewald, T. L. (2000). "Psychological Resources, Positive Illusions, and Health", American Psychologist, 55(1), pp 99–109.
Turnbull, A. P., Patterson, J. M., Behr, S. K., Murphy, D. L., Marquis, J. G., and Blue-Banning, M. J. (Eds.) (1993), Cognitive Coping, Families, and Disability, Paul H. Brookes.
Westby, C., Chen, K. M., Cheng, L., Jithavech, P., and Maroonroge, S. (2024), "Autism in Taiwan and Thailand: Influences of Culture", Neuropsychiatric Disease and Treatment, 20, pp 1523–1538.
Wolff, M., et al. (2023), "Individual-Level Risk and Resilience Factors Associated with Mental Health in Siblings of Individuals with Neurodevelopmental Conditions: A Network Analysis", Developmental Neuropsychology, 48(3), pp 112–134.

8 Systemic reasons to assess and diagnose childhood disorders

The journey taken by families with disabled children is long, confusing and fraught with roadblocks, changes and "transitions" – pivotal moments in the life of children and families where they are confronted by significant changes imposed externally, often by "systems". The first is the process of seeking clarity of diagnosis for a young child, generally followed soon after by the need to seek support for their children either through entry to programmes, therapies or services, or financial assistance to defray the costs of these. Most developed countries have long and proud histories of supporting people with disabilities, and increasingly "developing" nations are following suite. Either through direct service provision such as special education, or through financial support for participants such as government benefits and allowances, there is an increasing expectation of support. There will always be the need for bureaucratic oversight and accountability for provision of these services, sometimes leading to confusion, anger, frustration and dissatisfaction.

Access to services and funding

One reason for assessment and diagnostic services to produce precise "diagnostic outcomes" is that government departments and agencies often require "specificity" of diagnosis or assessment outcomes for eligibility and access to specific early intervention programmes such as specialist preschools and schools, and specific financial, material or service-related assistance. A failure to provide precise information can simply block one's access to such services and supports.

Early intervention and therapy programmes are expensive, and without government assistance, many families would be unable to afford the treatments and resources their young children desperately need. Estimates vary depending upon country and national economic circumstances, average wages and of the specifics of disability types and severity; however, for many families, educational, therapeutic and other supports would be beyond their means without government or state subsidy. There are many different forms of financial support. Rules and regulation for funding and service access vary globally, as do the types of schemes. There can be:

- Direct financial grants to families.
- Tax concessions and rebates for costs incurred by families for such things as therapeutic interventions.
- Hybrid schemes incorporating financial support, direct service provision and planning support.

DOI: 10.4324/9781003565338-11

Table 8.1 Summary of Global Statistics on financial support schemes

- 92% of nations provide disability funding support schemes with periodic payments to eligible people with disabilities.
- Of these, 48% require no individual contributions from people with disabilities or their families.
- Of these nations, 15% of these beneficiaries are not subject to means-testing, but 33% are.
- 44% of the schemes require some level of personal contribution.

- Government-provided therapeutic and intervention programmes.
- National Health Insurance Schemes.

Some countries, such as Australia and Norway, have more than one source of financial support, some are long-standing schemes, and others are recent developments as nations begin to assume their responsibilities in the sphere of disability. Overall statistics are given in Table 8.1.

An extremely small proportion of nations give participants a lump sum payment, instead paying an allowance or benefit, but only 2% of nations provide no funding support for disability support. The variety of funding approaches may reflect the political, economic and social attitudes of countries. The following examples provide an overview of the types of support schemes, and those with particular or unusual characteristics.

Specific financial support schemes

Australia

The Australian Government provides support funding for families of young children with disabilities through two specific schemes, which are separate entities and completely different:

- **Centrelink Carers Allowance.**
- **National Disability Insurance Scheme (NDIS).**

The application procedure for families applying to Centrelink for the Carers Allowance is a two-tiered process, where diagnoses with "known aetiology" such as genetic disorder, are automatically accepted as "proof". There is an additional onus of proof required for eligibility on the basis of a diagnosis of neurodevelopmental disorders such as Global Development Delay. "Automatic entry" conditions are listed in Table 8.2.

When additional evidence is required, it is through the form of a hierarchical developmental skills questionnaire, for developmental domains such as fine and gross motor skills, expressive and receptive language skills, social interaction skills, early learning skills and daily living skills. It will be noted that this information can readily be sourced from standard developmental tests such as the Griffiths 3 or the Bayley-4, and adaptive behaviour questionnaires such as the Adaptive Behavior Assessment System 3 or the Vineland 3.

Australia's second scheme is the **National Disability Insurance Scheme**, originally mooted in 1974, legislated in 2013 but not fully implemented until 2020. This is a hybrid scheme encompassing financial supports, direct or contracted service provision, and future planning for families. For eligibility criteria there is reference to various assessment schedules and tests, and to DSM-5-TR criteria for various neurodevelopmental disorders. Considerable professional reporting is required to establish eligibility, with a preference

Table 8.2 Australian Centrelink Carers Allowance Eligibility Evidence

Automatic eligibility conditions	Additional proof required

• Physical disabilities such as cerebral palsy and spina bifida
• Uncontrolled epileptic conditions
• Chromosomal or syndromic conditions which also cause moderate to severe intellectual disability
• Metabolic degenerative conditions which also cause moderate to severe intellectual disability
• Neurodegenerative conditions which also cause moderate to severe intellectual disability
• Hearing and/or vision loss within specific parameters such as levels of visual acuity, and degree of hearing loss is measured in decibels
	• Autism spectrum disorder as defined by DSM-5-TR
	• Moderate, severe or profound intellectual disability, defined by IQ scores below 55
	• Global developmental delay, with additional information required in relation to:
	  • Receptive language
	  • Expressive language
	  • Feeding and mealtime skills
	  • Hygiene and grooming skills
	  • Dressing skills
	  • Social and community skills
	  • Fine motor skills
	  • Gross motor skills
	  • Behaviour

for descriptions of the impact of disorders upon daily functioning and independence. Funding and support are provided for three domains:

- **Core supports:** To help with costs of everyday living.
- **Capacity building:** To facilitate the building of independence.
- **Capital supports:** For assistive technologies and home modifications.

New Zealand

New Zealand is a small nation with two distinct population bases, the Mauri people and the Europeans who settled and colonised the two islands in the 18th and 19th century. Child development services are available through the Ministry of Health. These "non-medical, multidisciplinary allied health and community-based services" can:

- Provide specialist assessment for young children.
- Organise intervention and management services.
- Coordinate with other agencies to ensure integrated support.

There is also the Needs Assessment and Service Coordination Organisation, to ascertain whether people may be eligible for government-funded disability support services, to outline the types of relevant supports and services required, coordinate "facilitated needs assessments" and advise on the allocation of resources.

The United States of America

In the United States, there is the Supplementary Security Income Program (SSI), a financial assistance scheme administered jointly by the American Federal Government and individual states, require clear evidence that:

- A child has a medically determinable physical or mental impairment (or combination of impairments).

Systemic reasons to assess and diagnose childhood disorders 99

- The impairment results in marked and severe functional limitations.
- The impairment has lasted (or is expected to last) for at least one year or to result in death.

A medically determinable physical or mental impairment "must result from anatomical, physiological, or psychological abnormalities that are demonstrable by medically acceptable clinical and laboratory diagnostic techniques". "Acceptable medical sources" include:

- Licensed physicians (medical or osteopathic doctors).
- Licensed psychologists, including those in independent practice or in other settings.
- Qualified speech-language pathologists for speech or language impairments only.
- Licensed audiologists for impairments of hearing loss, and auditory processing disorders.

Information required for SSI applications includes qualitative descriptions of how effectively a child:

- Learns or acquires information.
- Uses the information he/she has learned.
- Is able to focus and maintain attention.
- Carries through and finishes activities in a timely manner.
- Initiates and sustains emotional connections with others.
- Develops and uses the language of his/her community.
- Cooperates with others.
- Complies with rules.
- Responds to criticism.
- Respects and takes care of the possessions of others.
- Moves his/her body from one place to another.
- Moves and manipulates things.
- Maintains a healthy emotional and physical state, including how well the child gets his/her physical and emotional wants and needs met in appropriate ways.
- Copes with stress and changes in the environment.
- Takes care of his/her own health, possessions, and living area.

Consideration is also given to the cumulative impacts of physical or mental impairments, and their associated treatments or therapies, on a child's functioning. SSI funding can be supplemented with other specific State and County financial aid packages, and fee reimbursement through individual family's health insurance schemes.

Canada

In Canada, there is the "Child Disability Benefit (CDB)", "a tax-free monthly payment made to families who care for a child under age 18 with a severe and prolonged impairment in physical or mental functions". Eligibility criteria refer to "marked restrictions" in functioning in:

- Walking.
- Hearing.
- Mental functions.
- Speaking.

- Dressing.
- Vision.
- Feeding.
- Life-sustaining therapy.
- Eliminating (bowel or bladder function).

There is also a distinction between "marked restriction" and the "cumulative effect of significant restrictions", for example when a child has more than one impairment. Eligible families receive a tax refund on expenses incurred in supporting their child.

The United Kingdom

In the United Kingdom, early identification and early intervention are "key themes" in the "Framework for the Assessment of Children in Need and their Families (2000)" and the "Special Educational Needs Code of Practice (2001)", described jointly by the United Kingdom Department of Education and Skills, and the Department of Health.

They are integral to government programme initiatives such as "Quality Protects" and "Sure Start". Guidelines for service providers stress the following:

- The variation in legal definitions of disability in very young children.
- For families, the sometimes daunting nature of language used to describe and define disability.
- Existing definitions of disability tend to rely upon the expectation of "long-term and substantial disadvantage", whereas in very young children, it is not necessarily possible to predict clearly whether "impairments" will be long-term. However, the following guides are used:

A child under 3 years of age shall be considered disabled if he/she:

i is experiencing significant developmental delays, in one or more of the areas of cognitive development, physical development, communication development, social or emotional development, and adaptive development.
ii has a condition which has a high probability of resulting in developmental delay.

The guidelines also recognise that "the assessment and diagnostic process does not always work effectively for young children and their families" but do expand upon the assessment process. "Assessment" may refer to the process of arriving at a diagnosis, to the process of identifying needs, or to both. "Assessment is also regarded as a process of gathering information about the health, education and social care needs of a child".

Assessments should:

- Identify any specific health needs of a child.
- Promote understanding and agreement about the potential developmental implications of a condition so that effective educational, behavioural, physical or communication strategies can be put in place to promote development.
- Address the needs of the child in the family context so that the family is empowered and feels confident to provide for the learning and care needs of their child at the same time as feeling that their own needs and those of their other children are also being addressed.

Singapore

In Singapore, the Enhanced Pilot for Private Intervention Providers (Enhanced PPIP) is a subsidy scheme that offers choices of early intervention programs for children who have already been referred for the State-provided Early Intervention Program for Infants and Children (EIPIC). Parents who choose to use selected Private Intervention Centres (PIC)'s receive financial subsidies to help defray the costs. Early Intervention Programme for Infants & Children (EIPIC) stipulate that children must be:

- 6 years old or younger (children below age 2 are placed in "EIPIC Under-2's" if these are offered at their Early Intervention Centre).
- Diagnosed with, or at risk of, developmental, intellectual, sensory or physical disabilities or a combination of disabilities.
- Recommended for EIPIC by a Doctor from the available local Child Development Assessment Centres at a number of hospitals, or a private Paediatrician.

Relevant information from various professionals and practitioners is collated by a doctor and recommendations made. As with the Australian Centrelink application, estimates need to be made as to a child's ability to reach and demonstrate specific developmental milestone, again raising the significance of standardised developmental assessments as credible and convenient sources of such information. The recommending doctor must also provide considerable background information about family members, including maternal and paternal reactions to and acceptance of diagnoses of developmental disorders or disabilities. Again, psychological assessments and reports are crucial in eliciting and describing such reactions as well as offering families ongoing emotional support.

Taiwan

The Protection of Children and Youths Welfare and Rights Act (2011) established an assessment and diagnostic mechanism and intervention services for children under age 6 years, with eligibility for access through developmental screening between 2 and 6 years of age. Eligible children are typically diagnosed with developmental disability. They are then able to receive speech and language services provided at hospitals or medical clinics covered by the Nationwide Health Insurance scheme (NHI) created in 1994. There is also the National Health Insurance Research Database (NHIRD), the purpose of which is to promote biomedical and behavioural research and research on healthcare utilisation.

Thailand

Thailand is described as having one of the world's best healthcare systems. The country began its health coverage programme in 2002, providing universal healthcare to all citizens. The Thai government provides a disability grant for people with disabilities. This is doubled at age 60. University tuition is waived for students with disabilities who qualify for admission. The Royal Thai family has a significant role in the field of disabilities, including a rehabilitation programme for children with physical disabilities and supporting foundations for sensory impairments intellectual disability. This commitment became even more evident when the King's grandson was diagnosed with autism spectrum disorder. A national universal developmental screening program (DSPM) was initiated in 2015.

South Africa

In South Africa, the support services available to young children with neurodevelopmental disorders reflect the long and complex political and cultural journey of the nation's history. At present, parents of young children with disabling conditions can apply for the Care Dependency Grant through the South African Government. This grant applies to parents of children who have severe disabilities and are in need of full-time and special care. Access to early childhood centres for children with disabilities has been a controversial issue in South Africa for decades, and limitations of access have two distinct impacts upon support for children with disabilities:

- Early childhood centres are described as deficient in their screening of young children who may be at risk of developmental compromise or delay.
- As access to early education centres remains limited, young children with disabilities and developmental delays have less opportunity to practise, apply and generalise the skills and processes that may be developing through therapeutic input.

Mainland China

Mainland Chinese research articles refer to the "rehabilitation" of children with disabilities. This has been included in the outlines of various "five-year plans". The Communist Party of China (CPC) in 2018 proposed to develop a "rehabilitation assistance system" for children with disabilities, to fill in gaps in China's rehabilitation service guarantee system. The Chinese government is the main policy and fund supporter of the rehabilitation of disabled children through its various projects. In previous project-based social support systems, the government directly provided financial support and purchased assistive devices for children with disabilities in "poverty-stricken" and low-income households, for example "Public Welfare Lotteries".

In the new rehabilitation assistance system for children with disabilities, the previous relationship between government and clients has been changed, where the government has become the supporter, coordinator and supervisor of rehabilitation programmes. As of 2023, no studies have been conducted or published to assess the efficacy of China's rehabilitation assistance system for disabled children. There have been studies however that focus on policy issues and "optimisation measures".

Japan

The Land of the Rising Sun provides a "Special Child Rearing" Allowance for caring for children with disabilities at home. This provides differential funding according to the severity of disability:

- Grade 1 "serious conditions".
- Grade 2 "moderate conditions".
- The "Welfare Allowance" for persons under 20 years of age with severe disabilities living at home and in need of specialist nursing care.

South Korea

As with many other countries, the Republic of South Korea provides financial support for families of children with disabilities, through the Korea National Disability Registration

System (KNDRS), established in 1989, based on predefined criteria for disability registration. There is:

- An objective medical examination conducted by a suitably qualified physician.
- A medical advisory meeting to review the degree of disability, including medical institutions and specialists for the diagnosis of specific disabilities, including medical records to support diagnoses.

Over the years, the number of disability types has gradually expanded to 15. Korea has a mandatory public health insurance system that covers the entire Korean population, and the National Health Insurance Services manages all eligibility information, including disability types and severity ratings. Several specific categories of disability are detailed statistically for ongoing reference, along with definitional criteria for:

- Brain injury.
- Visual disability.
- Hearing disability.
- Speech and language disability.
- Epilepsy.
- Intellectual disability.
- Autism.
- Mental disorders.

Norway, Sweden, Denmark and Finland

Scandinavian countries have a long history of providing government support for social welfare issues including childhood disability:

- The Norwegian Government provides more than one allowance. There is a direct financial payment to offset the costs of early intervention and therapeutic services, and an additional "nursing" or "attendance" allowance if the nature of a child's disability or chronic illness requires parents to stay at home for long periods of time caring for their child.
- In Sweden, children with disabilities and their parents or guardians can receive various benefits. Children covered by the "Act concerning Support and Service for Persons with Certain Functional Impairments (LSS)" can receive personal assistance from local municipalities, and an assistance allowance from the Swedish Social Insurance Agency. They can also receive a car allowance to purchase or adapt a vehicle suitable for their child's needs.
- Under the Danish Social Services Act and the "Denmark Child Guarantee National Action Plan 2022", there is a Care Allowance for children with disabilities, and also the Danish Disability Fund to support Danish disability organisations to cooperate and coordinate more effectively.
- Finland's Kela, The Social Insurance Institution of Finland, supports families through its "Disability Benefit for Under 16-year-olds".

India

In India, there is a disability allowance, and also financial assistance for "non-school going disabled children". This scheme was commenced in 2008 and financial support is provided for children with intellectual disabilities and not able to attend formal education, who are totally dependent on parents and relatives, and need constant supervision and care of their families. A recent direct support initiative, commencing in 2021, is the opening of "Cross Disability Early Intervention Centres" for children up to the age of 6 years, staffed by a range of professionals.

Disability support is very expensive, and it will be readily understood from these and many more examples that governments are expected to perform "due diligence" on applications for support funding. Every nation will have its own variation on funding, support and service coordination methodologies, but there is a universal requirement for proof and certainty of eligibility for such assistance. This can include follow-up reports when it may, for example, be necessary to confirm that a child continues to need the support he/she has been receiving, whether additional funding is required to bolster or change therapies and programmes to meet a child's changing needs, or to change or transition from one programme to another.

Knowledge of the relevant support schemes for families of young children with neurodevelopmental disorders is an essential component of a psychologist's service provision. Assessments are not conducted in a "vacuum". Assessments and reports need to have relevance to and appropriate influence upon bureaucratic processes and decisions. "System accountability" is a valid and important function in the governance of service provision and funding but can be a confusing and daunting process for many families, and it is a responsibility of the assessing psychologist to best "tell the story" according to the rules and procedures in play.

Educational access

Another common "systems-orientated" purpose of psychological assessment for young children relates to another "transition point" for young children and their families. This is when a young child with a disability or disorder approaches school enrolment age. Different schools and school systems function under different rules governing enrolment eligibility and support availability and provision. What the "school system" does have in common is that it is the first social "agency" which can offer or deny "entry" on the basis of a disabling condition. It is a major transition point, with a significant influence upon a child's future development. If the enrolment process for a young child is dependent upon psychological assessment information, there can be a dual "burden of proof" placed upon a psychologist's shoulders.

On the one hand, the truth of a child's diagnosis and its functional implications must be told. On the other hand, psychologists have an ongoing role to support and advocate for their clients and families, regardless of whether they entirely agree with a family's choice of educational setting.

There is considerable variation in "eligibility criteria" for schools, whether government run, or privately operated. For example, special education programmes may be offered on the basis of highly specific diagnostic criteria such as:

- Specificity of diagnosis such as autism spectrum disorder.
- Level of developmental delay or intellectual disability.
- Physical mobility skills.
- Emotional and behavioural regulation skills.
- Sensory disorders.

Depending upon individual national contexts, these descriptors can relate closely to the types of educational programmes offered in different cities, states, counties or boroughs. Some special schools may be delineated strictly on the basis of assessment outcomes and diagnostic "labels". For example, in the United States, these schools are often referred to as "Charter Schools" – such schools have a specific educational charter and raison d'etre.

Once again, there is an imperative for psychologists assessing young children to understand what information is required for service or school eligibility purposes, as this will influence the type of assessments to be conducted, tests used and the style and content of reports written. It may also require an understanding of the timeframes associated with some enrolment opportunities, such as cut-off dates for enrolment applications. Psychologists may not see their roles as being entirely sympathetic to the "systems needs" referred to in this section but need to appreciate that their role does involve supporting families at crucial times such as significant transition points.

There is another dimension to appreciating the importance of developmental assessments for young children, and that is the provision of accurate and comprehensive descriptions of what young children can do and cannot do in their early play educational and adaptive experiences. Parents, teachers and therapists who read assessment reports need considerably more than statistical psychometric test results and diagnostic pronouncements. They need to know what a child could or could not do, why it was easy or why it was difficult, what types of compensatory or adaptive behaviours the child used to complete tasks and activities even if such achievement was difficult or "inaccurate".

Practitioners of various professions speak sometimes of a "common language" for issues relating to assessments of young children and subsequent reports. This will be considered in more detail later in this publication, but it is important to assert that assessments and subsequent reports serve a range of purposes for different "audiences" – parents, government departments and non-government agencies, therapists, doctors and teachers. It is important to consider how information derived from assessments is reported, for the benefit of a child with a disabling condition, whether this "benefit" is therapeutic, systemic, educational or medical.

Reports for "evidential" purposes – migration

Sometimes a psychological report for a child with a neurodevelopmental disorder is required for other burdens of proof. One relates to the increasing levels of migration globally. People immigrate to flee conflict and war, poverty and disadvantage, political persecution and religious bigotry. They migrate for family reunion, and for job opportunities, whether short or long term. They may be seeking permanent residency in another country, or a short-term visa. If a family has a child with a disability or a neurodevelopmental disorder, they may well need to prove that their child's condition will not impose too great a financial burden on their country of choice.

Article 18 of the United Nations Convention on the Rights of Persons with Disabilities (2006) brooches the issue of "liberty of movement and nationality". It states that individuals with disabilities:

- Have the right to acquire and change a nationality and are not deprived of their nationality arbitrarily or on the basis of disability.
- Are not deprived, on the basis of disability, of their ability to obtain, possess and utilize documentation of their nationality or other documentation of

identification, or to utilize relevant processes such as immigration proceedings, that may be needed to facilitate exercise of the right to liberty of movement.
- Are free to leave any country, including their own.
- Are not deprived, arbitrarily or on the basis of disability, of the right to enter their own country.

This is not necessarily how families are treated when attempting to migrate to a country of choosing when they have a child with a disability. Relevant state or government medical officers may make assessments of the costs, which might accrue should such a family wish to migrate. There may be strict financial limits to how much individual nation states may be prepared to expend on such families for disability support, and respond accordingly. It is not uncommon for families in these circumstances to be disbarred from entry or even deported, to not be allowed access to any support services or funding, or even to be allowed entry without their disabled child. These decisions and processes are of course subject to appeal, with many families accessing the services of immigration lawyers and consultants.

In those circumstances, detailed psychological assessment and reports may be sought by families and lawyers to advocate where possible for a review of any adverse decisions made. This can require a psychologist to have some knowledge and awareness of the relevant rules and processes involved.

Reports for "evidential" purposes – divorce and property settlements

"Evidential" reports may also be required when there are family break-up and divorce procedures taking place. Such matters are frequently unpleasant and emotional, and there is often an emphasis upon the costs of caring for a child with a neurodevelopmental disorder and how those costs should be shared between carers. One party or another may dispute the reported or estimated costs of therapies, education, resources and supports for a young child with a disability, and it may be that evidential support is sought from a psychologist as part of the negotiations.

There is access to specific training and education for psychologists, often through psychological associations or societies or private providers, in relation to their legal obligations in such situations, for example report and record keeping, subpoena responses, and in-person court evidence. Printed and on-line materials are also available. It is important that psychologists placed in such circumstances have access to appropriate advice and support when drawn into legal proceedings such as these, both for their own professional protection, and for the appropriate provision of service to their" primary client", the young child.

Bibliography

Canadian Government Support Payments and Benefits, Government of Canada website/Benefits. www.Canada.ca.

Centrelink Carers Allowance Application Form (SA426.1809), Australian Government Services Australia. https://www.servicesaustralia.gov.au/sa426.

Chiang, L. H., and Hadadian, A. (2010), "Raising Children with Disabilities in China: The Need for Early Intervention", Internation Journal of Special Education, 25(2), pp 113–118.

Clark, B. J., Holness, W. A., Nyamadzawo, R. T., and Moogie, D. (2024), "Implementing Early Childhood Education for Children with Disabilities in South Africa and Kenya", African Journal of Disability, 13(1), pp 1–12.

Government of Denmark (2022), "Denmark - Child Guarantee National Action Plan Overview", Government of Denmark, https://www.denmark.dk/.

Government of India, M/o Social Justice and Empowerment Department of Empowerment of Persons with Disabilities (2021), "Inauguration of Cross Disability Early Learning Centres", https://www.india.gov.in.

Gu, Z., Tan, H., Zang, H., and Zhou, R. (2023), "Assessment of Chinese Rehabilitation assistance system for disabled children", Frontiers in Public Health, 11, https://doi.org/10.3389/fpubh.2023.1098908

Health of Disabled People Strategy (2024), New Zealand Ministry of Health Website/Disability, health.govt.nz.

Kim, M., Jung, W., Kim, S. Y., Park, J. H., and Shin, D. W. (2023), "The Korea National Disability Registration System", Epidemiology and Health, 45, pp 1–9.

Moodley, S. (2021), "Children with Disabilities in South Africa: Policies for Early Identification and Education", In Pearson Jr., W. and Reddy, V. (Eds.), Social Justice in the 21st Century: Research from South Africa and USA, Springer, pp 95–112.

National Disability Insurance Scheme Application Form (2020), downloaded from www.ndis.gov.au website.

National Disability Insurance Scheme, "Our History", National Disability Insurance Scheme, www.ndis.gov.au.

OECD Family Database, Social Policy Division (2022), "Disability Work and Inclusion", OECD, oecd.org.

Peñafiel, T. (2001), "Disability + Immigration: A New Planetary Reality", Document presented at the United Nations The ONU World Conference Against Racism, Racial Discrimination, Xenophobia and Related Intolerance By The Multi-Ethnic Association for the Integration of Persons with Disabilities.

Ramcharan, P. (2016), "Understanding the NDIS: A History of Disability Welfare from 'deserving poor' to 'consumers in control'", www.theconversation.com (retrieved from "The Conversation website of 8 July 2016).

Samaita, A. K. D. (2005), The Role and Effectiveness of Disability Legislation in South Africa, Disability Knowledge and Research.

Shinomiya, S. (2024), "The Role of Administrative Categories in the Globalisation of a Psychiatric Concept: Case Studies of Autism in Japan", Social Science & Medicine Journal, 367(C) pp 1–43.

Singapore Government Ministry of Social and Family Development, https://www.msf.gov.sg/.

Storbeck, C., and Moodley, S. (2011), "ECD Policies in South Africa–What about Children with Disabilities?", Journal of African Studies and Development, 3(1), pp. 1–8.

Swedish Government (2024), "Act Concerning Support and Service for Persons with Certain Functional Impairments (LSS)", https://www.government.se/.

UNICEF (2019), "A World Ready to Learn: Prioritizing Quality Early Childhood Education", UNICEF, www.unicef.org.

UNICEF (2023), "Global Report on Children with Disabilities: From the Margin to the Mainstream", www.unicef.org.

United Kingdom Department of Education and Skills/Department of Health joint statement (2002), "Together from The Start – Practical guidance for professionals working with disabled children (birth to 2) and their families", United Kingdom Department of Health.

United Nations Convention on the Rights of Persons with Disabilities (2006), www.un.org.

United Nations Department of Economic and Social Affairs Disability and Development Report (2018), United Nations Department of Economic and Social Affairs, www.un.org.

United States Social Security Administration, "Childhood Disability: Supplemental Security Income Program: A Guide for Physicians and Other Health Care Professionals", United States Social Security.

Part III
The assessment and diagnostic process

How are developmental assessments conducted with young children? What tests are used, and from where did they originate? This chapter details the different types of assessment instruments for neurodevelopmental disorders, their authors and researchers, development, formats, statistical properties and relevance to diagnostic criteria such as DSM-5-TR and ICD-11. Reference will be made to remarkable people who pioneered the theory and practice of developmental assessment, their lives and work, contributions and legacies.

9 Psychometric assessment of childhood development

John Dewey had much to say about life, education, schooling, and even about psychometric assessment. Never short of a pithy analogy, his homily in Figure 9.1 humorously illustrates that psychometric tests are not "direct" measures of ability – they are abstract mathematical processes many times removed from the reality of what people can and cannot do. Psychometric assessments provide voluminous numerical data. One need to look no further than the technical manuals for any standardised tests, to be either impressed with or overburdened by the sheer number of tables, graphs, charts, formulae, facts and figures, whether they relate to:

- General intelligence.
- Adaptive behaviour.
- Developmental quotients.
- Social or emotional maturity.
- Academic achievement.
- Specific neurodevelopmental disorders such as ADHD or autism spectrum disorder.

This is not to discredit psychometric assessments in any way, but to stress that in practice, metric outcomes are not necessarily the only priority of psychometric assessments. More importantly, psychometric assessment results need to be reported and explained, to parents and caregivers, government and non-government agencies, doctors and other health professionals, whose experience and understanding of statistics and psychometrics will vary enormously. Psychologists have the advantage of specific graduate and postgraduate training to understand the underlying concepts of psychometric results. Take for example the most basic principle of psychometric assessment – the Bell Curve (Figure 9.2).

On the left of the image is the Bell Curve, or Gaussian curve, as is familiar to all psychologists. On the right is the mathematical formula by which the normal curve is constructed and individuals assessed and categorised according to their "position" on the curve. Are they in the average range as are approximately 68% of the population, or above, or below? How far do they vary from the "normal population?" What does that mean for a family whose child has a disability or a neurodevelopmental disorder, or for service provision? How easily can such concepts be explained to families under immense emotional stress when their rationale for assessment is to learn "what is wrong" and "what to do" to help? How is this statistical information relayed to families and others who may not be familiar with the statistics of psychometric assessments, when the following statistical concepts are involved?

- Standard scores.
- Developmental quotients.

DOI: 10.4324/9781003565338-13

112 *Diagnosing Young Children with Neurodevelopmental Disorders*

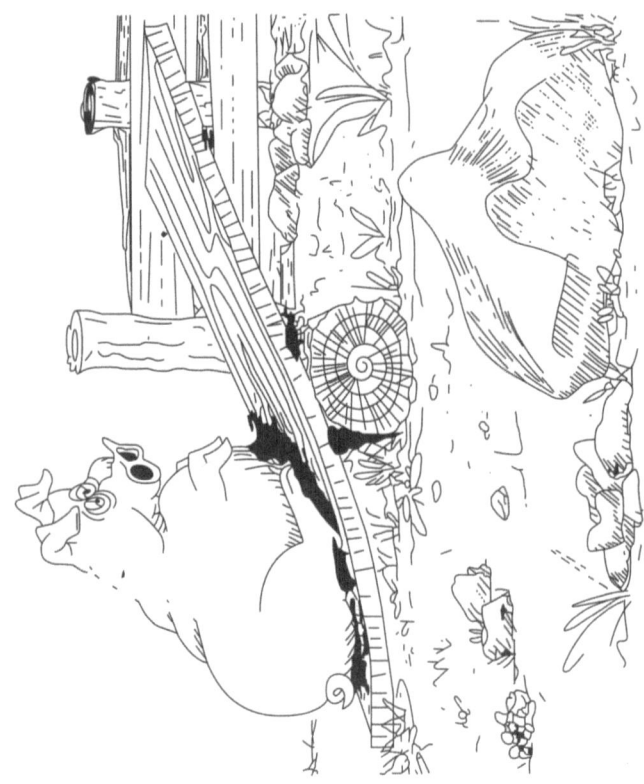

JOHN DEWEY 1859-1952

"This intelligence-testing business reminds me of the way they used to weigh hogs in Texas. They would get a long plank, put it over a cross-bar, and somehow tie the hog on one end of the plank. They'd search around till they found a stone that would balance the weight of the hog and they'd put that on the other end of the plank. Then they'd guess the weight of the stone."

Figure 9.1 John Dewey's reference to intelligence testing

Psychometric assessment of childhood development 113

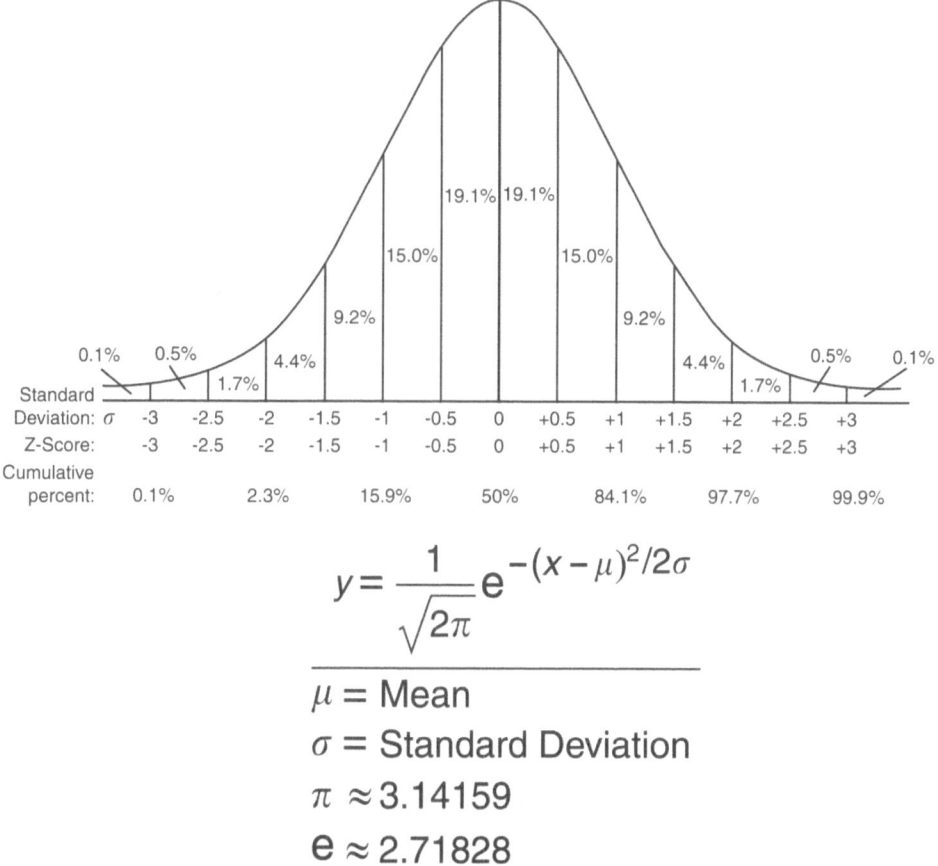

Figure 9.2 The normal or Gaussian curve

- General adaptive composites.
- Standard errors of measurement.
- Standard deviations.
- Percentile ranks.
- Stanines and quartiles.
- Measures of construct and predictive validity.
- Factorial analysis.
- Rausch models of item difficulty.
- T scores, eigen values and other statistical underpinnings.

These different scores often reflect the same or similar results but with slightly different emphases (Table 9.1).

Formal psychometric assessment of developmental milestones and skills in young children differs from psychometric assessment of cognitive skills, although there are clear parallels and areas of overlap. All psychometric assessments have to be valid, reliable and empirically sound. They need to be able to show empirically that they are actually assessing what they claim to be assessing. Let us focus upon the types of tasks and skills which

114 *Diagnosing Young Children with Neurodevelopmental Disorders*

Table 9.1 Standard scores, percentiles and standard deviations

STANDARD SCORE	50	55	60	65	70	75	80	85	90	95	100	105	110	115	120	125	130
PERCENTILE				1	2	5	9	16	25	37	50	63	75	84	91	95	98
STANDARD DEVIATIONS		−3			−2			−1						+1			+2
		Moderate			Mild			Borderline				Average					

are assessed by developmental tests, how these are converted from "real-world" skills to numerical concepts, and how this process should be explained and reported. Formal assessments of intelligence such as the various Weschler and Stanford-Binet Intelligence Scales are appropriately taught and supervised in relevant graduate, postgraduate and "in-career" courses and workshops, but the same does not apply to developmental assessments, which are generally taught and trained "on request" for specific career purposes.

Earlier in this book, the rise of awareness of the need to conceptualise, measure, compare and categorise the thinking and problem-solving skills of people was outlined, and it was a natural extension of this quest that assessments of the very young were explored and developed. However, for a considerable period of time, abilities of younger children took a "back seat" to the development of psychometric assessments of intelligence. Chapter 1 outlined some of the social, cultural and political influences, which revitalised interest in the assessment of young children, but consideration first needs to be given to the way young children grow and learn, as this is the key to developmental assessment.

Learning in the very young

Young children begin learning from the moment they are born, in fact even before their birth. No two young children will learn and develop in exactly the same way or at the same rate. Just ask any parent with more than one infant! They do however have many learning schema in common. Early on they learn through imitation, play and exploration. Chapter 1 made reference to the environmental factors associated with imitation, prediction, exploration and play in young children, for example Ruth Griffiths' "Avenues of Learning", through which children learn the consistency and regularity of environmental stimuli, human contact, nurturing and response to need. And this is where the first point of differentiation may occur – the context in which a young child is born and raised.

There are the impacts of poor diet and subsequent malnutrition, illnesses such as chronic colds and ear infections, with the consequence of possible hearing difficulty and even loss, which can then lead to delayed language acquisition. There are also the impacts of an unstimulating environment, compromised early bonding experiences or even abandonment.

Studies from both Sub-Saharan Africa and parts of India have indicated that early malnourishment of infants is associated with poorer overall development, later literacy skills and mortality rates.

Regardless, children begin to "problem-solve" from an early age. They begin to learn that their needs will be met if they cry or grizzle, that responses to their needs will occur in an orderly and predictable fashion, including time of day, level of need, and in response to their own behaviours. Children gradually begin to learn that they can apply a degree of influence to these circumstances to express their needs and have them met. Once again, disruptions to this process can impact upon early learning, behaviour and development.

Later, children begin to learn they can move and manipulate their bodies and body parts, sometimes to satisfy their needs, but also quite simply to explore. They gradually learn to manipulate objects and to move about in their environment. They begin to learn and appreciate that such manipulation and movement is both fun and a means of problem-solving. They learn that their vocal sounds are a source of fun and entertainment for caregivers, as well as being a means of inducing response from them. They begin to learn therefore that there is a communicative function to their vocalisations. They begin to learn early stages of "theory of mind" whereby they appreciate the fact that their movements, sounds and interactions bring joy to other people.

They also begin to appreciate that imitating the sounds and actions of adult caregivers brings about positive social response from parents and other family members. They learn about humour, for example through "mock attack" ("gotcha") games, and they learn about anticipation and surprise. They learn about object permanence and early "cause-and-effect" actions.

Soon, young children begin to appreciate that notions of the world can be created, and that early symbolic forms of communication such as pointing can be substituted for vocalisations if necessary. They begin to develop formalised language, and that they can compensate for a lack of appropriate vocabulary through other symbolic means such as gestures. They begin to understand the complex social dimensions of the world through symbolic role play, both imitated and self-generated. They begin to understand that although their immediate needs such as feeding, toileting and emotional comfort will be met by parents and loved ones, they too can begin to take increasing responsibility for some of these tasks.

Babies and toddlers increasingly develop independence in movement, emotional control, self-help, play and learning. They begin to learn that they can amuse themselves and take care of themselves independently of their parents for increasing periods of time, including managing complete separation such as attendance at childcare, without undue anxiety.

For those young children fortunate enough to commence childcare or preschool, these skills can be practised and applied in different settings and with different carers. They learn that they can separate from parents in the morning, who will return in the afternoon. They learn that they can play with others, take turns, negotiate, bargain and even argue. They begin to learn how to make friends, and to apply social rules set by adults other than their parents, and that there are sanctions for disobeying. They learn and practise care and empathy skills with others, and they also learn that they can control unpopular or unpleasant situations through such behaviours as refusal, lying, bargaining or rationalising. They eventually begin to learn pre-academic and early academic skills such as writing and reading, counting and calculating.

It has been pointed out previously however that access to childcare and early learning opportunities is not in any way universal, that many young children from "Lesser Developed Countries" do not have access to the toys and equipment, skilled teaching and caring, or the opportunity to socialise and play with others beyond the immediate bounds of their family, kinship or localised cohort.

Many early learning experiences can be conceptualised as developing "direct" skills – a child learns to pick up and release objects, to vocalise, to run and jump. These are not "extrapolated" or "indirect" skills as would tend to be included in formal psychometrical measures of intelligence for older children.

Prior to school entry, learning is exploratory and imitative. In the early years of formal schooling, there is an emphasis upon skills development and practice. Upon entry to primary school, usually 8 years of age, the curriculum focus has shifted dramatically to the application of acquired skills to abstract and hypothetical situations and concepts. Child development in that respect may be seen as a gradual but non-linear progression from the "concrete" to the "abstract" and "symbolic".

It is this complex developmental trajectory, from reflexes to purposeful action, from manipulation to problem-solving, from total dependence to relative independence, non-symbolic play to creativity, "sound play" to speech and language, that developmental tests endeavour to compress into 90 minutes of assessment.

In that sense, developmental assessment of young children is a parallel of their early socialising and learning experiences, whether at preschool or daycare, or family life. Standardised tests of developmental milestones however are, as with tests of intelligence, predicated upon comparisons of rates of skills development within specific populations, and these usually focus upon normative data from the countries in which the assessments were developed and published. Most are American or European, and even if attempts are made to include normative data from different ethnic, social and language groups, these attempts still relate to sample populations within the countries from which the tests originate. There is therefore implicit "assessment bias" in Western developmental tests.

A United Nations UNICEF report from April 2019 reviewed the educational opportunities for preschoolers around the world. In summary:

- Only half of the world's preschool-age children were receiving preschool education.
- One hundred and seventy-five million children were not enrolled in pre-primary education during their early years.
- In lesser developed countries, nearly 78% of children were missing out on preschool opportunities.

A previous but similar report from UNICEF opened with a quote from José Ortega y Gasset: "I am I and my circumstance", referring to the disparate opportunities young children had to even attend preschool programmes in developing countries. This disparity of opportunity not only entrenches inequities and inequalities in later learning for children but also raises questions about how truly representative of the "normal population" developmental tests actually are. When exploring the statistical information included in any technical manual for a standardised test, it is a worthwhile exercise to focus on the normative population data-where the sample children came from, whether efforts were made to "control for" cultural and language issues, socio-economic background. Some developmental tests even indicate normative population data based on a rigid "social class" hierarchy and other demographic limitations such as the exclusion of children from non-English speaking backgrounds.

American assessment tools need to incorporate many cultural and language groups-Hispanic, Mexican and Afro-American origins-as well as smaller "minority" groups such as Native Americans, but they are rarely entirely "culture-free". Assessment tools, generally emanating Great Britain or the United States, are sometimes adapted for specific test

Table 9.2 Standardisation sample demographics

Assessment	Griffiths 3	ABAS 3	ASRS
Normative Sample n=	208	7,700	1,280
SAMPLE ORIGIN	English Republic of Ireland Northern Ireland Scotland Wales 40% Rural 60% Urban	• American Asian • American African • Hispanic Origin • Native Hawaiian/Pacific Islander • American Indian • White • Other	• American Asian • African American • Hispanic • White • Multiracial/other

"markets", for example the Australian "norming" of the Bayley-4, and sometimes simply through language translations, for example into Spanish for certain American tests and other European languages such as Swedish for the early Griffiths tests emanating from the United Kingdom.

Let us consider three widely used assessment protocols from the United States and the United Kingdom for which such background information is readily available and compare them with the lack of opportunity experienced by many "Lesser Developed Countries" (Table 9.2).

Developmental tests are expensive to create and develop, manufacture and market. Although considerable effort is made to "standardise" and control for as many cultural and linguistic variables as possible, there will always be concerns about whether a particular test of development will mirror the cultural and linguistic conditions of all countries.

In a later chapter, a number of specific assessment adaptations to meet "local" cultural, ethnic and linguistic needs will be highlighted and discussed, ranging from language and instruction translations, substitutions of test items and materials, locally developed normative data and culturally adapted administration protocols. These projects tend to be either "local" initiatives, or research projects conducted by others, reflecting genuine concern and care for the betterment of societies other than their own.

Developmental assessments

Young children are less predictable in their social, behavioural and emotional responses to the demands of formal assessment procedures than children of school age. They may be more or less cooperative, less able to concentrate for long periods of time, and less able to understand the "social agenda" in play during a formal assessment.

At a statistical level, reference has been made to the reduced predictive validity of psychometric assessments of child development. A psychometric assessment of a young child's developmental status is often conceptualised as a "snapshot" of the child's performance "on the day" of assessment. This is an important concept for psychologists to grasp as they commence their career journeys through early childhood assessments. Despite this reduced predictive validity, there are some generalisations which can be made:

- A normally developing child will progress at a rate of approximately 12 months development for each 12 chronological months, in other words a 1:1 correlation between chronological and developmental age. There will of course be variations depending

118 *Diagnosing Young Children with Neurodevelopmental Disorders*

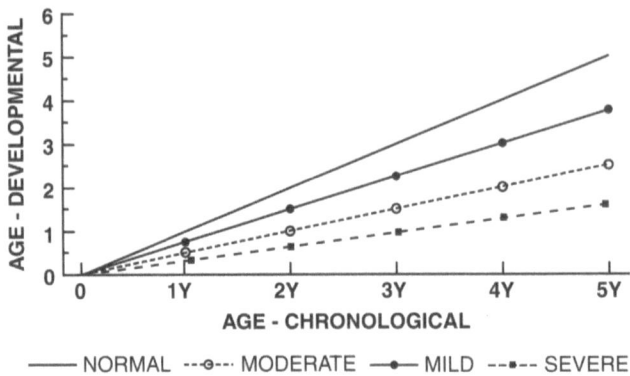

Figure 9.3 Rates of developmental growth by level of developmental delay

upon the sub-skills being assessed, for example a child may develop more rapidly in fine motor skills than in language skills at certain ages.
- A child with a mild developmental delay will progress at approximately 70% of that rate; in other words, 8–9 months' progress will be made every 12 months. Again, individual sub-skill variation should be expected.
- A child assessed as having a moderate developmental delay will perhaps gain only 6 months developmental skill every 12 months, and a child with a severe developmental delay even less so. This is simplistically represented in Figure 9.3.

This is of course an approximated theory of child development, but part of the clinical understanding that practitioners develop over time with repeated exposure to young children. Another such "clinical" view which psychologists may develop over time is that children who are developing in a typical fashion will have reached milestones on time and be striving to master the "next level" of skill, whereas a child with delayed developmental milestones is striving and sometimes struggling to attain age-appropriate skills.

An important discussion point from this concept is that a child will appear to be falling further and further behind the trajectory of "normal development" over time-the gap "widens". Explaining this to families is important, as there will be misunderstandings when a "delay" is understood to mean a simple need to "catch up". In test and "retest" situations, there is a need to explain that "new skills" are in fact being practised, learned and consolidated, albeit at a slower rate than expected.

Currently, the Griffiths III and the Bayley-4 Scales are the most frequently used and readily available developmental tests in English-speaking countries. They are the "gold standard" for developmental assessments, and come from a long history of research, development, usage and revision. Although originating from different countries, their similarities far outweigh their differences in philosophical underpinnings, research findings, internal structure and psychometric properties. This publication implies no preference for either of these tests and emphasises that the rigid training processes required of psychologists to administer these assessments is as much about learning and discovering the processes of "child development" as of learning the tests themselves. Both the Griffiths III and the Bayley-4 originate from the dedicated research, observation and theorisation of two particular women whose contributions to the world of child psychology are under-recognised and under-rewarded.

Sequences of development

Developmental tests are essentially an attempt to standardise and objectify the behaviours and skills observed in young children, but in a controlled and contrived assessment context. Young children develop in a number of specific developmental domains:

- Gross motor skills such as physical movement.
- Fine motor skills such as manipulation, coordination and planning.
- Language and communication skills.
- Problem-solving skills.
- Social and emotional skills.

Within these domains, there is a gradual progression from exploration, to imitation, through to purposeful action, application and generalisation of skills across tasks and settings. This is often referred to as "sequences of development", and although the Griffiths III and the Bayley-4 may have subtly different perspectives on these sequences, their similarities lie in the observation, conceptualisation and assessment of these skills.

It needs to be appreciated that the Griffiths III and the Bayley-4 attempt to cover all major areas of development but do not substitute for specific in-depth assessments provided by physiotherapists, speech pathologists or occupational therapists. They are in essence "comprehensive screening assessments".

The sequence of gross motor skills

Children begin to move early in life, as a means of exploration, stimulation, problem-solving, play and satisfaction of need (Figure 9.4). There are several clear developmental sequences associated with movement at a gross motor level, which commence from "reflex" actions and gradually progress through to various intentional movement patterns and skills:

- Early postural strength and stability skills such as lifting chin, holding head erect, sitting with firm back, pivoting, rolling, crawling, standing, side-stepping, climbing.
- Mobility and balance skills such as walking, stooping and squatting, kneeling, purposeful climbing and descending skills such as those on steps, and independent sitting at a table.
- Applied mobility and balance skills such as walking up and down steps, running, riding on ride-on toys or tricycles, jumping and throwing.
- Recreation-based skills such as throwing balls, kicking, throwing into or at targets and sequences of coordinated movements such as star jumps and hopscotch, dancing and imitating rhythmic patterns.

The sequence of fine motor coordination and planning skills

This sequence begins with involuntary reflex behaviours such as early grasping behaviour (e.g. the Palmar grasp), and onwards through the development of grasp and release (fine prehension) skills, and ending with the purposeful use of these skills to solve problems and engage in early pre-academic activities (Figure 9.5):

- Eye and head tracking skills such as following a moving light.
- Grasping skills and "take to the mouth" skills.

120 *Diagnosing Young Children with Neurodevelopmental Disorders*

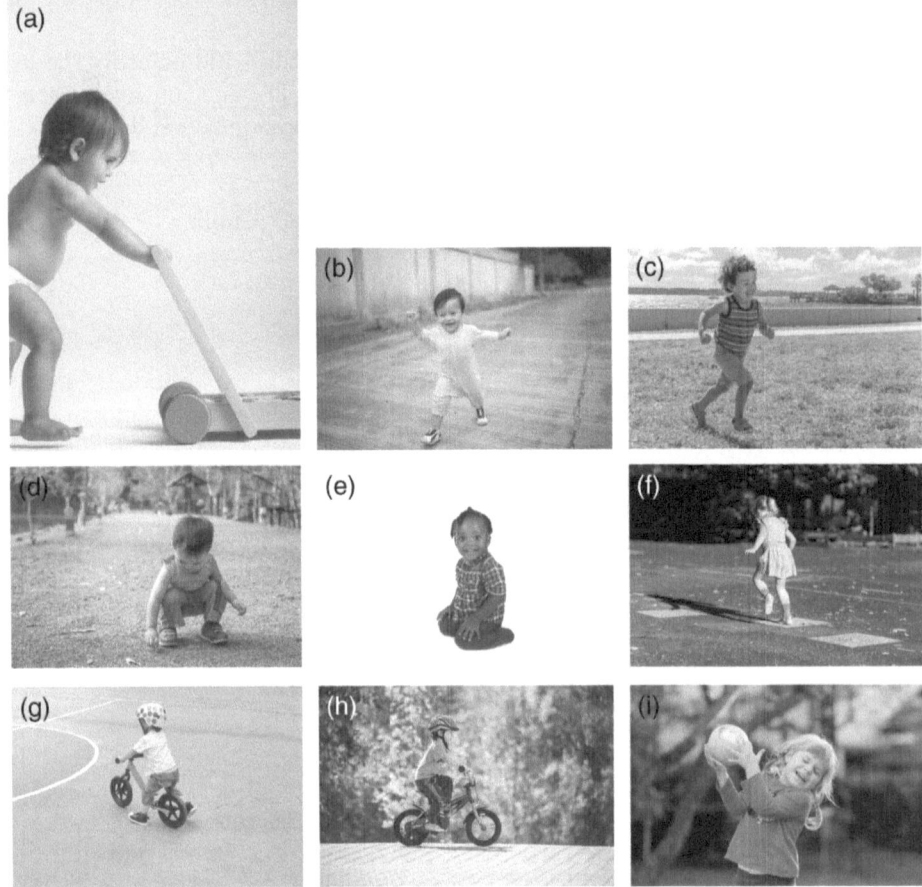

Figure 9.4 Examples of the sequence of gross motor skills

- Hitting, banging and dropping skills.
- Partial "specialisation" of thumb and forefinger skills such as picking up small objects.
- Fine prehension skills such as involving the tips of finger and thumb to pick up small objects more effectively.
- Complete "thumb opposition", for example the ability to hold a glass or drinking bottle.
- Putting and placing skills, such as making towers of blocks.
- Exploration skills with the forefinger, leading to the ability to point.
- "Transfer skills" such as tipping an object from one container to another.
- Crayon or pencil holding skills, leading to the development of a genuine "tripod grip" to facilitate the learning of writing and drawing.
- Page-turning skills.
- Opening and closing skills, for example manipulating a screw-top jar.
- Transition into self-help skills such as undoing buttons, removing shoes and other items of clothing.
- Cutting skills, for example with scissors.
- Complex utensil use such as eating and constructive play.
- Purposeful use of drawing and writing skills such as drawing circles, squares and triangles, letters, names and numbers.

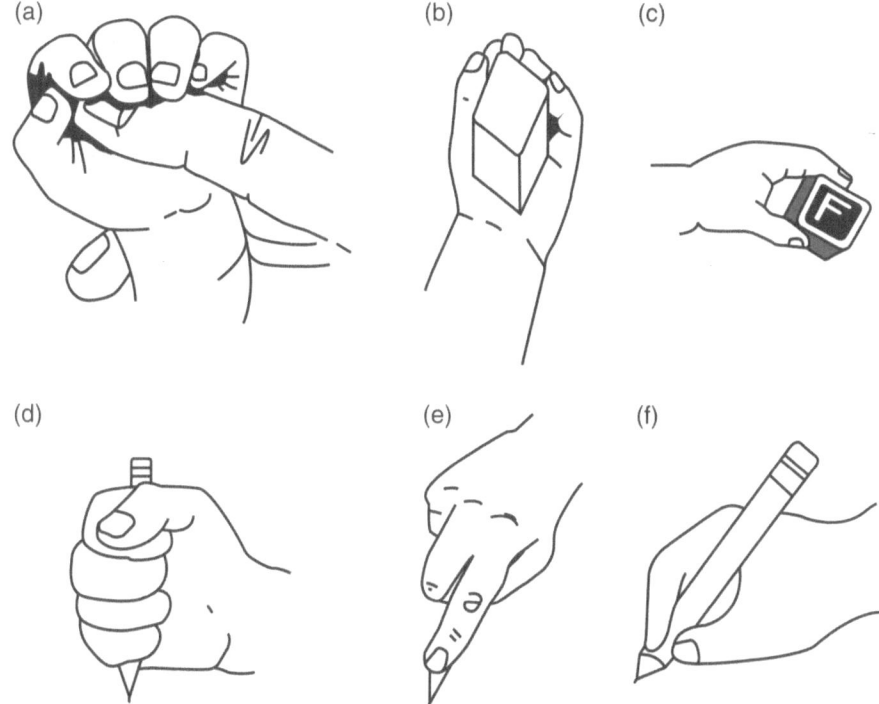

Figure 9.5 Examples of the sequence for fine motor skills

The sequence of speech, language and communication skills

The Griffiths III Scales do not attempt to clearly differentiate between expressive and receptive language skills, although the Bayley-4 does. In the case of Griffiths III, when one examines individual items from the associated subscale, this delineation can be inferred, but there are no separate scoring protocols for these. The various speech and language sequences follow below:

- Attention to the language and sound environment, for example "stilling" to a rung bell, searching for sounds, making eye contact with someone speaking, "following" the conversations of others, and enjoying music.
- Sound-making and babbling, including the presence of vowel and consonant sounds heard either alone or in combination, and the "prosodic" or tuneful quality of vocalisations.
- The development of spoken vocabulary, starting from the imitation of a single word through to the spontaneous, purposeful use of words to name people, objects and pictures. This sequence develops through word combinations, sentences and sequences of conversation, including the use of descriptive vocabulary (adjectives, adverbs, prepositional terms and terms denoting expressions and emotions).
- The development of listening skills, for example following simple and eventually multi-step instructions, with or without physical gesture or cues.
- Early use of language and communication to engage in pleasurable activities such as scanning books for fun and for information, extracting information and following simple storylines.
- The development of short-term memory skills such as the ability to remember and repeat words and sentences.

The sequence of personal/social development

This domain emphasises the need to involve parents in the formal assessment process, as they possess a depth of knowledge and understanding about the social, emotional and self-help skills of their children which cannot be adequately or conveniently assessed in a formal assessment session. Both the Griffiths III and the Bayley-4 make clear reference to when "parental report" can be used to score particular items. A more recent development in these "gold standard" assessment tools is the inclusion of tasks associated with the development of personal identity and the development of "theory of mind":

- Recognition of caregiver and the nature and quality of social response.
- Recognition of "self", for example in mirrors.
- Early social engagement skills such as social smiling and making anticipatory movements prior to being lifted.
- Early displays of affection.
- Social greeting and farewell skills such as waving goodbye.
- Self-introduction skills and demographic information such as giving of name, age, address and telephone number.
- Recognition and naming of body parts, both on the child him/herself and external agents such as dolls.
- The development of emotional regulation skills such as self-calming.
- Awareness of others, including interest in other children, and the development of "theory of mind skills" such as "false beliefs", and other perspective-taking activities such as showing concern for the well-being of others, to recognise and express emotions appropriately, and engage in social play involving cooperation and compromise.
- The development of independence in toileting awareness and successful completion skills, dressing and undressing, eating and utensil skills.

The sequence of early learning and reasoning skills

In this domain, there is overlap between Griffiths III and Bayley-4. Subscales associated with early learning skills were not originally included in developmental tests but were added to the upper age levels through successive revisions as the popularity of these tests expanded.

The 1970 edition of the Griffiths Mental Development Scales introduced a "Practical Reasoning" subscale, which included many tasks found in standardised assessments of cognitive abilities. It is a matter of ongoing professional discussion as to whether a child who is capable of successfully negotiating these domains is better assessed on the Griffiths III or Bayley-4, or a formal psychometric assessment of intelligence. These skills generally relate to the final stages of preschool education and are in many respects "school readiness" tasks. They include:

- Puzzle-solving and practical applications of fine motor coordination and planning skills as a means to demonstrate early reasoning capabilities.
- Pattern recognition and sequence completion skills.
- Number, numeration and early mathematical skills and concepts, commencing from counting, and including number memory and manipulation skills.
- The purposeful use of drawing and writing skills, such as word and numbers, human figure and other symbolic drawings.

- Enhanced memory and retention tasks, including delayed response items.
- "Clerical accuracy" tasks such as matching, finding and sorting.
- Contextual understanding tasks such as similarities and differences activities.
- Associative learning and matching tasks.
- Enhanced imitation and creation skills.

The activities in this sequence are generally a combination of verbally and non-verbally presented information. They involve sub-skills from other developmental sequence domains such as fine motor coordination and planning skills, listening skills, verbal expression and explanation skills, instruction-following skills, matching and memory skills.

Both the Griffiths III and the Bayley-4 require training and accreditation. Training can be undertaken at formal courses over a number of days, with an emphasis being on the theoretical assumptions underpinning the tests, explanation and demonstration of test items and procedures, and "hands-on" supervised practice with young children ranging from babyhood through the "toddler" age, to early preschool and beyond. Increasingly, there is provision for video training modules. Both tests can be used by trained and accredited psychologists and paediatricians, and some other allied health professionals.

It is generally recommended that upon "graduation", course participants should undertake an initial period of supervised practice through paired or supervised assessments whilst they master the complexities of assessing young children. Many psychologists undertaking Griffiths or Bayley training find it daunting at first, particularly when not accustomed to establishing and maintaining rapport with young children. Children below 5 years of age can be unpredictable in their response to the formal assessment context, and when the complexities of manipulating toys, paper, scissors, stop-watches, pictures and other materials are added, it can be a challenging process to master. Add in that assessments of young children are usually conducted with at least one parent present, and it can be even more character-building, particularly for psychologists who have only assessed children of school-age.

There are also organisational and administrative differences when assessing young children. Older children can generally be expected to "work through" assessments of intelligence in a predetermined order as prescribed by the test. This is not the case with babies, toddlers and young pre-schoolers. Considerable flexibility and adaptability is required of assessing psychologists to adapt to the whims of young children, to change preplanned assessment routines "on the run", to "follow the child's lead" in task selection, and sometimes to abandon formal "table-top" assessment procedures altogether and instead allow the child to sit on the floor, play with equipment, and be assessed through observation.

The presence and participation of parents in these circumstances can be most valuable at these times. They may be able to "find a way" to help engage or encourage their child, or to judge if particular tasks are simply beyond child's capability.

Young children have less patience when tasks are too demanding for them but can lack the communication skills to say so. Instead, they may "communicate" their displeasure through behavioural responses such as refusal or reluctance, physical agitation, distress or attention-seeking, and parents may be best able to "read" such behaviours for what they are. But research studies are in fact equivocal about parental expectations and estimations of their children's abilities on assessment tasks, and such parental involvement is best kept to a minimum.

Learning to master these assessment and "child maintenance" skills is a part of the "art" of developmental assessments. Every child and every assessment is different, and is another "learning experience" for the practitioner. It is the challenge of the psychologist or medical practitioner to negotiate each assessment situation on its merits, with as few preconceived notions as to its course and outcomes as possible.

Developmental assessments can therefore take differing amounts of time to complete. Sometimes young children will respond best if they are able to take short breaks, for toileting or a quick snack. A psychologist can take advantage of these pauses, to discover for example whether a child can subsequently return to task.

Bibliography

Bayley, N., and Aylward, G. P. (2020), Bayley-4: Bayley Scales of Infant and Toddler Development (4th Edition), Pearson Clinical.

Connell, P. (1984), "Language and the Preschool Child", Queensland Preschool Curriculum Project, Division of Preschool Education, Department of Education Queensland.

Dewey, J., and Miscellaneous quote in Fisher, D.C., (1953), Vermont Tradition: The Biography of an Outlook on Life, Little Brown.

O'Brien, C. C. (1982), Movement and the Preschool Child, Queensland Department of Education.

O'Brien, C., and Ziviani, J. (1984), "Fine Motor Development and the Preschool Child", Queensland Preschool Curriculum Project, Division of Preschool Education, Department of Education Queensland.

UNICEF (2019), "A World Ready to Learn: Prioritizing Quality Early Childhood Education", www.unicef.org.

10 The Griffiths scales of mental development

In the field of psychometric developmental tests for the comprehensive assessment of young children, two tests stand out as the current "gold standard" for developmental assessment: The Griffiths III and the Bayley-4 Scales. One is English and the other is American, and neither are new, although both have been significantly revised over the decades to accommodate changes in expectations of development progress in children, and the manner in which children's play and learning have evolved over time.

Doctor Ruth Griffiths was born in London in 1895, lived and studied in Australia, graduating with a degree in psychology from the University of Queensland in 1925. She held a Queensland Government training fellowship between 1927 and 1930, before obtaining further degrees at Somerville College Oxford and University College London. She subsequently held a research post with the Australian Council for Education Research Ltd between 1931 and 1933, and in 1935, published her first book, "Imagination in Early Childhood".

During the 1930s, Doctor Griffiths worked as a Psychologist at St George's Hospital, London, the Burdun Mental Research Trust in Bristol, and the Somerset County Education Committee, and as Director of the Child Development Research Centre in London. In 1957, Doctor Griffiths and Doctor Brian Burne co-founded the Association for Research in Infant and Child Development (ARICD), which is the custodian of the Griffiths Scales. In honour of her contributions to the field of child development, Doctor Griffiths was awarded an OBE. She died in 1973 at age 78 years.

Whilst working at the Maudsley Hospital in London after World War II, Griffiths designed an assessment instrument to evaluate the treatment outcomes of children with phenylketonuria (PKU), based on her "Avenues of Learning" theory (Figure 10.1). Her original test, "The Abilities of Babies", was so highly regarded that in 1970, it was extended in age range to 8 years and renamed "The Abilities of Young Children". The five "Avenues of Learning" corresponded to five subscales:

- Locomotor.
- Personal-social.
- Hearing and speech.
- Eye and hand co-ordination.
- Performance.

Griffiths' theory dictated that the "Avenues of Learning" were of equal value in child development and reflected the "environment" within which children were raised. This equivalence was expressed in the number of individual test items, and the rapid

126 *Diagnosing Young Children with Neurodevelopmental Disorders*

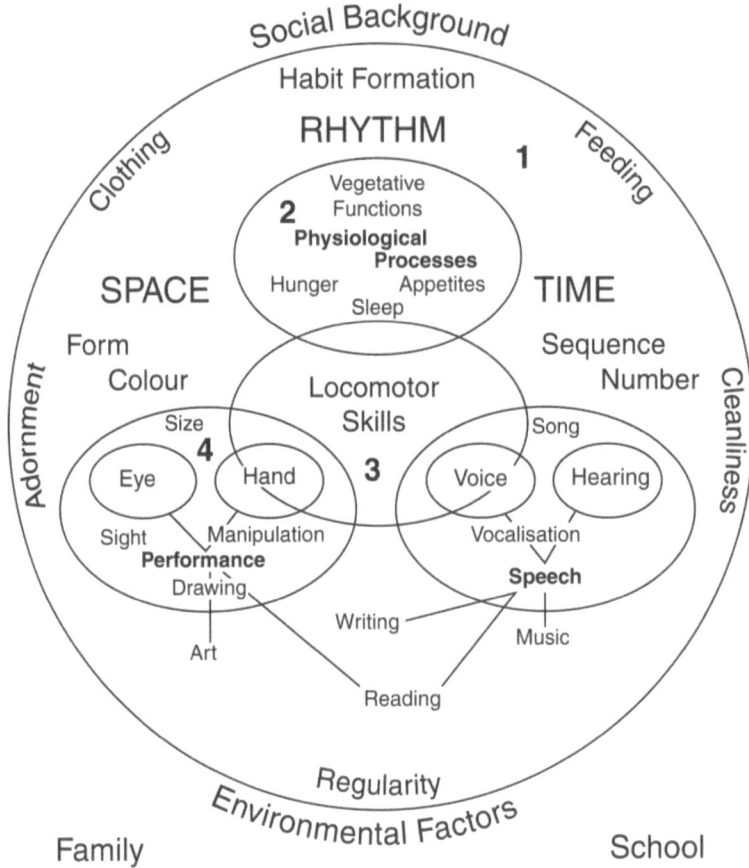

Figure 10.1 Griffiths' original "Avenues of Learning"

rate of developmental progress in the first 12 months was reflected by there being more test items per than in the second year. Results were calculated in two forms: Developmental age equivalents ("Mental Age") in each of the five subscales as well as an overall "Global Developmental Age", generally reported in months, and being the mean of the five subscales. A "General Quotient" was derived from a simple mathematical formula:

$$\frac{MA}{CA} \times 100 = GQ$$

This simplistic formula proved to be popular for ease of diagnosis; however, Griffiths was well aware of the flaws associated with the general quotient concept, particularly for very young children, stemming from:

- Individual differences between children of the same age.
- The maturity of children at birth, particularly in the context of prematurity.
- Difficult or traumatic births.
- Postnatal illnesses.

Intensive specialist training, initially conducted by Griffiths herself and a small circle of colleagues, was required for both psychologists and paediatricians to use the Griffiths. She also produced a training film for this purpose, sponsored by the British baby food manufacturer Cow and Gate.

The 1970 "Extended" version of the scales ("The Abilities of Young Children") covered the age range birth to 8 years, with additional test items for children 2–8 years of age. A "Practical Reasoning" subscale was introduced with formal pre-academic tasks such as counting and computation, conceptualisation of thought and ideas, and generalisation of skills into to problem-solving strategies.

In 1996, the original "Baby Scales" were revised by Doctor Michael Huntley, then Chief Psychologist at the Wolfson Centre, Institute of Child Health, London, and the "Extended" Scales were updated by Professor Dolores Luiz (University of Port Elizabeth, South Africa). It was released as the "Griffiths Mental Development Scales-Extended Revised" in 2006.

"Griffiths III" was released in 2016, marking a significant departure from previous versions of the test. There was new content, materials and statistical qualities. It was developed in both the United Kingdom and South Africa and included changes to Griffiths' original "Avenues of Learning" model. It is now "three-dimensional" and included reference to "socio-environmental" factors such as cultural background, religion, geographic location, socio-economic status, technology, political and educational influences (Figure 10.2).

The Griffiths III comprise five subscales:

- Foundations of learning.
- Language and communication.
- Eye and hand co-ordination.
- Personal-social-emotional.
- Gross motor.

The "Foundations of Learning" scale is derivative of the previously used "Practical Reasoning" scale. The Griffiths III has more "traditional" statistical properties than its predecessors. Although developmental age equivalents remain available for both subscales and overall "General Development", there are also developmental quotients for both, with means of 100 and a standard deviation of 15. Scaled scores from 0 to 20 are also provided, with a mean of 10 and standard deviation of 3.

An important addition to the test is a series of "Theory of Mind" and "False Belief" tasks, enhancing the test's potential in the assessment of children with suspected autism spectrum disorder. Materials are bright, colourful, sturdy, washable and "child-friendly". Additionally, new resources relating to the Griffiths III, for example technical reports, standardisation statements, and revised normative data, are now available.

Training on the Griffiths III continues to require mandatory course attendance and certification, including evidence-based practice prior to certification. The Griffiths III is published and distributed by Hogrefe, under the auspices of the Association for Infant and Child Development (ARICD), which offers annual on-line "scientific meetings" covering issues pertinent to child development trends.

Statistical information

The Griffiths III Manual Part 1: Overview, Development and Psychometric Properties, provides intercorrelation data between the various subscales at different age levels, ranging from .29 to .94, and states that there is "moderate to moderately high"

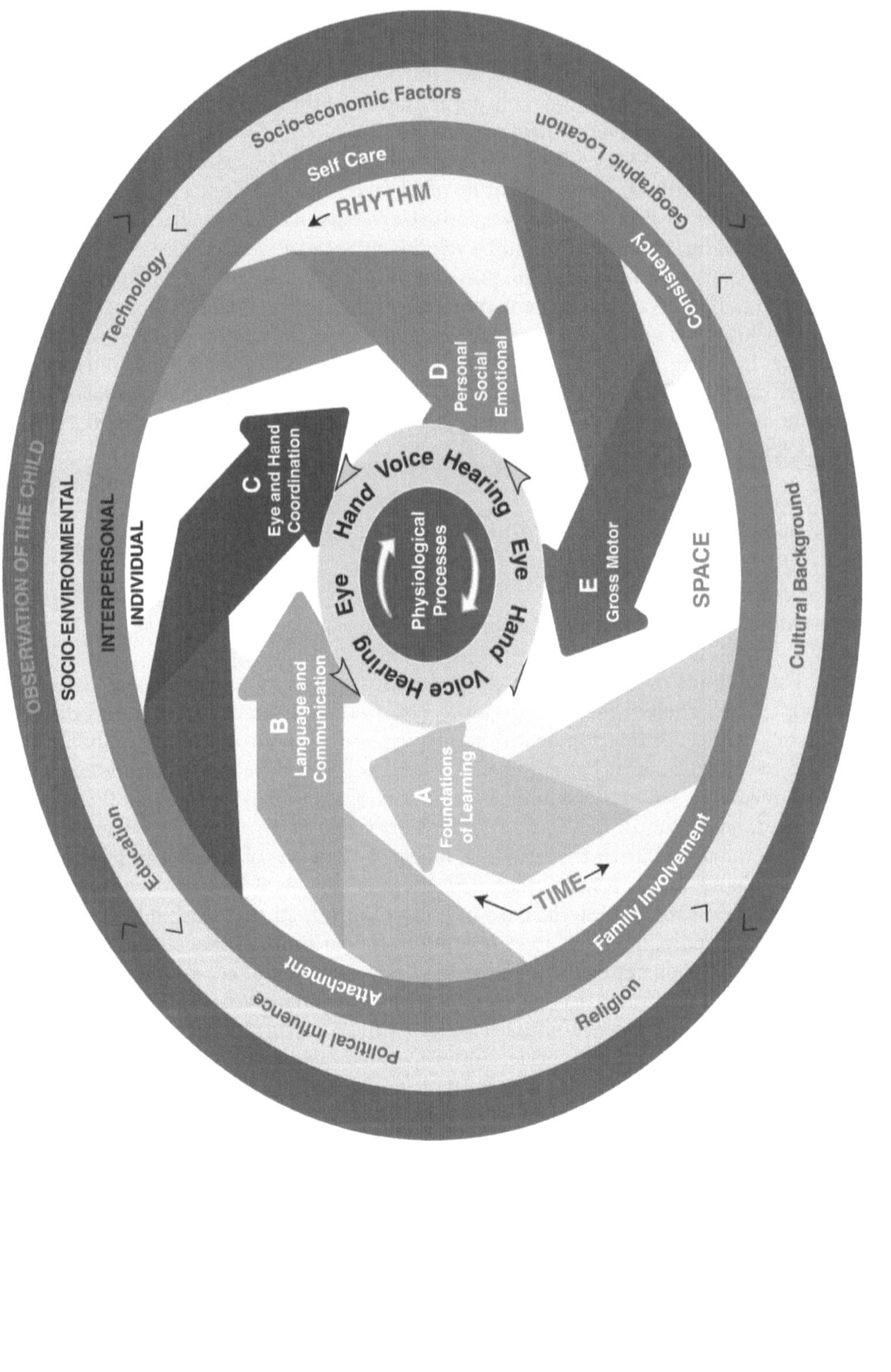

128 *Diagnosing Young Children with Neurodevelopmental Disorders*

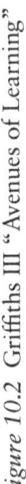

Figure 10.2 Griffiths III "Avenues of Learning"

intercorrelations, and this supports the generation of a total developmental score. Also reported are reliability coefficients ranging from .80 to .84, which is described as "acceptable for a standardised test".

Bibliography

Association for Research in Infant and Child Development (ARICD) (2020), Biography of Doctor Ruth Griffiths, www.aricd.ac.uk.

Griffiths, R. (1954), The Abilities of Babies, University of London Press.

Griffiths, R. (1970), The Abilities of Young Children: A Comprehensive System of Mental Measurement for the First Eight Years of Life, ARICD and University of London Press.

Huntley, M. (1996), Griffiths Mental Development Scales from Birth to 2 Years, ARICD.

Luiz, D. (2006), "The Griffiths Scales of Mental Development: A Factorial Validation Study", South African Journal of Psychology, 36(1), pp 192–214.

Luiz, D., et al. (2006), Griffiths Mental Development Scales-Extended Revised (GMDS-ER), ARICD.

Stroud, L., and Green, E. (2022), Griffiths III: A Case Study Book for Practitioners, Hogrefe Ltd.

Stroud, L., Foxcroft, C., Green, E., Bloomfield, S., Cronje, J., Hurter, K., Lane, H., Marais, R., Marx, C., McAlinden, P., O'Connell, R., Paradice, R., and Venter, D. (2016), Griffiths III: Griffiths Scales of Child Development (3rd Edition), Technical Manual, Hogrefe Ltd.

11 Bayley scales of infant and child development

Nancy Bayley (born 1899) was an American Psychologist best known for her work on the Berkeley Growth Study and the subsequent Bayley Scales of Infant Development. Bayley was the fourth of five children of a pioneer family. Until the age of 8, Bayley was described as a "sickly" child who could not attend school, but then recovered and advanced rapidly. In 1922, she completed her Bachelor of Science in Psychology, followed by a Master of Science (Psychology) in 1924. At the University of Washington, she worked as a laboratory assistant in the Gatzert Foundation for Child Welfare. Bayley earned her Doctoral Degree at the University of Iowa in 1926. She started her career in 1926 as an instructor at the University of Wyoming, publishing her first of almost 200 papers.

In 1928, she moved to the University of California, Berkeley, to work in the Institute of Child Welfare on the Berkeley Growth Study. Bayley's work there included the assessment of physical, motor, mental and physiological development. Assessments were repeated at regular intervals and included measurements of reflexes and bodily dimensions, blood pressure and breathing rates. Background information was collated about maternal and prenatal history. Follow-up assessments were conducted through home visits, paediatric centres, and field group outings. Mental measurements included the California First-Year Mental Scale, the California Pre-school Mental Scale, tests of vocabulary, and Stanford-Binet intelligence tests. Motor assessments included speed, dexterity, and reflexes.

Participants completed the California Infant Scale of Motor Development and examinations of footprint records. Physiological tests assessed exercise and exertion abilities, galvanic skin reflex, and metabolism. There were also x-ray assessments, and tests of emotion and personality.

Bayley's research led her to believe that intelligence was not "set" at birth but evolved over the span of child development. It was impacted by environmental factors and social influences such as poverty, parenting attitudes and behaviours, rather than merely psychological influences. Bayley discovered no gender differences in terms of physical and psychological development. Examinations of x-rays and physiological growth earned Bayley the reputation as the first scientist to recognise the predictability of adult height based on infant size.

Bayley's research led in 1933 to the publishing of the California First-Year Mental Scale and the California Infant Scale of Motor Development in 1936, both precursors to her later Bayley Scales of Infant Development. In 1954, Bayley moved to the National Institute of Mental Health in Bethesda, Maryland, where she worked in the Laboratory of Psychology. In 1964, she returned to Berkeley and published the original Bayley Scales of Infant Development.

Bayley retired in 1968, then lived in Carmel, California, until she died at age 95. For her efforts in the field of Psychology, Bayley received honorary awards, including becoming the first woman to receive the Distinguished Scientific Contribution award from the American Psychological Association (APA), of which she was a Fellow. Bayley was also a member of the American Association for the Advancement of Science.

The original Bayley Scales of Infant and Toddler Development were published by Nancy Bayley in 1969 and have been revised through the Bayley Scales of Infant Development II, and more recently the Bayley-3 and Bayley-4. The original Bayley Scales were the amalgam of three previous scales:

- The California First-Year Mental Scale.
- The California Preschool Mental Scale.
- The California Infant Scale of Motor Development.

Prior to its release, Bayley undertook research to determine which important variables should be included in a cumulative developmental test for infants, including the development of mental processes in the second year of life, followed by a study of the reliability of her previous exploration scale of mental and motor development during the first year of life. These findings implicated early diagnosis of neural malfunctioning. Bayley also conducted a test on infant vocalisations and their relationships to mature intelligence, correlating them with language skills of the same individual over childhood and adolescence, into early adulthood. The results indicated that vocalisations significantly correlated with girls' later intelligence, increasingly so with age, and more highly with verbal then performance scores.

Prior to the publishing of the second edition published in 1993, it was found that the Bayley Scales may have led to underestimations of cognitive abilities in infants with Down syndrome, leading to test revisions and a scale which provided a meaningful and stable measure of cognitive functioning in infants with Down syndrome.

The most significant revision for the Bayley-3 released in 2003 was the development of five distinct scales rather than three scales in the second edition, rendering the test more consistent with areas of appropriate developmental assessment for children from birth to age 3. Thus, the Bayley-3 revision included

- Cognitive Scale.
- Language Scale.
- Motor Scale.
- Social-Emotional Scale.
- Adaptive Behaviour Scale.

At face value, these five scales mirror the format of the Griffiths III, but there are important differences. For example, two distinct subtests are included: The Language Scale: The Receptive subtest and the Expressive subtest. The Motor Scale similarly divides into fine motor and gross motor subtests.

The Cognitive Scale includes relational and representative play items, information processing, number concepts and counting, sensorimotor skills, exploration and manipulation, object relatedness, concept formation, and memory. The previously used Bayley-3 recognised that "vital aspects of emotional functioning are best observed in naturalistic settings rather than in clinical or controlled experimental settings", and therefore, a Social-Emotional questionnaire was included for parents or primary caregivers to complete.

Similarly, the Bayley-4 Adaptive Behaviour Scale includes a simplified version of the Vineland-3 Adaptive Behavior Scales, again to be completed by parents and caregivers.

The Bayley-4 covers the age range birth to 42 months and conforms to typical psychometric assessment properties, with a mean standard score of 100 and a standard deviation of 15. These statistics are calculated for overall composite scores and individual scale scores, and can be reported at either the 90% or 95% level of confidence. The Technical Manual advises that although age equivalent scores can be calculated, these can be misinterpreted and are best not used literally. It is also noted that the Bayley-4 should not be the sole determinant of diagnostic certainty in any one specific area of functioning, rather it should contribute to the overall process of assessment and diagnostic formulations. Changes in format include

- Provision of partial item scoring for "emerging" skills.
- Simplified administration and reduced administration time.
- Local normative data for Australia and New Zealand census material.
- Further inclusion of parents in the scoring and evaluation process.
- Changes to specific items to reduce redundancy.
- Inclusion of specific neurodevelopmental items.
- Specific cultural adaptations.
- Normative data from disability groups, including autism spectrum disorder, Down syndrome, global developmental delay, fetal alcohol spectrum disorder, cerebral palsy, language disorders and significant prematurity.

The Bayley-4 requires specific training and appropriate qualifications and experience in early childhood assessments, including on-line as well as face-face training options. Testing duration, as with the Griffiths III, varies considerably depending upon the age and nature of the children being assessed, with estimates ranging from 50 to 90 minutes. The Bayley-4 is distributed by Pearsons.

Statistical information

Statistical information provided by Pearson Clinical indicates internal consistency scores between .85 to .99, test-retest reliability ranging from .72 to .87, and inter-rater consistency scores of .67 to .81.

Bibliography

Balasundaram, P., and Avulakunta, I. D. (2024), "Bayley Scales of Infant and Toddler Development", In StatPearls. StatPearls Publishing.

Bayley, N. (2006), Bayley-3: Bayley Scales of Infant and Toddler Development (3rd Edition), Pearson Clinical.

Bayley, N., and Aylward, G. P. (2020), Bayley-4: Bayley Scales of Infant and Toddler Development (4th Edition), Pearson Clinical.

Kinsella-Ritter, A., Gibson, F. L., and Wyver, S. (2009), "The Clinical Use of the Bayley Scales of Infant and Toddler Development, Third Edition (Bayley-3) in Australia", The Australian Educational and Developmental Psychologist, 26(2), pp 154–164.

O'Connel, A. (1990), Women in Psychology: A Bio-bibliographic Sourcebook, Greenwood Publishing Group.

12 Mullen scales of early learning
(Eileen M. Mullen)

Born in 1926, Eileen Mullen attended Rhode Island College in the American state of Rhode Island, graduating with a degree in education in 1948. She was also a semi-professional singer. She originally taught in Rhode Island before receiving her doctorate in Developmental and School Psychology from Boston University in 1974. She was the founder and president of TOTAL Child, Inc. For twenty years, she was the Vice President and Director of Clinical Services at Meeting Street School in Providence, Rhode Island. She also worked in private practice and as a consulting school psychologist at a number of schools in Rhode Island and was a charter member of the American Psychological Society. She died in 2018 at the age of 81. The Mullen Scales of Early Learning were originally published in 1995, and the test is described as "a developmentally integrated system that assesses language, motor, and perceptual abilities", for children aged up to 68 months. It is comprised of five scales, namely:

- Gross motor.
- Visual reception.
- Fine motor.
- Expressive language.
- Receptive language.

It is described as a measure of cognitive function rather than a developmental assessment but incorporates elements of both in each scale. A composite score referred to as an estimate of overall intelligence is generated, along with T scores and age-equivalent scores. Separate and distinct scales of learning are preferred rather than a single measure of intelligence, to recognise that young children tend to develop unevenly across the various domains assessed. As with many American tests of development and intelligence, strengths and weaknesses profiles are reported as a guide to specific interventions. The Mullen Scales are often used in research projects and are often used in relation to children with autism spectrum disorder. The Mullen Scales of Learning are marketed through Pearson Assessments.

Statistical information

Internal consistency scores between .74 and .90 are reported for the Mullen Scales, and test-retest reliability scores of .83–.99.

Bibliography

Akshoomoff, N. (2006), "Use of the Mullen Scale of Early Learning for the Assessment of Young Children with Autism Spectrum Disorders", Child Neuropsychol, 12, pp 269–277.

Staples, K. L., and Zimmer, C. (2012), "Assessment of Motor Behavior among Children and Adolescents with Autism Spectrum Disorder", International Review of Research in Developmental Disabilities, 42, pp 179–214.

Stein, M. T., and Lukasik, M. K. (2009), Frequently Used Standardized Tests for Developmental Assessment (4th Edition), Developmental-Behavioral Pediatrics.

13 Other notable assessments for young children
The McCarthy scales and the Miller scales

The 19th-century American poet John Greenleaf Whittier wrote many quotable quotes, including the following from his poem "Don't Quit":

For all sad words of tongue and pen,
the saddest of all is "it might have been".

McCarthy scales of children's abilities (1972)

Doctor Dorothea McCarthy was a child psychologist who taught in Fordham University's Graduate Department of Psychology for 40 years. She completed her scales at age 64 after two decades of research but did not survive to see them published. She died aged 68 years in 1973. She originally graduated from the University of Minnesota. In 1942, she was the Director of a child-guidance clinic at Fordham's Psychology Department for training Clinical Psychologists. The McCarthy Scales were highly regarded and frequently used during the 1970s and 1980s, but have since faded into obscurity.

The McCarthy Scales measured "cognitive ability" rather than "intelligence". The scoring protocol referred to "strengths" and "weaknesses" compared through T-scores with a mean of 50 and standard deviation of 10 so they could not be interpreted as IQ scores. The McCarthy Scales were for children from ages 2 to 8. They were regarded as psychometrically and structurally sound, but possibly lacking in validity data. The scales produced a variety of composite scores, allowing analysis of both individual sections as well as overall results. Fifteen of the 18 subtests combined to produce a general cognitive index (GCI), with a standard score mean of 100 and standard deviation of 16. The scales were separated into two main sub-parts. In the GCI were:

Verbal scale: Including pictorial memory, word knowledge, verbal memory, verbal fluency and opposite analogies.
Perceptual-performance: Including block building, puzzle solving, tapping sequence, right-left orientation, drawing tasks and conceptual grouping.
Quantitative: Including number questions, numerical memory, counting and sorting.

The additional scales included:

Memory: Including pictorial memory, tapping sequence, verbal and numerical memory.
Motor: Including leg and arm coordination, imitative action and drawing tasks.

Miller assessment for preschoolers (1988)

Lucy Miller was an occupational therapist, research scientist, Professor of Paediatrics at Rocky Mountain University and Associate Clinical Professor in the Departments of Rehabilitation Medicine and Paediatrics at the University of Colorado. She published "Sensational Kids: Hope and Help for Children with Sensory Processing Disorder". Doctor Miller obtained her Bachelor of Science degree in Psychology from Lewis and Clark College in Portland, Oregon, a Master of Science degree (Occupational Therapy) from Boston University and a Doctorate in Special Education from the University of Denver. Her awards are numerous and include

- The Award of Merit from the American Occupational Therapy Association, the highest award offered in her profession.
- The Martin Luther King Jr. Humanitarian Award from the State of Colorado for her lifetime commitment to children with special needs.

Her work has been featured on American television, as well as in the New York Times, TIME Magazine and other media outlets. She was founder and Executive Director of the Sensory Processing Disorder Foundation and of STAR (Sensory Therapies And Research Center), in Denver, Colorado. Doctor Miller announced her retirement in October 2019.

The Miller Assessment for Preschoolers was published in 1988 and provides an overview of a child's developmental status relative to his/her peers. It provides a separate form for each of six age levels, each evaluating five performance areas:

Foundations Index: Assesses basic motor movements sensory awareness.
Coordination Index: Assesses complex gross, fine and oral motor abilities.
Verbal Index: Focuses on memory, sequencing, comprehension, association and expression.
Nonverbal Index: Examines memory, sequencing, visualisation and the performance of nonverbal mental manipulations.
Complex Tasks Index: Measures sensorimotor abilities in conjunction with cognitive abilities that require interpretation of visuospatial information.

The Miller Assessment for Preschoolers is still available. It has generally been used by occupational therapists and is less well known outside of that profession, despite its child-friendly format and equipment. It is perhaps best understood for providing considerable and rich qualitative information about the manner in which young children learn and develop through play.

Bibliography

Hunt, T. V. (1978), "Review of McCarthy Scales of Children's Abilities", In Buros, O. K. (Ed.), The Eighth Mental Measurements Yearbook (Vol. 1), Gryphon Press.
McCarthy, D. (1972), McCarthy Scales of Children's Abilities, Psychological Corporation/Pearson.
Miller, L. J. (1988), Miller Assessment for Preschoolers, Western Psychological Services.
Miller, L. J. (2014), Sensational Kids: Hope and Help for Children with Sensory Processing Disorder, Penguin Random House.
O'Connel, A. (1990), Women in Psychology: A Bio-bibliographic Sourcebook, Greenwood Publishing Group.

Schnell, R. R., and Workman-Daniels, K. (1992), "Intellectual Assessment of Preschoolers", In Nuttall, E. V., Romero, J., and Kalesnik, J. (Eds.), Assessing and Screening Preschoolers- Psychological and Educational Dimensions, McCarthy Scales of Children's Abilities.
Biography of Doctor Lucy Miller (2019), STAR Institute, www.sensoryhealth.com.
Whittier, J. G., and Whittier, E. (2018), The Complete Poetical Works of John Greenleaf Whittier, Scholar Select.

14 Checklist and questionnaire-based assessments

Many psychologists, medical practitioners, therapists and teachers, and increasingly parents, are familiar with "brief" or abbreviated versions of tests, developmental screening checklists and questionnaires, either as an adjunct to direct "hands-on" assessments or as convenient substitutes for such methods. Questionnaires and checklists have a number of attractive qualities which would encourage their use:

- They are far less expensive than formal "hands-on" psychometric tests such as Griffiths III and Bayley-4.
- They are more convenient and time-effective in use. It takes a matter of minutes to complete a questionnaire or checklist as opposed to the 90 minutes of administration time, followed by parental follow-up and report writing.
- They are less restrictive in user qualifications and licencing requirements. A broader range of professionals can request that questionnaires and checklists be completed.

But there are questions to be asked about the use of such "pen and paper" assessment techniques:

- Do they provide accurate and useful information?
- Do they encompass a sufficiently broad array of developmental skills to understand the profile of a young child without engaging with him/her directly?
- Are they statistically sound?
- Are they subject to any potential "response bias" which may compromise or invalidate results?
- Do they accurately reflect a parent's or teacher/caregiver's perception of a young child? Do they allow for emerging skills or "light and shade" in quality of performance?
- Are they best utilised for obtaining background information prior to formal assessment?
- Are they considered appropriate as a basis for diagnostic confirmation?
- Can questionnaires be administered as "structured interviews"?

Checklists and screening questionnaires are used by many differing professions. Paediatricians' use of developmental questionnaires and screening tests has been found to have increased significantly in recent years. There are many questionnaires and checklists available for purchase and use. Some are focused upon developmental milestone screening and evaluation, others on adaptive behaviour skills.

There are "disability-specific" questionnaires for accumulating evidence of "symptoms" for conditions such as autism spectrum disorder, language delay and disorder.

DOI: 10.4324/9781003565338-18

Others focus upon the strengths and weaknesses associated with disabling conditions for therapeutic prioritisation and case management, or to suggest the "likelihood" of a specific disability. Some can be administered through clinical interview, whilst others are simply for completion. All of these questionnaires and checklists can demonstrate sound psychometric properties, so choice-making is complex. A number of these tools are described below.

Developmental screening tests

The Ages and Stages Questionnaires, 3rd edition (ASQ-3) (Squires and Bricker)

The Ages & Stages Questionnaires 3rd Edition is designed to "pinpoint developmental progress in young children". It is intended for use by early educators and healthcare professionals but with a "parent-centric" approach. The ASQ-3 is not merely questionnaire-based. It also requires direct play and engagement with young children and includes specific toys and equipment. It is the most widely used developmental screening tool. It features:

- Age range from birth to 6 years.
- Ease and portability of administration, including in-person or telephone explanation and use. Administration is described as taking as little as 3 minutes for professionals and 10–15 minutes for parents.
- Consideration as to whether children are "at risk" of developmental delay.
- Pinpointing of strengths and weaknesses in developmental profiles.
- The ability to inform and teach parents about child development and their own child's skills.

The ASQ-3 assesses five areas of development:

- Communication.
- Gross motor.
- Fine motor.
- Problem solving.
- Personal social.

It includes instructional material for parents, such as printed materials, on-line support and a CD-ROM. Stimulus and learning activities are also included, as well as specific activities designed to foster the development of early language and literacy skills. Follow-up monitoring of children considered to be in the "monitoring zone" is also included. A "Materials Kit" includes approximately 20 toys, books and other items designed to encourage a child's participation in learning activities.

Empirical research comparing the ASQ-3 with the "Parents' Evaluation of Developmental Status" (PADS) indicated that the ASQ-3 appeared to have higher sensitivity and specificity across a range of age groups. The ASQ-3 lends itself to creative usage such as on-line Zoom or Skype training and administration, particularly for families in regional and remote areas with limited access to formal assessment services. Reference will be made later in this publication to such applications during the Covid-19 pandemic and subsequent "lockdown" in 2020.

Developmental Profile 4 (DP-4) (Alpern)

The 4th edition of the Developmental Profile (DP-4) retains core elements of its predecessor, the Developmental Profile 3. New features have also been added. The DP-4 includes the following functional aspects:

- Identification of a child's strengths and weaknesses.
- Comparison of a child's development in key areas.
- Planning of interventions, including "item-by-item" teaching activities.
- Determining eligibility for special education programmes, although this function is primarily related to the United States.
- Preparation of goals for individual education plans.
- Determining specific areas for further assessment.
- Monitoring progress over time.

The DP-4 has an extended age range, from birth to 21 years 11 months. The 190 individual items are described as having been updated to "reflect changes in society, technology, and culture". Normative data for children with hearing impairments have been added. A new growth score allows monitoring of progress over time. The DP-4 can be administered in 20–40 minutes. Robust psychometric qualities are reported, and on-line scoring and administration are available. Five areas of functioning are assessed:

Physical: Including large-and small-muscle coordination, strength, stamina, flexibility and sequential motor skills.
Adaptive behaviour: The ability to cope independently with the environment, through eating, dressing, working, using current technology and taking care of self and others.
Social–Emotional: Including interpersonal skills, social-emotional understanding, functionality in social situations and peer and adult relating skills.
Cognitive: Including intellectual abilities and skills necessary for academic achievement.
Communication: Including expressive and receptive communication skills, written, spoken and gestural language.

Item Questions follow a simple "yes" or "no" response format based on a child's mastery of a skill. The three forms of the profile (Parent/Caregiver Interview, Parent/Caregiver Checklist and Teacher Checklist) provide both standard scores and growth scores. The Clinician Rating provides growth scores for monitoring progress.

Developmental Assessment of Young Children-2 (DAYC-2) (Voress, Maddox and Hammill)

This is the second edition of this test, which identifies developmental delays and deficits in children from birth through age 5. The test is composed of five subtests, each focusing on a separate domain: Adaptive Behaviour, Cognition, Communication, Physical Development, Social–Emotional Development. The test format allows the collection of information about children through observation, parent/caregiver interview and direct assessment. Any combination of the five subtests can be administered, thus tailoring it to the particular needs of a child. Administration of each individual domain takes approximately 10–20 minutes, and results are reported in standard scores, percentile ranks and age-equivalent scores. It is intended for use by psychologists experienced in psychometric assessment.

Adaptive behaviour questionnaires

The assessment of adaptive behaviour skills or "activities of daily living" is not new, but in recent decades has assumed increasing significance in assessments of neurodevelopmental disorders, intellectual disabilities and other category of functional impairment. Adaptive behaviour scores are now increasingly sought for any consideration of eligibility for:

- Funding and resources.
- "Proof of need" when there are inter and intra-assessment discrepancies.
- Transitional information, such as movement from one school programme to another.
- Efficacy of therapeutic and educational interventions.

As with other psychometric assessment modes, the measurement and categorisation of adaptive behaviours has a long history, but one individual stands out above all others as the well-spring for adaptive behaviour assessments. His name was Edgar Doll, author of the original Vineland Social Maturity Scales, and no appraisal of adaptive behaviour assessments is complete without reference to his extraordinary contributions.

Edgard Doll was born in Cleveland, Ohio, in 1889, and educated at Cornell University, New York University and Princeton University. Doll's career was dedicated to services for children with special needs. He was long associated with The Training School at Vineland (New Jersey), first as a clinical psychologist. Doll also worked for the State of New Jersey's Department of Institutions and Agencies, but returned to Vineland in 1925 as a Research Director, remaining there until 1949.

Doll published the original Vineland Social Maturity Scale in 1936. It was translated into dozens of languages. Doll left Vineland in 1949 to become Coordinator of Research for the Devereaux Schools in Devon, Pennsylvania, before becoming Consulting Psychologist to the Public Schools of Bellingham, Washington in 1953. His professional affiliations included the Clinical Division of the American Psychological Association, the American Orthopsychiatric Association and the American Association on Mental Deficiency.

In 1938, Doll married Sarah Geraldine Longwell, also renowned for her work in the field of special education. Longwell was educated at Denison University, Radcliffe College and Cornell University, gaining her PhD in Experimental Psychology in 1937. From 1930 to 1938, she worked at Vineland, first as a Research Fellow and later as a Clinical Psychologist. Upon the Doll's relocation to Washington, Longwell taught at Western Washington College and established her own career as a Psychologist in the public school system of Bellingham. Together, Longwell and Edgar Doll established an innovative system of special education, emphasising individual placement, practical training and lifetime planning.

Ms Longwell continued this work after her husband's death in 1968. She retired in 1972 but continued to publish and speak to parent organisations and educators interested in innovations in special Education until her death in 1983.

The original Vineland Social Maturity Scales (1936) were designed to measure "social competence", defined as a "functional composite of human traits that subserve social usefulness and are reflected in self-sufficiency and in service to others". The original scales spanned the ages from birth to 30 years of age and measured eight categories of behaviour:

- Self-help general.
- Self-help eating.
- Self-help dressing.
- Locomotion.

142 *Diagnosing Young Children with Neurodevelopmental Disorders*

- Occupation.
- Communication.
- Self-direction.
- Socialisation.

It was interview-based, conducted with a parent, sibling or other third party familiar with the person being assessed. Scores were assigned according to the behaviours reported to be customarily exhibited, deriving scores of social age or social quotient. Its first major revision in 1984 included a change of name to the Vineland Adaptive Behaviour Scales, and this title has been maintained in subsequent revisions (Vineland II in 2005 and the current Vineland III).

Vineland Adaptive Behavior Scales III (Vineland-III) (Sparrow, Cicchetti and Saulnier)

This latest iteration of the Vineland Scales follows closely from Vineland-II but with updated item content and normative data. The introduction of "basal and ceiling" rules has streamlined test administration, and the test can be administered and scored either with paper protocols or digital versions. Scores from adaptive domains and the overall adaptive behaviour composite are aligned to DSM-5 requirements for diagnosing intellectual disability. There are both "interview" and questionnaire-completion forms. The assessment covers the age range 3 years to adult for interview and parent/caregiver forms, and from 3 to 21 years for the teacher form. The interview form can be administered in approximately 20 minutes and approximately 10 minutes for parent/caregiver and teacher forms. The Vineland-III consists of the following domains and sub-domains (Table 14.1).

Subdomain scores are reported with a mean of 15 and a standard deviation of 3, whilst domain and composite scores have means of 100 and standard deviations of 15. Descriptive categories based on composite scores are also provided. Items are scored by parents, caregivers and teachers on the basis of their experience with and observations of a particular child in their care, on the likelihood that certain skills will be demonstrated reliably or only occasionally, or not at all.

Some psychologists prefer the interview version, as it allows more thorough exploration of a child's strengths and weaknesses, emerging skills and clarification of contextual

Table 14.1 Vineland-III assessment domains

Domain	Subdomains
COMMUNICATION	Receptive
	Expressive
	Written
DAILY LIVING SKILLS	Personal
	Domestic
	Community
Socialisation	Interpersonal relationships
	Play and leisure
	Coping skills
Motor skills (Optional)	Fine
	Gross
Maladaptive behaviour (Optional)	Internalising
	Externalising

information. This has proven to be useful for regional and remote assessments by telephone, Skype or Zoom when face-to-face assessment has not been possible, and assessments conducted in this manner most certainly align with DSM-5-TR requirements for diagnoses of global developmental delay. Although not mandatory, some service providers have organised and conducted systematic training programmes in the use of the Vineland III, particularly the interview form, so that specific interview and questioning techniques can be learned and practised when seeking detailed information about a child.

Statistical information

Pearsons Clinical provides the following statistical information regarding internal consistency scores, test-retest reliability scores and inter-rater reliability scores:

- Internal consistency scores range from .90 to .98, depending upon domain, age group and rater.
- Test-retest scores range from .73 to .92 depending upon age group and rater.
- Inter-rater reliability scores range from .70 to .81 depending upon domains.

Adaptive Behavior Assessment System, 3rd edition (ABAS-3) (Harrison and Oakland)

The ABAS-3 is similar in format to previous versions, and with Vineland-3, except without a dedicated interview form. The age range 0–89 years is covered in specific protocol questionnaires:

- Parent/Primary Caregiver Form (Ages 0–5).
- Teacher/Daycare Provider Form (Ages 2–5).
- Parent Form (Ages 5–21).
- Teacher Form (Ages 5–21).
- Adult Form (Ages 16–89).

The Adult Form allows for either self-report or third-party rating of skills, and in general, the ABAS-3 encourages "multiple ratings" from parents, family members, teachers, daycare staff, supervisors, counsellors or others who are familiar with the individual being evaluated. The ABAS-3 covers three broad adaptive domains:

- Conceptual.
- Social.
- Practical.

Eleven adaptive skill areas are assessed within this structure, each form assessing 9 or 10 skill areas based on age range, but these different skills are not internally differentiated as in the Vineland-3, for example, overall communication skills and not expressive or receptive language (Table 14.2).

The ABAS-3 is aligned with DSM-5-TR criteria for intellectual disability. Scaled scores and test-age equivalents are reported for the 11 skill areas. There are also standard scores, confidence intervals, and percentile ranks for the three adaptive domains and overall general adaptive composite. Scores can be categorised descriptively as "Extremely Low", "Low", "Below Average", "Average", "Above Average" and "High". The ABAS-3 is essentially a

Table 14.2 ABAS 3 assessment domains

Adaptive domain	Parent/primary caregiver 0–5 yrs	Teacher/daycare provider form 2–5 yrs	Parent form 5–21 yrs	Teacher form 5–21 yrs	Adult form 16–89 yrs
Conceptual	Communication Functional pre-academics	Communication Functional pre-academics	Communication Functional academics	Communication Functional academics	Communication Functional academics
Social	Self-direction Leisure Social	Self-direction Leisure Social	Self-direction Leisure Social	Self-direction Leisure Social	Self-direction Leisure Social
Practical	Community use Home living Health and safety Self-care	School living Health and safety Self-care	Community use Home living Health and safety Self-care	Community use Home living Health and safety Self-care	Community use Home living Health and safety Self-care Work
Age-specific	Motor	Motor	Work	Work	

questionnaire-completion test, and guidelines are provided for parents and caregivers to complete the questionnaires. Some services supply additional "in-house" guidelines for completion, and the ABAS-3 can be used as the basis for a structured interview.

Statistical information

Considerable reliability, validity and consistency statistics are provided in the ABAS-3 Manual:

- Reliability coefficients for the General Adaptive Composite (GAC) range from .96 to .99.
- Reliability coefficient scores varied depending upon age bracket, domain and questionnaire responder (Teacher, Parent or self-report), but ranged from .72 to .99.
- Similarly, Test-Retest correlations varied depending upon age and responder, but ranged from .70 to .89

Bracken School Readiness Assessment 4th edition (Bruce Bracken)

Assessing a young child's readiness to enter formal schooling or otherwise is a vexatious issue, with so many variables to consider – age, social and/or emotional or physical maturity, pre-academic skills and of course the requirements and expectations of specific school systems and philosophies. And these factors apply equally to children with no apparent developmental difficulties, delays or disorders. However, psychologists may be called upon to assist parents, and indeed schools, to make determinations of "readiness".

The Bracken School Readiness Assessment-4 includes six subtests to assess basic concepts such as colour recognition and naming, letters, numbers and basic counting, concepts of size and shapes, and self and social awareness skills. There is a concept development guide, which may assist in targeting areas of perceived delay or weakness. It is brief in administration and as with many modern assessment tools, computer scorable. The Bracken School Readiness Assessment is available through Pearson Clinical.

Assessments of attention deficit hyperactivity disorder (ADHD)

Conners 4th edition (Conners 4) (C. Keith Conners)

The Conners 4 provides for assessment of symptoms and impairments associated with attention deficit hyperactivity disorder and common comorbid problems and disorders. It is for children and youth aged 6–18 years. In its latest version, it provides:

- A "Severe Conduct and Self-Harm Critical Items and Sleep Problems Indicator".
- Evaluation of new content areas and common co-occurring problems such as emotional dysregulation, depressed mood and anxious thoughts.
- Synchronisation with the DSM-5-TR ADHD Total Symptoms index.
- An enhanced Parent Feedback Handout.
- Improved gender and cultural normative data.

The Conners 4 is 100% digital and offers digital scoring only. It is published by Multi-Health Systems and distributed worldwide by Pearson. Three forms are available: Parent report, teacher report and self-report.

BRIEF2 (Behavior Rating Inventory of Executive Function second edition) (Gerard A. Gioia, Peter k. Isquith, Steven C. Guy and Lauren Kenworthy)

The BRIEF2 screens for executive function impairment in ages 5–18 years. There are parent and teacher forms, and a self-report form for older students. It is designed for a broad range of children when there are concerns about self-regulation, for example in autism spectrum disorder, learning disabilities, attentional disorders, traumatic brain injuries, depression and range of other developmental, neurological, psychiatric and medical conditions. The BRIEF2 features:

- Three indexes-behavioural, emotional and cognitive.
- An "infrequency" scale for unusual responses.
- An "Interpretive Report", which includes all information on the score report as well as interpretive text for the BRIEF2 clinical scale, index and composite scores and validity indicators.
- An optional ADHD score profile, interpretive text, for the parent/teacher form.

The BRIEF2 is published by PAR and dates from 2015. A Spanish-speaking version available via PARiConnect, and also a Russian version which has been researched for validity. Results confirmed that the BRIEF2 Teacher Form was valid for 5- and 6-year-old children but not sufficiently valid for 7-year-olds.

"Special population" questionnaires and checklists

Certain disabilities can require specific information for diagnosis, derived through observation and reporting, for example autism spectrum disorder where the presence of tightly defined symptomatology needs to be confirmed. This has led to many "special population" questionnaire and checklist tests. Three are outlined here, and many others deserve mention. The level of specificity of some questionnaires reflects the unique behaviours and problems associated with certain disability types. For example, maladaptive behaviours can occur with significant intellectual disability or developmental delay, whether associated with genetic factors, or other neurodevelopmental causes.

Observing and monitoring symptomatic behaviours is an integral component of behavioural management planning and programmes, both for diagnostic confirmation and for assessment of program efficacy and symptom reduction. Many professionals engaged in behavioural support programs create their own measures of "intervention success", but formal "test-retest" psychometric evidence is of considerable value. One such measure is described below.

Developmental Behavior Checklist 2 (DBC 2) (Einfeld, Tonge, Gruber and Klein)

Standardised assessment tests, checklists and questionnaires are generally written and published through either American or British corporations. A notable exception is the Griffiths III which although originally British, now owes its success to South African and British expertise, and German-based publishers. Australian tests are virtually unheard of due to the complex "business" dynamics of test development, standardisation, publication, mass distribution and market penetration. One Australian assessment and monitoring tool, which has experienced international success, is the Developmental Behavior Checklist (Einfeld and Tonge).

Now in its second edition, and published and distributed through Western Psychological Services, the DBC-2 has its origins in the ground-breaking research of Professors Bruce Tonge, Stewart Einfeld and others, into the mental health status of people with intellectual and other disabilities. The DBC was originally produced and distributed "in-house" by Professor Stewart Einfeld (Faculty of Health Science & Brain and Mind Research Institute, University of Sydney) and Professor Bruce Tonge (Centre for Developmental Psychiatry and Psychology, Monash University) in 1992. It was a "suite of instruments for the assessment of behavioural and emotional problems of children, adolescents and adults with developmental and intellectual disabilities".

The DBC shared a similar structure to the Child Behaviour Checklist (Achenbach & Edelbrock, 1983). Parents, teachers or caregivers completed and repeated questionnaires over a 6-month period. Questions related to the likelihood of certain behavioural or emotional traits being "true" at a particular point in time. Normative data was derived from approximately 7000 clinical case records, relating to children, adolescents and young adults from 4 to 18 years of age. This data was based on levels of intellectual disability (mild, moderate, severe or profound). The DBC scoring algorithms were, and remain, computer-based, and categorised problem behaviours into five domains, as well as a "Total Behaviour Problem Score", reported as a T-score, which could be compared with a clinical cut-off score. The categories were:

- Total behaviour score.
- Disruptive/antisocial.
- Self-absorbed.
- Communication disturbance.
- Anxiety.
- Social relating.

Scores from these domains were used for an internal "Autism Screening" measure. Scoring produces an inbuilt bar graph presentation as well as statistical information.

The strength of the DBC lies in its ability to monitor reduction or change in symptomatology over time, facilitating programme evaluation and further planning. The DBC was revised by Christian Gruber and Amber Klein from Western Psychological Services. DBC-2 maintains its original Australian format, scoring criteria and software output and although the test has been re-normed in the United States, the original normative data proved to be sufficiently robust and reliable to be retained in the Technical Manual for reference and comparison. The DBC is often used in special schools to measure pre- and post-behavioural presentations when specific problem behaviours are being "targeted" for intervention.

Developmental Assessment for Individuals with Severe Disabilities, third edition (DASH-3) (Mary Kay Dykes and Daniel W. Mruzek)

As the name would imply, the third edition of this test is primarily designed to assess individuals from 6 months to adulthood with severe to profound intellectual disabilities, although it can also be used for young children up to the age of 6 years who have moderate intellectual disabilities. Its primary purpose is to give an estimate of developmental levels when clients are too intellectually disabled, physically incapacitated or sensorily impaired, to be assessed using formal assessments of intelligence or development. It can be administered directly, or through observations, or via structured interviews with parents or caregivers. The DASH-3 can also be used to analyse developmental strengths and weaknesses and to consider plans for targeting areas of support.

The DASH-3 consists of five subscales:

- **Sensory motor:** Receiving and responding to environmental stimuli, and moving reflexively and voluntarily.
- **Language:** Understanding and using communicative behaviours and purposeful language.
- **Activities of daily living:** Feeding, dressing, toileting, travel.
- **Social-emotional:** Awareness and understanding of self and others.
- **Academics:** Learning and using information, concept formation, basic reading and number skills.

The DASH 3 is published through Western Psychological Services.

Bibliography

Achenbach, T., and Rescorla, L. (2000), Child Behavior Checklist, ASEBA Publishing.
Alpern, G. D. (2020), DP-4: Developmental Profile (4th Edition), Western Psychological Services.
Center for the History of Psychology, "The guide to the Edgar A. and Geraldine Longwell Doll papers, 1932-1983", Center for the History of Psychology website Center for History of Psychology, www.uakron.edu.
Dykes, M. K., and, Mruzek, D. W., Developmental Assessment for Individuals with Severe Disabilities, Third Edition (DASH-3), Western Psychological Services.
Einfeld, S. L., and Tonge, B. J. (1989), "Developmental Behaviour Checklist", TEACCH Program, www.teacch.com.
Einfeld, S. L., Tonge, B. J., Gruber, C., and Klein, A. (2018), DBC-2: Developmental Behaviour Checklist (2nd Edition), Western Psychological Services.
Harrison, P. L., and Oakland, T. (2015), Adaptive Behavior Assessment System (3rd Edition), Western Psychological Services.

Limbos, M. M., and Joyce, D. P. (2011), "Comparison of the ASQ and PEDS in Screening for Developmental Delay in Children Presenting for Primary Care", Journal of Developmental & Behavioral Pediatrics, 32 (7), pp 499–511.

Meisels, S., and Atkins-Burnett, B. (2005), Developmental Screening in Early Childhood: A Guide (5th Edition), National Association for the Education of Young Children.

Radecki, R. P. (2011), "Trends in the Use of Standardized Tests for Developmental Screening," Paediatrics, 128, p 14.

Sparrow, S. S., Balla, D. A., and Cicchetti, D. V. (1998), Vineland Social-Emotional Early Childhood Scales, AGS Publishing.

Sparrow, S. S., Cicchetti, D. V., and Saulnier, C. A. (2016), Vineland-II Adaptive Behaviour Scales, AGS Publishing.

Squires, J., and Bricker, D. (2009), "ASQ-3: Ages and Stages Questionnaire (3rd Edition), Brookes Publishing.

Tamm, L., Day, H., and Duncan, A. (2022), "Comparison of Adaptive Functioning Measures in Adolescents with Autism Spectrum Disorder without Intellectual Disability", Journal of Autism and Developmental Disorders, 52(3) pp 1247–1256.

Voress, J. K., Maddox, T., and Hammill, D. D. (2012), DAYC-2: Developmental Assessment of Young Children (2nd Edition), Pearsons Clinical.

15 Cross-cultural adaptations of developmental assessments

There is an increasing awareness in relation to neurodevelopmental disorders of the need to take cultural factors into account. The assessment and diagnostic practices, processes and tools associated with autism spectrum disorder emanate in the majority of instances from "Western" cultures. This can give rise to "cultural bias" in assessment. In its simplest form, cultural bias in assessment can be defined as the tendency of people to assess others on the basis of their own background and culture, ethnicity or other social constructs. In many respects, this bias may be unconscious on the part of those undertaking the assessing, and an artefact of their backgrounds, studies and qualifications, experiences and readings.

The fact that the overwhelming majority of developmental assessment tools for neurodevelopmental disorders emanate from "first world" Western countries is a pervasive element of this bias. Test translations and adaptations are a vital means of lessening the impact of cultural bias. They are an example of the difference between "equality" and "equity". "Equality" refers to laws, statutes and practices whereby governments and agencies treat everyone the same, irrespective of their circumstances. "Equity" means that, in some circumstances, people need to be treated differently to provide meaningful equality of opportunity.

In assessment contexts, "equality" stipulates that in clinical practice, everyone is assessed under as far as possible the same conditions and protocols, whereas "equity" refers to the fact that some people and population groups will be unable to be given "due process" in psychometric assessments unless specific adaptations are made (Figure 15.1).

There are historical examples "equity" in specific test adaptations:

- Jerome Sattler's adapted subtests for the Stanford-Binet LM Test of Intelligence so that children with limited or no hand function were not required to attempt physical tasks such as block stacking and puzzles.
- Translated test instructions such as the Swedish version of the Griffiths Mental Development Scales.
- There have even been specific tests designed for "special" populations, for example:
- The Snijders-Oomen Nonverbal Intelligence Test for children with severe hearing difficulties, in which instructions were mimed by the assessing psychologist.
- The Queensland Test (QT), which was an Australian attempt at non-verbal assessment of Indigenous Australians, again using visual and mimed instructions. This test had five non-verbal subtests, including one, the "Knox Cubes," from the procedures used by Howard Knox at Ellis Island.
- The Slosson Test 4th Edition (SIT-4), originally created by Richard Slosson but revised in 2017, is a screening measure of cognitive ability for individuals with visual impairments or blindness and features large colour stimulus items.

DOI: 10.4324/9781003565338-19

150 *Diagnosing Young Children with Neurodevelopmental Disorders*

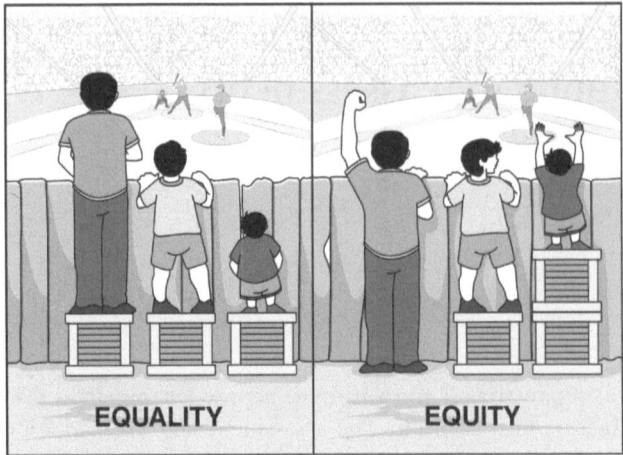

Figure 15.1 Equality and equity

Cultural bias in psychometric assessment

In its simplest form, "cultural bias" in assessment can be defined as the tendency of people to assess others on the basis of their own background and culture, ethnicity or other social construct. In many respects, this bias may be unconscious on the part of those undertaking the assessing, and an artefact of their backgrounds, studies and qualifications, experiences and readings. Although the developmental processes and sequences for young children may be universal, there are considerable differences in the opportunities children have to grow and learn, the environments they inhabit, the toys and materials with which they can play, their access to formal or informal early learning opportunities, and indeed the relative value placed on different developmental milestones and the manner in which these skills are utilised.

First, as already mentioned, children living in "developing" countries are subject to more early "developmental compromise" due to such factors as lack of expert medical care and follow-up, malnutrition, illness and disease.

Second, there is in "developing" countries far less opportunity for young children to attend early childhood programmes such as day care centres, nurseries, preschools or kindergartens. The statistics from the previous chapter are worth repeating. In 2019, only half of the world's preschool-age children were receiving preschool education. One hundred and seventy-five million children were not enrolled in pre-primary education during their early years. In under-developed countries, 78% of children were missing out on preschool opportunities.

This leaves the responsibility of facilitating early learning to parents who may themselves not have had access to optimal educational and learning opportunities, who are living with financial constraints or who are "time poor" as they carry out their other daily chores and responsibilities.

Third, young developing children do not readily have access to the quantity, quality, range and sophistication of toys and equipment, which developed nations tend to take for granted. In developed countries, children are used to playing with a rich variety of toys, for example puzzles, blocks, scissors, cars, trains, dolls, picture books, crayons and pencils. Young children in "developing" countries may instead play and learn through whatever materials they have access to, such as "found" objects from their local surroundings: Rocks and pebbles, sticks and domestic items. Modern developmental tests, such as the Griffiths III or Bayley-4, are redolent with materials which stimulate the child's imagination, mirror the purposeful nature of play learning experiences with which they are already familiar, and which are specifically designed to reflect the developmental progressions and hierarchical milestones. Children in "lesser developed" countries who are assessed on such developmental tasks will not necessarily be familiar with such games and activities, materials and requisite skills.

Fourth, modern "Western" developmental assessments also make assumptions about a developing child's place in society, their ability to make friends, to cooperate with others, to imagine and create, and to move towards greater independence and competence. These assumptions do not necessarily hold true for young children in "developing" nations, where young children may be required to take on very different social roles and responsibilities and allegiances, chores and duties which restrict opportunities to play and socialise, learn and create in the same manner as young children from more affluent backgrounds.

How then are young children from developing nations, from low to middle-income backgrounds and reduced opportunity, assessed for their developmental status and support needs? This introduces the concept and practice of test adaptations such that standardised assessment tools from the developed "Western" world are made more suitable for use in low to middle-income "developing" nations. The process of adapting tests for specific populations is detailed in guidelines published by The International Test Commission in 2016 and included in the Appendices section of this book. These adaptations may entail:

- "Re-norming" standardised tests on local populations without changes to test items or materials.
- Changes to language and instructions to suit indigenous languages.
- Substitution of equipment such as toys with more familiar materials.
- The introduction of more culturally appropriate and valid test items based around the lives and circumstances of particular populations.
- The development of entirely new assessment tools for specific populations.

Thus, adapted assessments tend to fall into a number of categories:

- **Adoption**: Whereby there is a close translation of an instrument in a target language.
- **Adaptation**: This generally involves a combination of a close translation of some stimuli and a change of other stimuli (for example test materials) when a close translation would be inadequate for linguistic, cultural or psychometric reasons.
- **Assembly**: The compilation of a new test instrument. An assembly maximises the cultural suitability of a test but precludes easy numerical comparisons of scores across cultures.

"Task equivalence" or "task substitution" is achieved when individual test items from standardised developmental assessments are replaced by equivalent tasks using materials more familiar to a child's repertoire of activities, effectively assessing the same fundamental skill in a more contextually appropriate manner (Table 15.1). Examples include:

- Tasks requiring the naming of objects and toys are replaced with a focus on common household utensils.
- Formal counting tasks utilising commonly found and used objects such as pebbles to be counted into jars.

Table 15.1 Substitute test items from Malawi

Gross motor	Fine motor	Language	Social	Learning and reasoning
• Carries basket or water pitcher on head • Can ride an animal, e.g., donkey • Can chase an animal • Can kick a ball made of bound or bundled rags or cloth	• Can peel a banana • Sorts out maize or beans • Shelling nuts • Uses chopsticks • Pours water from pitcher	• Shrugs in disapproval • Names common household objects, e.g., cups, animals, foods • Plays local language games	• Plays clapping games e.g. "Chipapa" • Copies parents' chores, e.g., washing • Helps gather or harvest • Shares food with others • Fetches water for house • Goes on errands • Shows tribal leadership • Spreads arms for hug	• Makes a car out of wire • Makes toys from mud • Can count bottle tops • Puts stones in a jar • Makes rattle toys from beans • Makes patterns with coloured bottle tops • Makes own toys

Source: Professor Melissa Gladstone.

- Making a baby's rattle out of "found" materials such as crisp packets filled with beans.
- "Localised" gross motor tasks such as carrying a bucket or basket on one's head.
- Specific changes to test instructions and wording to reflect local dialects.
- The use of leadership/responsibility tasks such as fetching water to measure social maturity.

Adapted standardised tests and locally "normed" tests consist of commercially available measures of developmental skills and milestones which are modified to suit local contexts. This does not necessarily occur with all standardised developmental tests, due to the cost of "legal" and production logistics associated with such issues as copyright. Alternatively, assessment tools remain the same, but a local normative sample is derived to act as a "benchmark" for specific population groups. Specific examples of such tests will be detailed in the next section of this book, again relating to sub-Saharan Africa in particular. These adaptations form the framework for more culturally appropriate of assessment tools, and have been referred to as "**ECLECTIC**", standing for:

E: Education and literacy.
C: Culture and acculturation.
L: Language.
E: Economics.
C: Communication.
T: Testing situation, comfort and motivation.
I: Intelligence conceptualisation.
C: Context of immigration.

Specifically designed tests, incorporating "local" materials and tasks, normative population data and instructional protocols, are less common because of the expense of such projects. Examples of such specialised tests will be detailed in the next section of this book. Reference is made below to several specific projects exploring, researching and quantifying neurodevelopmental status of young children through item substitution and test adaptations, locally "normed" and adapted versions of existing developmental tests, and new "global" developmental scales in regions as diverse as sub-Saharan Africa, the Sub-Continent, China, Japan, Australia, South America and South-East Asia.

The Global Scales for Early Development (GSED) for children aged 0–3 years

An initiative of the World Health Organization, the Global Scales for Early Development (GSED) is intended to provide developmental measures of early childhood from 0 to 3 years which are valid, reliable and have psychometrically stable performance across geographical, cultural and language contexts. Initial development involved the adaptation of two subtests (pattern reasoning and story completion) from the Kaufman Assessment Battery for Children-2nd edition (KABC-II).

After initial assessments of face validity, extra test items were substituted and added to the test battery through a co-design process with fieldworkers and child development practitioners. Eight hundred and seven psychometrically "best-performing" test items were selected from an Early Childhood Development (ECD) measurement databank consisting of over 2000 test items from 32 countries.

The resulting assessment questionnaire comes in "short form" (SF) via a caregiver report, and "long form" (LF) by direct administration. Both versions of this assessment can be administered in paper-based and tablet-based formats. A validation study is intended to be conducted in seven countries (Bangladesh, Brazil, Côte d'Ivoire, Pakistan, The Netherlands, People's Republic of China, United Republic of Tanzania).

The Malawi Developmental Assessment Tool (MDAT)

Originally adapted from the Denver II, which is widely used in many countries, the Malawi Developmental Assessment Tool (MDAT) is intended for use in rural African settings. Item substitution and addition was again undertaken through research and local consultation, and then validated on a sample of children with neurodevelopmental disorders and children with delayed developmental milestones from the impact of malnutrition. It was found to be a "culturally relevant" assessment tool, but it was stressed by the researchers that further research was necessary to test its applicability to other countries and settings.

The Kaufman Assessment Battery For Children II (KABC-II) adapted for use in rural Zimbabwe

This project again adapted two subtests from the KABC-II (pattern reasoning and story completion), and again added and substituted more "culturally appropriate" test items. The KABC-II planning domain was described as "successfully adapted to improve cross-cultural validity". This pilot project has since been applied to a follow-up study.

The Developmental Disorder-Children Disability Assessment Schedule (DD-CDAS), for use in Pakistan

The Developmental Disorder-Children Disability Assessment Schedule (DD-CDAS) is an adaptation of the World Health Organization's Disability Assessment Schedule for Children (WHODAS-child), which itself is described as a "lay health worker administered functioning-related" assessment tool. A "mixed-method" approach to adapting the

WHODAS-child was utilised, through initial translation into Urdu, followed by selective rephrasing of test items. To render them more comprehensible for parents, the DD-CDAS was trialled and normed on children up to 12 years of age already diagnosed with neurodevelopmental disorders and their caregivers. Study results indicated that the DD-CDAS was a "pragmatic measurement tool, easy for 'lay' health workers to learn, and of short an simple administration". Psychometric properties included "high reliability", responsiveness to different developmental difficulties and adequate sensitivity to change over time. However, caution in interpretation with children under 5 years was raised, as the DD-CASD was not specifically adapted for this age group.

The Kilifi Developmental Checklist (KDC) and the Kilifi Developmental Inventory

The Kilifi Developmental Checklist (KDC) in its original form consists of four subscales:

- Locomotor.
- Eye and hand coordination.
- Hearing, speech and language.
- Social-emotional.

Adaptations and refinements were undertaken to provide a measure of psychomotor development in Kenyan infants aged 6–35 months, whereas the original edition was appropriate for children aged 12 months to school entry age. Its item content was drawn from several standardised developmental assessments such as an earlier edition of the Griffiths Mental Development Scales, the Merrill Palmer Scales of Tests and the Movement Assessment Battery for Children, and some of these items were retained or modified for the development of the Kilifi Developmental Inventory, which consists of 69 test items.

A study of 319 children was undertaken and "acceptable" levels of reliability were reported. There was a significant association between performance level and chronological age and anthropometric status, and a lack of association with gender. A significant correlation was also found with levels of parental report. The acceptability of the measure to the community was further evaluated through a series of focus group discussions. For example, mothers reported "high face validity" in that their children's performance on psychomotor tasks adequately characterised their developmental level.

The adaptation of the Ages and Stages Questionnaire For mainland China: The ASQ-C

In 2013, the Chinese government announced Guidelines for the development of a national system for early detection of disability among children under 6 years of age. To meet the needs of this agenda in a timely and economical manner, the Ages & Stages Questionnaires: Inventory (ASQ:3) was translated into Simplified Chinese, and validated on a regional sample of 812 Chinese children from 1 to 25 months of age.

Mainland China has an enormous population, and in 2013, it was estimated that the number of children in China from birth to 6 years with a documented disability was 1.68 million. Under the Law of the Protection of Persons with Disabilities 2008, access to government-funded intervention services require official proof of disability. This usually entails a diagnosis from a qualified physician using standardised procedures and assessment tools, including the Chinese Denver Development Screening Test (DDST) for screening, and the Beijing Gesell Developmental Schedule (Beijing GDS).

In China, assessment for developmental status and eligibility for intervention services is the responsibility of paediatricians, who often lack appropriate clinical training and who can provide only very brief clinical consultations. Training in child development and assessment skills for medical practitioners is described as a recent phenomenon in China. For all of these reasons, it was necessary to adapt an existing, brief and easy to use developmental assessment tool, the Ages & Stages Questionnaires-Third Edition (ASDQ-3).

Instructions and prompt questions were translated into Simplified Chinese, and a national Chinese normative sample was obtained (Bian, Xie, & Squires, 2014). The ASQ-C was pilot tested on 8372 subjects in the Shanghai metropolitan area between 2007 and 2008 and cross-referenced with rural samples. Internal consistency scores ranging from 0.51 to 0.68 were reported, and inter-rater reliability scores of 0.79–0.89. Parents participating in the study reported that the questionnaires were easy to understand and helpful to their parenting practices. After its publication in China, the ASQ-C was widely adopted by over 50 child health organisations in 10 provincial regions.

Adaptations of developmental tests in India

India has long used a range of adapted and modified developmental screening tests, particularly since the 1990s, but academic literature about these adaptations is scarce. Two adaptations are particularly highlighted however: The Developmental Assessment Scale for Indian Infants (DASII) is an adaptation of the Bayley Scales of Infant Development, and despite it being derived from the second edition of the Bayley Scales, it is still widely used in India. There are the "Baroda norms", which emanate from Professor Arun Phatak from KGP Children's Hospital in Vadodara, who collated data from a "door-to- door" survey in the Baroda slums by community workers. From this data, he chose a number of motor and "mental" items for his test, the Trivandrum Development Screening Chart.

The LEAP-CP prospective cohort study protocol Australia

This study is an example of how a variety of test instruments, including adapted tests, can be used together to collate invaluable population statistics. The LEAP-CP prospective cohort study is intended as a means of investigating the effectiveness of early developmental screening programmes in Queensland, Australia, a large state with immense areas of remote land. The aim is for earlier identification of Aboriginal and Torres Strait Islander infants who are at risk of adverse or suboptimal neurodevelopmental outcomes, including neurodevelopmental disorders.

The context of the study is the alarming statistics, which emanate from the ongoing intergenerational trauma, systematic displacement from traditional lands, and loss of culture and racism experienced by Australian Indigenous people, manifesting in socio-economic disadvantage, marginalisation, reduced education and employment opportunities, and poorer health outcomes than the national average:

- Indigenous Australians are nearly twice as likely to experience disability, twice as likely to have a severe disability and less likely to access appropriate supports compared with non-Indigenous Australians.
- Inequities and inequalities in accessing culturally appropriate health and disability support services further exacerbate this disadvantage.

A battery of assessment protocols is planned for use, including:

- General Movements Assessment (GMA).
- Hammersmith Infant Neurological Examination (HINE).
- Rapid Neurodevelopmental Assessment (RNDA).
- Ages and Stages Questionnaire-Aboriginal adaptation second edition (ASQ-TRAK2).
- Peabody Developmental Motor Scales.
- Functional capabilities (Paediatric Evaluation of Disability Inventory-Computer Adaptive Test).
- Behaviour (Infant Toddler Social and Emotional Assessment).

Infants will be classified as typically developing or "at risk" of adverse neurodevelopmental outcomes including specific neurodevelopmental disorders based on symptomology using developmental and diagnostic outcomes such as autism spectrum disorder and fetal alcohol spectrum disorder. The study will investigate the effects of perinatal, social and environmental factors, caregiver mental health on child development, and clinical neuroimaging of suboptimal neurodevelopmental outcomes will be investigated.

The Ages and Stages Questionnaire-Talking about Raising Aboriginal Kids Second Edition (ASQ-TRAK2) is a culturally adapted developmental screening tool for Aboriginal and Torres Strait Islander children, currently the only culturally appropriate developmental screening tool for this context. Fourteen age intervals have been adapted and the revised for the second edition, (ASQ-TRAK2), which now covers all 21 age intervals equivalent to the ASQ-3. The original ASQ-TRAK communication, gross motor, fine motor and problem-solving domains were moderately correlated with the corresponding domains on the Bayley-III. Overall sensitivity for the ASQ-TRAK was 71% and specificity was 92%. Overall percentage agreement between the ASQ-TRAK and the Bayley-III was 90%. No statistical data is currently available for the second edition. The ASQ-TRAK2 is available for purchase from the Royal Children's Hospital in Melbourne.

BRIEF2 Russian adaptation

This study was designed considering the specific characteristics of Russia's cultural and educational context. The multilingual nature of Russia was thought to potentially limit the validity evidence of the Russian-language version of BRIEF2. The study involved children aged 5–7 years old to assess the applicability of the Russian-language version of BRIEF2 over existing differences in the age period of the transition from early childhood to primary school.

One hundred and seventy-eight typically developing children were included in the study. Internal consistency for 5-year-old children was described as "good" or "acceptable", and the same was found for 6-year-olds except for the "Initiate" subscale. However, for the sample of 7-year-old children, the internal consistency was, in general, lower than that in the previous two age groups. The interrater reliability analysis results indicated the level of agreement between teachers decreased slightly as the children aged.

The Children Neuropsychological And Behavior Scale (CNBS-R2016), China

The Children Neuropsychological and Behavior Scale (CNBS) is a diagnostic assessment tool developed by the Capital Institute of Pediatrics in China that is widely used in China to assess the developmental level of children aged 0–4 years. It consists of five subscales: Gross Motor, Personal-Social, Language, Fine Motor and Adaptive Behavior. It was restandardised in 2005, completed in 2016 and was renamed the Children Neuropsychological and Behavior Scale-Revision 2016 (CNBS-R2016). In a study comparing the CNBS-R2016 with the Griffiths Mental Development Scale 1996 revision with a sample population of children with autism spectrum disorder, obtained results showed the proportion and distribution of the two tests for the detection of developmental delays in different domains were consistent.

However, this finding was not true for overall diagnoses of developmental delay, where the CNBS-R2016 identified less children a diagnosable developmental delay. One hypothesis for this outcome was that the CNBS-R2016 was a locally normed assessment, therefore detecting a child's optimal ability. It should also be noted that this research study was conducted using the previous edition of the Griffiths Scales, and not the current Griffiths III.

The Griffiths Development Scales-Chinese (GDS-C)

The same methodological issue also pertains to this adapted version of the 1996 Griffiths Mental Development Scales for Chinese use, and thus, caution needs to be used in any consideration of the efficacy of this adapted measure. However, the survey results are of interest in that the Chinese developmental curves obtained from the GDS-C were similar in some respects and different in others to the developmental curves from the original British normative data. It was recommended that the adapted Chinese test was preferrable for the assessment of urban Chinese children due to its more culturally appropriate nature.

The Child Development Assessment Questionnaire (QAD-PIPASS), Brazil

In response to the World Health Organisation, Early Childhood Development Index (ECDI2030), which aims to determine whether children aged 24–59 months are developmentally appropriately, the Regional Project on Child Development Indicators (PRIDI) was initiated in Brazil. Resulting from this is the Caregiver Reported Early Development Index (CREDI), a 21-item questionnaire, a population-level measure for assessing the overall development of children aged 0–35 months across the motor, language, cognition, socio-emotional and mental health. From this in turn came the PIPAS Project (Early Childhood for Healthy Adults) and an easy-to-use assessment instrument, the QAD-PIPAS.

To validate this instrument two studies were undertaken, in 2017 and 2018. The QAD-PIPAS showed evidence of construct validity and reliability to be used in population studies involving children aged 0–59 months. The QAD-PIPAS was described as "sensitive to risk and "protective factors" based on the "Nurturing Care Framework". (The Nurturing Care Framework is a World Health Organisation "roadmap for action", to help children survive and thrive to transform health and human potential.) The chance of being classified as a suspected developmental delay was higher in children experiencing risk factors than others, as opposed to children with "protective factors" who were less likely to be suspected of developmental delay.

Thus, children exposed to unfavourable socio-economic conditions, such as low maternal education and not having children's books, were more likely to have suspected developmental delays, whereas children receiving one or more developmental stimuli at home over the course of a week (a "protective factor") lowered the chances of children presenting with signs of developmental delay. Internal consistency was "acceptable" across all age groups, but it was noted that reliability and consistency were better when the questionnaire was administered in a "uniform" manner.

The Child Development Review (CDR) questionnaire, survey of Surinamese children in the Caribbean

The Child Development Review (CDR) was originally developed by Dr. Harold Ireton in 1990 for identifying preschool children enrolled in special education Minnesota, USA. It is a screening tool for use in routine paediatric checkups, taking into account parental concerns for their child's development and behaviour as well as direct observation by paediatricians. It is quick and convenient to use, but there is little be way of research data to evaluate and judge this measure.

For this study of Surinamese children, an adapted version of the CDR was administered along with the Dutch adaptation of the Bayley Scales of Infant and Toddler Development (Bayley-III), perhaps the first time the CDR has been evaluated in a detailed manner. Moderate levels of reliability were reported, with an "acceptable" level of internal validity. Sensitivity and specificity values were highly vulnerable to fluctuations, and it was concluded that sensitivity and specificity of the CDR in Suriname should be interpreted carefully.

New Zealand Well Child Tamariki Ora Programme

This review of a mass screening programme for pre-school aged children illustrates the complex policy and bureaucratic decision-making process which needs to occur, particularly in a small nation with distinctly different cultural groups. New Zealand has a population of approximately 5 million people, of whom approximately 18% have Mauri or Polynesian Island ancestry and heritage. There are discrepancies in health and educational outcomes for the two primary demographics, and sufficient statistical information to suggest also that this figure underestimation for Māori and Pacific peoples. The New Zealand Well Child Tamariki Ora Programme is intended as a screening, data gathering and policymaking process for the treatment and remediation of young children with neurodevelopmental disorders or sub-optimal development.

To develop this comprehensive screening programme, five areas of developmental concern were prioritised:

- Language development and hearing.
- Fetal alcohol spectrum disorder.
- Autism spectrum disorder.
- Global developmental delay.
- Motor disorders such as cerebral palsy.

A preliminary list of 25 possible assessment protocols were identified over these five diagnoses, and specific criteria was applied to which of these would be suitable for population screening:

- Primary purpose-discrimination, prediction or evaluation.
- Validity.
- Reliability.
- "Clinical utility", for example cost and availability.

In respect to "utility", it was projected that most of the chosen screening instruments would be administered by health professionals "such as GPs, Paediatricians, Developmental Paediatricians, Nurses, Occupational or Speech and Language Therapists". Psychologists were not mentioned in this list. Reference was made to a dual process where the above process was "primary screening", and that "secondary screening" would also be necessary, using PEDS Developmental Milestones (PEDS: DM), which comprises six to eight items per age and aims to predict the developmental status of children accurately in the domains of fine motor skills, gross motor skills, expressive language, receptive language, self-help, social–emotional development. Also used was the Brigance Early Childhood Screen and the Ages and Stages Questionnaire (ASQ).

An issue of concern arising from the use of screening instruments was that of "false positive" and "false negative" results. Another concern was the perceived need to use language assessment tools, which were culturally appropriate for the Mauri population. Further, the recommended screening tests were described through literature review as having wide ranges of sensitivity and specificity when compared with "reference standards" such as Bayley-III (at the time of the report's publishing), M-CHAT and the Battelle Developmental Inventory Screening Test (BDI II).

Recommendations from this study included:

- Translation of the screening tools into commonly spoken languages in New Zealand.
- Determination of the ages at which infants and children should be screened for neurodevelopmental disorders to be coordinated with information from the rapid evidence reviews for other domains.
- Screening instruments should be selected on the basis of the best ways of coordinating the varying screening processes.

Bibliography

Abubakar, A., Holding, P., Van Baar, A., Newton, C. R. J. C., and Van De Vijver, F. J. R. (2008), "Monitoring Psychomotor Development in a Resource-Limited Setting: An Evaluation of the Kilifi Developmental Inventory", Annals of Tropical Paediatrics, 28(3), pp 217–226.

ASQ-TRAK Practitioner Training Procedure Guide (2023), Supporting the Implementation of the ASQ-TRAK Developmental Screening Tool, University of Melbourne.

Chaudhari, S. (1996), "Developmental Assessment Tests: Scope and Limitations", Indian Pediatrics, 33, pp 541–555.

Faruk, T., et al. (2020), "Screening Tools for Early Identification of Children with Developmental Delay in Low- and Middle-Income Countries: A Systematic Review", BMJ Open, 10, pp 1–17.

Gavrilova, M. Aslanova, M., Tarasova, T., and Zinchenko, Y. (2023), "Russian Version of BRIEF2 Teacher Forms: Validation Study in Typically Developing Children Aged 5 to 7 Years Old", Frontiers in Psychology, 21, pp 1–8.

Gladstone, M. Lancaster, G., Umar, E., Nyirenda, M., Kayira, E., van den Broek, N., and Smyth, R. L. (2009), "Perspectives of Normal Child Development in Rural Malawi-A Qualitative Analysis to Create a More Culturally Appropriate Developmental Assessment Tool", Child Care, Health and Development, 36(3), pp 346–353.

Gladstone, M., Lancaster, G. A., Umar, E., Nyirenda, M., Kayira, E., van den Broek, N. R., and Smyth, R. L. (2010), "The Malawi Developmental Assessment Tool (MDAT): The Creation, Validation, and Reliability of a Tool to assess Child Development in Rural African Settings", PLoS Medicine, 7(5), pp 1–14.

Hamdani, S. U., Huma, Z., Wissow, L., Rahman, A., and Gladstone, M. (2020), "Measuring Functional Disability in Children with Developmental Disorders in Low-Resource Settings: Validation of Developmental Disorders-Children Disability Assessment Schedule (DD-CDAS) in Rural Pakistan", Global Mental Health, 7, pp 1–12.

International Test Commission (2016), ITC Guidelines for Translating and Adapting Tests (2nd Edition) Version 2.4, International Test Commission.

Kearney, G. E., and McElwain, D. (1976), Aboriginal Cognition: Retrospect and Prospect, Australian Institute of Aboriginal Studies.

Kinsey, M., et al. (2024), "The Utility of the Child Development Review in Suriname: Validating a Neurodevelopmental Screener for Use in a Low- to Middle- Income Country", Global Pediatrics, 9, pp 1–9.

Li, H. H., et al. (2019), "Comparison of The Children Neuropsychological and Behavior Scale and the Griffiths Mental Development Scales When Assessing the Development of Children With Autism", Psychology Research and Behavior Management, 12, pp 973–981.

Luke, C. R., Benfer, K., Mick-Ramsamay, L., Ware, R. S., Reid, N., Bos, A. F., Bosanquet, M., and Boyd, R. N. (2022), "Early Detection of Australian Aboriginal and Torres Strait Islander infants at High Risk of Adverse Neurodevelopmental Outcomes at 12 Months Corrected Age: LEAP-CP Prospective Cohort Study Protocol", BMJ Open, 12, pp 1–18.

Madaan, P., Saini, L., and Sondhi, V. (2021), "Developmental Assessment Scale for Indian Infants: A Systematic Review and Perspective on Dwindling Cutoffs", Indian Journal of Pediatrics February, 88(9), pp 918–920.

McGray, G., et al. (2023), "The Creation of the Global Scales for Early Development (GSED) for Children Aged 0-3 Years: Combining Subject Matter Expert Judgements with Big Data", BMJ Global Health, 8(1), pp 1–11.

New Zealand Ministry of Health (2019), Brief Evidence Reviews for the Well Child Tamariki Ora Programme, New Zealand Ministry of Health.

Sattler, J., and Tozier, M. A. (1970), "Test Modifications Used with Children with Cerebral Palsy and Other Handicapped Groups", Journal of Special Education, 4(4).

Simpson, S., D'Aprano, A., Tayler, C., Khoo, S. T., and Highfield, R. (2016), "Validation of a Culturally Adapted Developmental Screening Tool for Australian Aboriginal Children: Early Findings and Next Steps", Early Human Development, 103, pp 91–95.

Slosson, L., Erford, B., T., Larsen, S., L, and Slosson, S. W. (2017), SIT-4: Slosson Intelligence Test (4th Edition), Slosson Publications.

Snijders, J. T., Tellegen, P. J., and Laros, J. A. (1997), Snijders-Oomen Nonverbaler Intelligenztest SON-R 5.5-17, Hogrefe.

Tso, W., et al. (2018), "The Griffiths Development Scales-Chinese (GDS-C): A Cross-Cultural Comparison of Developmental Trajectories between Chinese and British Children", Child Care Health and Development, 44, pp 1–2.

Venancio, S. I. (2021), "Psychometric Properties of the Child Development Assessment Questionnaire (QAD-PIPAS) for Use in Population Studies Involving Brazilian Children Aged 0-59 Months", Jornel de Pediatria, 97(6), pp 637–645.

Vorster, C., Kritzinger, A., Lekganyane, M., Taljard, E., and van der Linde, J. (2022), "Cultural Adaptation and Northern Sotho Translation of the Modified Checklist for Autism in Toddlers", South African Journal of Childhood Education, 12, pp 1–10.

Xie, H., Clifford, J., Squires, J., Chen, C, Y., Bian, X., and Yu, Q. (2017), "Adapting and Validating a Developmental Assessment for Chinese Infants and Toddlers: The Ages & Stages Questionnaires: Inventory", Infant Behavior and Development, 49, pp 281–295.

Yankowitz, L. D., et al. (2020), "Evidence against the 'Normalization' Prediction of the Early Brain Overgrowth Hypothesis of Autism", Molecular Autism, 11(51), pp 1–17.

16 Assessing autism spectrum disorder in young children

Interest in and knowledge surrounding the broad spectrum of autistic disorders has expanded enormously in the last quarter of a century, and autism spectrum disorder is now clearly understood and accepted as a neurodevelopmental disorder occurring with considerable frequency. Incidence rates such as 1 per 100 and 1 per 160 children are often quoted, and with its increased acceptance and recognition have come a plethora of support services through therapies, educational programmes, literature and training programmes. Support funding through various government agencies has increased significantly, but access to these services requires accurate diagnosis of the condition. There has consequently been a proliferation of new assessment tools for autism spectrum disorder, and updates to other, older assessments tools.

Autism spectrum disorder is classified as a neurodevelopmental disorder by both DSM-5-TR and ICD-11, and despite clear evidence of heritability factors, no genetic foundation to autism has been confirmed. Assessment and diagnosis are ideally undertaken through detailed observation and case history, and autism spectrum disorder often requires more than one assessment technique for confirmation. There are three broad assessment genres for autism spectrum disorder:

- Questionnaire and checklist-based assessments.
- Interview-based assessments with parents, caregivers and teachers.
- "Direct interaction" and observation-based assessment.

These three modes of assessment are frequently undertaken concurrently for individual children. This triumvirate of methods often functions in a "cascade" model. Early concerns about possible autism spectrum disorder are often raised and recorded through questionnaire and checklist-based case histories, followed by parental or caregiver interview, and then by direct observation and interaction-based assessments. Parents may therefore be gradually exposed to the possibility of a diagnosis of autism spectrum disorder. It is also worth noting that "direct observation" assessments are not limited to assessment sessions in a clinic or office, but can also include observations made at preschools and childcare centres, home visits and through video recordings or on-line technologies.

The following section provides a review of autism spectrum disorder assessments from each of the three categories. Some have been known for considerable periods of time and subject to review. Some are very new. There are those with an emphasis upon research-based outcomes, and others based more on clinical observations made by practitioners.

DOI: 10.4324/9781003565338-20

Screening checklists for autism spectrum disorder

Social responsiveness Scale-2 (SRS-2) (John Constantino)

The Social Responsiveness Scale-2 (SRS-2) is a 65-item questionnaire covering the age range 2 years 6 months to adulthood. It is specifically described as a screening instrument with the ability to identify social symptoms associated with autism spectrum disorder. Despite its brevity, it is claimed to have sufficient sensitivity to detect autistic-type symptoms.

Administration time is reported as being between 15 and 20 minutes, and both hand and software scoring options are available. For young children, there are preschool-aged forms covering the range 2.5–4.5 years. School-age forms commence at 4 years and extend to 18 years of age. Both parent and teacher forms are available. Raters evaluate symptoms using a quantitative scale representing a range of severity. Because the SRS-2 does not have a binary "yes-or-no" response format, it is described as being able to detect even subtle signs of autism spectrum disorder. As is required of all American-based assessment tools, the SRS-2 is described as providing "treatment subscales", which can be used to monitor programme and intervention effectiveness in the following areas:

- Social awareness.
- Social cognition.
- Social communication.
- Social motivation.
- Restricted interests and repetitive behaviour.

As well as the Treatment Subscales, the SRS-2 provides two DSM-5 compatible subscales:

- Social communication and interaction.
- Restricted interests and repetitive behaviour.

These scores are described as "clearly informing diagnosis" and are an aid to determining whether an individual meets the most current diagnostic criteria for autism spectrum disorder.

Modified checklist for autism in toddlers, revised (M-CHAT-R) (Robins, Fein and Barton, 1999)

This brief screening questionnaire consists of 20 questions about a child's behaviour, covering the age range 16–30 months. When scored, the results are intended to determine whether further assessment may be needed, and whether further discussion is needed with primary healthcare providers.

It is intended to assess the risk of possible autism spectrum disorder. Often used in medical and child health settings, the M-CHAT-R can be administered and scored as part of a "well-child" check-up.

As a primary goal of the M-CHAT-R was to maximise sensitivity, there is a high "false positive" rate, meaning that not all children who score in the "at risk" range for autism spectrum disorder will later be diagnosed with autism spectrum disorder. A structured follow-up interview format is available following administration, including discussions as to whether children "not at risk" of developing autism spectrum disorder may continue to be "at risk" for other developmental disorders or delays. Scoring the M-CHAT-R can

Eric Schopler's contributions to the understanding of autism spectrum disorder

Eric Schopler was born in 1927 in Fürth, Germany, and with his Jewish parents fled Nazi Germany and emigrated to the United States, settling in Rochester, New York. In 1970, he married his second wife, Margaret Lansing. He died of cancer in 2006. Together, Schopler, Lansing and Gary Mesibov radically changed the manner in which autism spectrum disorder is diagnosed and treated, through educational and therapeutic programmes and techniques which are still used today. In 1949, Schopler earned his Bachelor's Degree from the University of Chicago, followed in 1955 by a Graduate Degree in Social Service Administration, and then in 1964 a PhD in Clinical Child Psychology.

After initially working as a Family Counsellor, Schopler was employed at the Emma P. Bradley Hospital at Rhode Island as Acting Chief Psychiatric Social Worker, followed by employment at the Treatment and Research Center for Childhood Schizophrenia in Chicago. Subsequent employment and research at the University of North Carolina at Chapel Hill led to the development of the Treatment and Education of Autistic and Related Communication Handicapped Children (TEACCH) programme in 1971, with Schopler assuming directorship in 1972.

The TEACCH Programme led to many advances in knowledge of Autism. Schopler disapproved of the then current theory that most autistic children suffered from "mental disorders". He also highlighted the role of parents as effective collaborators in the treatment and education of their children. He remained Director of the TEACCH programme until 1993, as well as being the Associate Chair for Developmental Disabilities until 1996.

The TEACCH programme is still employed across the world. Schopler worked at the University of North Carolina's TEACCH programme until 2005. He is associated with two assessment systems for children and adults with autism spectrum disorder, both reviewed in this section.

Childhood Autism Rating Scale 2nd edition (CARS-2) (Eric Schopler, Mary E. Van Bourgondien, Glenna Janette Wellman, and Steven R. Love)

The Childhood Autism Rating Scale was originally developed by Eric Schopler, Robert Reichier and Barbara Rochen Renner and published in 1988. It has been widely used ever since in a variety of clinical, educational and research settings. This 2009 revision marks Eric Schopler's final contribution to this instrument and is a means of differentiating between children with mild to severe autism spectrum disorder, and also between autism spectrum disorder and children with cognitive deficits.

The CARS-2 allows practitioners to rate children according to the following functional areas:

- Relating to people.
- Body use.
- Visual response.
- Listening response.
- Taste, smell and touch response and use.
- Verbal communication.

- Nonverbal communication.
- Level and consistency of intellectual response.

The CARS 2 includes three forms:

- **Standard Version CARS 2 ST Rating Booklet:** This is equivalent to the original CARS, and is for use with individuals younger than 6 years of age and those with communication difficulties or below-average estimated IQs.
- **High Functioning Individuals CARS 2 HF Rating Booklet:** This is described as an alternative for assessing verbally fluent individuals, 6 years of age and older, with IQ scores above 80.
- **Questionnaire for Parents or Caregivers CARS 2 QPC:** This is an unscored scale that allows the collection of information for use in making CARS 2-ST and CARS 2-HF Ratings. Sub-skills assessed include
  - Relating to people.
  - Imitation.
  - Social-emotional understanding.
  - Emotional response.
  - Emotional expression and regulation of emotions.
  - Body use.
  - Object use.
  - Object use in play.
  - Adaptation to change and restricted interests.
  - Visual response.
  - Listening response.
  - Taste, smell and touch response and use.
  - Fear or nervousness, or anxiety.
  - Verbal communication.
  - Nonverbal communication.
  - Activity level.
  - Thinking and cognitive integration skills.
  - Level and consistency of intellectual response.
  - General impressions.

Children are rated on each item, using a 4-point response scale, based on frequency of occurrence of behaviours, as well as intensity, peculiarity, and duration. The result is a Total Raw Score, which is converted to a standard score or percentile rank. The Questionnaire for Parents or Caregivers allows exploration of a child's early development, including social, emotional, and communication skills, repetitive behaviours, play and routines, and unusual sensory interests. A typical administration of the CARS-2 is of some 15 minutes duration.

Gilliam Autism Rating Scale, 3rd edition (James E. Gilliam, 2013)

The Gilliam Autism Rating Scale was originally released in 1995 and is now in its third edition. It is widely used as a screening instrument for the assessment of autism spectrum disorder and covers the age range 3–22 years. The 56-item questionnaire is based on the DSM 5 criteria for autism spectrum disorder and is essentially a "pen and paper" completion task, which takes approximately 10 minutes for parents, teachers and other caregivers. The GARS-3 yields standard scores, percentile ranks, severity level, and a "probability of Autism" rating. Items are categorised into six subscales:

- Restrictive/Repetitive behaviours.
- Social interaction.
- Social communication.
- Emotional responses.
- Cognitive style.
- Maladaptive speech.

This structure incorporates considerably more individual items than previous editions to encompass DSM 5 criteria for autism spectrum disorder, and there is an additional "diagnostic validation form" to ensure linkage with DSM 5. The brevity and convenience of administration of the Gilliam Autism Rating Scales has long been seen as advantageous for its usage as a screening instrument.

Autism Spectrum Rating Scales (ASRS) (Sam Goldstein, and Jack A. Naglieri, 2010)

The Autism Spectrum Rating Scales (ASRS) are an "easy-to-use, norm-referenced assessment designed to identify symptoms, behaviours, and associated features of the full range of Autism Spectrum Disorders". Parents and teachers complete questionnaires to evaluate how often they observe specific behaviours associated with possible autism spectrum disorder, including

- Socialisation.
- Communication.
- Unusual behaviours.
- Behavioural rigidity.
- Sensory sensitivity.
- Self-regulation.

The ASRS was designed to identify symptoms, behaviours, and associated features of autism spectrum disorders in children and adolescents aged 2–18 years. It was initially released before the advent of DSM 5, and therefore, findings were aligned to DSM IV-TR criteria for the various autistic presentations defined therein, but a 2013 revision included links to DSM 5 symptom criteria for autism spectrum disorder. Scoring software or hand-scoring options are available. There are full-length and short-form versions of the instrument. The full-length version consists of 71 items, whilst the short version is 15 items only. Full-length scores are reported for the following domains:

Core symptoms

- Social/Communication.
- Unusual behaviours.
- Self-regulation.
- Total score.
- DSM 5.

Treatment scales

- Peer socialisation.
- Adult socialisation.
- Social/Emotional reciprocity.
- Atypical language.
- Stereotypy.
- Behavioural rigidity.
- Sensory sensitivity.
- Attention.

There are minor variations in this format depending upon the age of the subject, and specific alternative instructions are provided in cases where respondents are reporting on non-verbal children. The short-form version provides only Total Score information. Scores are reported in T scores, percentile ranks, and descriptive categories such as "very elevated," "elevated", "slightly elevated", "average", and "low". The ASRS is designed to "help guide diagnostic decisions," and also to contribute to treatment plans and ongoing monitoring of progress through via the included "Treatment Scales". Considerable statistical data is provided, illustrated by a number of individual case examples.

All psychological assessment tools are subject to intense and at times critical review, and the ASRS is no exception. In 2022, a study by Hong et al. concluded that the ASRS did not necessarily perform well as a valid measure for detecting autism spectrum disorder in children who had been referred to a specialist assessment and diagnostic clinics. It suggested that the ASRS was limited in its ability to accurately differentiate autism spectrum disorder from other clinical disorders, as has been found in other screening instruments, which similarly possess difficulties associated with "false positive" results.

It is therefore important to thoroughly read the ASRS technical and Users' Manual, which explicitly makes reference to the need to integrate information derived from the ASRS with other sources of information for diagnostic decision-making, and "interpretative guidelines provided should be carefully examined to avoid inaccurate interpretations". This advice should apply to any assessment procedure for possible autism spectrum disorder. Checklists and questionnaires should never take precedence over direct observation of, and interaction with, young children. They are a valid means of gaining background information from a variety of sources and contexts (Table 16.1).

Statistical information

- The ASRS Technical Manual reports internal reliability scores of .97 for Total Scores.
- Inter-rater reliability scores range from .73 to .92 for Parent responders and .59 to .73 for Teacher responders.

Table 16.1 Diagnostic statement, Autism Spectrum Rating Scale

"The assessor must combine ASRS scale score information with information gathered from other sources and measures, including that obtained through interviews and discussions with the individual and other informants. The ASRS results should be interpreted within the context of any factors that may influence results. The ASRS should, therefore, not become a substitute for a trained and experienced assessor's overall judgement regarding diagnosis, treatment planning, and treatment outcome." (ASRS Manual pp 3-4)

Autism Diagnostic Interview-Revised (ADI-R) (Michael Rutter, Ann LeCouteur, and Catherine Lord)

This is an in-depth interview-based assessment of possible autism spectrum disorder, with a long history of usage as a clinical research tool. Michael Rutter will be remembered for his association with the revised Griffiths Mental Development Scales in the 1990s. Catherine Lord has long been associated with research into autism spectrum disorder. The ADI-R is often used in conjunction with the ADOS 2, making for a lengthy but detailed assessment process. This dual technique has its roots in the work of Eric Schopler, and the psychoeducational profile (PEP) with which he was involved.

In the ADI-R, specific interview questions are asked of a parent or caregiver familiar with the developmental history and current behaviour of the individual being evaluated, whether child, adolescent, or adult, provided the assessed or assumed mental age of the subject is at least 2 years. There are 93 test times focusing upon three broad areas of functioning:

- Language/Communication.
- Reciprocal social interactions.
- Restricted, repetitive, and stereotyped behaviours and interests.

It is recommended that only skilled and experienced clinicians conduct these interviews, which follow standardised procedures but allow for individual styles of responding. The responses when coded consider eight different content areas:

- The subject's background, including family, education, previous diagnoses, and medications.
- Overview of the subject's behaviour.
- Early development and developmental milestones.
- Language acquisition and loss of language or other skills.
- Current functioning in regard to language and communication.
- Social development and play.
- Interests and behaviours.
- Clinically relevant behaviours, such as aggression, self-injury, and possible epileptic features.

The aim of the ADI-R is to standardise the clinical interview procedure into a "template" for considering responses at an empirical level. A formal ADI-R interview can take from 90 minutes to 2 and a half hours, and is sometimes conducted with one parent whilst the individual in question is formally assessed using the Autism Diagnostic Observation Schedule-2 in another room. Sometimes such an assessment procedure is conducted over 2 days. Scored results emanate from The Comprehensive Algorithm Form, which allows calculation and interpretation of any one of five age-specific ADI-R algorithms:

- Two diagnostic algorithms based on developmental history for formal diagnosis.
- Three current behaviour algorithms which focus on present functioning. These can be used for treatment and educational planning.

The ADI-R focuses on behaviours that are rare in unaffected individuals. For this reason, it provides "categorical" results rather than scale scores or normative data. These

"Direct interaction" assessments of autism spectrum disorder

These types of assessment are similar in nature to standardised developmental assessments such as Bayley-4 and the Griffiths III, except for their emphasis upon symptoms of autism spectrum disorder. They are play-based interactions between assessor and child, usually with parental participation. They are often described as being "planned social activities", to observe, explore, and examine the core social and communication deficits in children with autism spectrum disorder. Two such protocols will be discussed, and it will be noted that as with the Bayley-4 and the Griffiths III, specialised training is mandatory for certification and usage.

Psychoeducational profile, 3rd edition (PEP-3) (Eric Schopler, Margaret D. Lansing, Robert J. Reichler, and lee M. Marcus)

The original PEP was published in 1970, followed by the PEP-R in 1990, the PEP-2 in 2004, and now the PEP-3. It was always intended to be a means of assessing the skills and behaviours of children with autism spectrum disorder and other communication-based disorders, and particularly to assuage concerns that tests based on "normal curve" normative populations did not reliably capture the sometimes unique skills of children with autism spectrum disorder. The PEP-3 is for children as young as 6 months through to 7 years, with assessment duration from approximately 45 minutes to approximately 90 minutes.

Because it charts "uneven and idiosyncratic development", emerging skills, and autistic-type behaviours, the PEP-3 is often used for planning individualised education programmes (IEPs) for young children. The PEP-3 measures 11 specific domains, especially in the areas of social functioning and communication:

- Visual–motor imitation.
- Affective expression.
- Social reciprocity.
- Characteristic motor behaviours.
- Characteristic verbal behaviours.
- Cognitive verbal/preverbal.
- Expressive language.
- Receptive language.
- Fine motor.
- Gross motor.
- Maladaptive behaviours.

Additionally, the PEP-3 includes a new caregiver report, which allows parents or caregivers to estimate their child's developmental levels compared with typical children. This report examines:

- Problem behaviours.
- Personal self-care.
- Adaptive behaviour skills.

The inclusion of this feature is interesting when one considers research suggesting that the ability of parents to accurately estimate in this manner is equivocal. The transition from PEP-2 to PEP-3 has included revised items and normative data, in particular, data from a control group of "neurotypical" children. It is stressed that the PEP-3 "assesses the developmental level of young children with Autism, who may be non-verbal, have limited attention skills and poor concentration, and who are not used to a formal testing situation".

As well as identifying a child's special learning strengths and "teachable" skills, the PEP-3 describes the severity of a child's autistic symptoms. This information can be useful in clarifying the diagnostic status of a child with autism spectrum disorder. It is stressed as well however that "this test alone should not be used as a diagnostic tool". What may have been forgotten over time is that Eric Schopler suggested often that the PEP was the ideal vehicle to observe children with suspected autism spectrum disorder as a means of then administering the Childhood Autism Rating Scale.

Autism diagnostic observation schedule 2nd edition (ADOS 2), (Catherine Lord, Michael Rutter, et al)

The Autism Diagnostic Observation Schedule is often spoken of as the "gold standard" for comprehensive assessment of autism spectrum disorder. The second edition (ADOS-2) was published in 2012 and as such is still influenced by the then used DSM IV-TR criteria for the various pervasive developmental disorders, but co-author Catherine Lord was an Editorial and Coding Consultant for Neurodevelopmental Disorders for the DSM 5 publication, and her intensive research into autism spectrum disorder is reflected in both DSM-5-TR and ADOS-2. Michael Rutter is also peerless in his knowledge of autistic-type disorders.

The ADOS-2 is described as a "semi-structured, standardised assessment of communication, social interaction, play/imaginative use of materials, and restricted and repetitive behaviours for individuals who have been referred because of possible autism spectrum disorders". It is a revision and extension of the original ADOS published in 1999, particularly the addition of a Toddler Module, which extends the age range of the ADOS from as young as 12 months through to adulthood. There are now five modules, based on a combination of age and verbal expression skills, and only one selected module is administered at an assessment:

- **Toddler Module** for infants aged 12–30 months who do not consistently use phrase speech.
- **Module 1** for children 31 months and older who do not consistently use phrase speech.
- **Module 2** has no age restriction, and is for children who use phrase speech but not verbally fluent.
- **Module 3** for children and adolescents who are verbally fluent.
- **Module 4** for use with verbally fluent older adolescents and adults.

Given the focus of this book on the assessment of young children, focus will be on the Toddler Module and Modules 1, 2, and 3.

Scoring criteria for Module 1, in particular, require an understanding of a young child's ability to speak, as there are different outcomes for children who are essentially non-verbal or only have a few single words, compared with children who may be demonstrating an increasing vocabulary of single words and short communicative phrases.

The ADOS contains a series of semi-structured social and play activities, sometimes referred to as "social occasions". Some of these require scoring of a child's response to various social overtures or "presses" (a term used by H.A. Murray in 1938), for example a child's response to the call of his/her name. Modules 1 and 2 focus on much the same areas for analysis:

Language and Communication, including:

- Overall level of non-echoed speech.
- Frequency of directed spontaneous vocalisation.
- Speech anomalies such intonation, volume, and rhythm.
- Immediate echolalia and other stereotypic or idiosyncratic speech.
- Use of another's body to communicate.
- Nonverbal communicative gestures such as pointing.

Reciprocal Social Interaction, including:

- Frequency and quality of eye contact and gaze.
- Responsive social smile and response to call of name.
- Range and frequency of directed facial expressions.
- Responsive/reciprocal smile.
- Integrated use of eye gaze and gestures in social engagement.
- Shared enjoyment.
- Initiation and response to joint attention.
- Pro-social acts such as showing and giving.
- Frequency and context of social engagement, including establishment and maintenance of rapport.

Play, including:

- Functional play with toys and objects.
- Imaginary play.
- Unusual sensory interests and responses.
- Stereotypic movement patterns.
- Repetitive interests and non-functional routines and rituals.
- Maladaptive behaviours such as self-injury, temper tantrums, and aggression.
- Over or under-activity.

Modules 1, 2, and 3 are scored on normative data related to age and levels of spoken language. Th scoring algorithm is clear and logical. Children can reach threshold for diagnoses of Autism, Autism Spectrum, or Non-Spectrum. Additionally, ratings of severity of Autism are provided, ranging from "Minimal to No Evidence, Low, Moderate and High". Different behaviours are "weighted" at different ages, reflecting the influence of normal stages of development. For example, a young non-verbal child is not adversely scored if he/she does not engage in purposeful pointing or engages in babble which may be considered to be "stereotyped".

The Toddler Module was added for the 2012 revision, and although it is very similar in format, equipment, and activities to Modules 1 and 2, the diagnostic outcomes are quite different, and clearly reflect the understanding that children between 16 and 30 months are frequently too young for definitive diagnoses of autism spectrum disorder, particularly as they are entering a dynamic phase of development at that stage, may not have experienced any sustained social interaction opportunities such as day care or child care, and may not have had access to early therapeutic interventions such as speech pathology or occupational therapy. Thus, following test administration, the scoring algorithm makes reference to the following score categories:

- Moderate to severe concern about possible autism.
- Mild to moderate concern.
- Little to no concern.

Apropos the ADOS 2 predating DSM 5, these categories were quite logical and in fact reflected the DSM-IV-TR diagnostic label "Pervasive Developmental Disorder" (Not Otherwise Specified) and the ICD 10 "Pervasive Developmental Disorder, Not Specified". Both these terms were colloquially referred to at various times as "Atypical Autism" or the "Wait and See" diagnosis. Whether agencies determining eligibility for funding and services such as Australia's National Disability Insurance Scheme appreciate this nuanced approach to assessment and diagnosis is not entirely clear.

The ADOS-2 is a test requiring specialist training and accreditation, and is often administered by multi-disciplinary teams whereby one parent is present for the ADOS assessment whilst the other may be engaged in the ADI-R. Experienced users of assessment tools such as the Griffiths III or Bayley-4 will adapt with ease to the assessment activities and format, and some will even administer both ADOS-2 and other developmental tasks concurrently.

Bibliography

American Psychiatric Association (2013), Diagnostic and Statistical Manual 5, American Psychiatric Association.
American Psychiatric Association (2022), Diagnostic and Statistical Manual 5 TR, American Psychiatric Association.
Constantino, N. (2012), SRS-2: Social Responsiveness Scale (2nd Edition), Western Psychological Services.
Goldstein, S., and Naglieri, J. A. (2010), Autism Spectrum Rating Scales (ASRS), Manual, Multi-Health Systems.
Hong, J. S., Perrin, J., Singh, V., Kalb, L., Cross, E. A., Wodka, E., Richter, C., and Landa, R., (2022). "Psychometric Evaluation of the Autism Spectrum Rating Scales (6–18 Years Parent Report) in a Clinical Sample", Journal of Autism and Developmental Disorders, 54(3), pp 1024–1035.
Lord, C., Rutter, M., DiLavore, P., Risi, S., Gotham, K., Bishop, S., Luyster, R., and Guthrie, W. (2012), Autism Diagnostic Observation Schedule (2nd Edition) Manual, Western Psychological Services.
Mesibov, G., Shea, V., and Schopler, E. (2004), The TEACCH Approach to Autism Spectrum Disorder, Springer Science and Business Media.
Murray, H. A. (1938), Explorations in Personality, Oxford University Press.
Robbins, D., Fein, D., and Barton, M. (2018), "M-CHAT-R: Modified Checklist for Autism in Toddlers-Revised", M-Chat/screen.

Rutter, M., Le Couteur, A., and Lord, C. (2003), ADI-R: Autism Diagnostic Interview-Revised, Western Psychological Services.

Schopler, E., and Lansing, M. D. (2005), PEP-3: Psychoeducational Profile (3rd Edition), Western Psychological Services.

Schopler, E., and Mesibov, G. (2013), Diagnosis and Assessment in Autism, Springer Science and Business Media.

Schopler, E., Van Bourgondien, M. E., Wellman, G. J., and Love, S. R. (2010), CARS-2: Childhood Autism Rating Scale (2nd Edition), Western Psychological Services.

TEACCH Autism Program (2017), "Remembering Dr. Eric Schopler, Founder of TEACCH" www.teacch.com.

World Health Organisation (1993), The ICD-10 Classification of Mental and Behavioural Disorders: Diagnostic Criteria for Research, World Health Organisation.

17 Cross-cultural assessment and diagnosis of autism spectrum disorder

Do all cultural groups, language groups, ethnicities and societies understand the complexities, subtleties and variations within the broad spectrum of autistic disorders? Are the symptoms of autism spectrum disorder universally understood and regarded as problems? Are there societal attitudes and values in some areas of the world, which make it more or less likely that autism spectrum disorder will be diagnosed and treated? As with other neurodevelopmental disorders, there is increasing awareness of the need to take such factors into account, and to adapt Western and "Euro-centric" assessment protocols for autism spectrum disorder to avoid as far as possible "cultural bias" in assessment.

There are many factors which can influence the understanding and acceptance of autism spectrum disorder in "lesser developed" nations. A medical specialist or and psychologists might ponder, "how can one be sure if my assessment results genuinely reflect the traits of Autism Spectrum Disorder, or do they reflect a cultural difference?" The cultural context within which a diagnostic assessment of autism spectrum disorder may occur can include such factors as:

- The educational and literacy levels of a young child's family.
- The relevance of test items to a given family.
- The language and idioms used in specific assessment tools compared with the communication, grammar and idiomatic references common to specific cultures.
- The assessment situation itself, including setting, timing, ambience and format.
- The relevance or otherwise of specific characteristics of autism spectrum disorder to families from diverse cultural, linguistic and socio-economic circumstances.

This last point is of particular importance, because it underpins the nature of what an assessment of autism spectrum disorder is attempting to explore-the presence or otherwise of symptomatology, and its impact upon daily functioning for a young child. There are many examples of the conundrums posed by what may or may not be considered a "symptom":

- In some cultures, avoiding eye contact may be a sign of "respect" towards adults.
- Traditional greeting gestures may be misinterpreted as "scripted", ritualistic or repetitive.
- Not being able to interpret idiomatic language and jokes may be a cultural difference based on specific language usage.
- Non-verbal gestural communication such as pointing is not necessarily a universal construct.

- Lack of or restricted pretend play may in some cultures be an artefact of the types of toys available and the nature of local play.
- Some language styles are more precise and structured than others, raising possible impressions of being overly pedantic.

There may also be "administrative" decisions as to the manner in which autism spectrum disorder is assessed, diagnosed and supported in specific cultures. In Japan for instance, the manner in which the Japanese government and autism spectrum support services have used "Japanese-specific" administrative categories, rather than emphasising a "medical" concept of autism spectrum disorder, to avoid the possibility of debate and obfuscation in relation to the nexus between scientific and medical concepts of aetiology, and the autonomous administrative process of providing funding and support.

Whatever the cause and mechanism of autism spectrum disorder were, the priority instead was a clear description of the problem that government and jurisdictions needed to address. The mention of the causal mechanisms and factors for autism spectrum disorder raised the risk of conceptual controversies among doctors and bureaucrats. By avoiding such debate, administrators were described as being more able to argue in favour of funding supports in their areas.

In a further example, in Israel, it has been reported that there is a lower prevalence of autism spectrum disorder and fewer requests for services in the peripheral regions of Israel and among minority groups, including religious sectors. Underdiagnosis of autism spectrum disorder in minority groups was thought to be accounted for by low awareness of autism, limited accessibility to services, physical, linguistic, cultural, social barriers related to community norms, and the meaning of diagnosing autism and associated stigmas.

An erroneous assumption that needs to be dispelled is that when people migrate to other countries, joining a new community or even becoming part of the diasporas that form around the commonalities of language, background and experience, that such families and groups will assume the beliefs, attitudes and values of their adopted countries. Research suggests otherwise, for example the "Latine" populations in the United States or the South East Asian communities in Australia, where different understandings of conditions such as Autism Spectrum Disorder can result in under-diagnosis of disability. This may be associated with language barriers, mistrust in or lack of service providers, misunderstanding of the assessment and diagnostic process, particularly if they do not experience "culturally affirming" support processes.

Exploring cross-cultural stigma surrounding autism spectrum disorder: The Autism Stigma and Knowledge Questionnaire Second Edition (ASK-Q-2)

From these cycles of suspicion, misunderstanding, disbelief, reluctance and unintended neglect surrounding autism spectrum disorder in various cultures, and the subsequent "flow-on" effect to acknowledged incidence rates, policy and budgetary decisions for service provision, came the Autism Stigma and Knowledge Questionnaire (ASK-Q) (2017). Its primary purpose is to explore attitudinal and educational issues surrounding autism spectrum disorder as a guide for promoting better societal understanding of the condition.

The original 2017 edition of ASQ-Q was later re-evaluated and modifications made. Eighteen questionnaire items were either removed or refined and the overall measure shortened. Statistical data derived from a Mongolian-based study indicated "adequate" internal consistency and reliability.

The Societal Attitudes Towards Autism Questionnaire (SATA) (Flood, L., N., Bulgrin, A. And morgan, B., L)

With the increasing incidence of autism spectrum disorder and exposure to individuals with the diagnosis, community interest and acceptance of autism spectrum disorder is also changing, but at attitudes towards autism spectrum disorder remain relatively understudied. Hence, the need for an attitudinal scale, which may delve into societal attitudes towards autism spectrum disorder. The Societal Attitudes Towards Autism Questionnaire (SATA) was originally developed in 2012 and changed and enhanced through various samples and trials, mainly involving American College students. Validity analysis suggested that attitudes towards autism spectrum disorder differed from attitudes towards disability in general. Since its development, the SATA has been translated and adapted for language and cultural groups such as Portuguese and Greek.

Modification and adaptations of autism spectrum disorder assessments

As has already been illustrated, there are many projects globally where standardised "Western" tests have been adapted to suit specific cultures and languages, and the same applies to assessments of autism spectrum disorder, both through checklists and surveys, interview schedules and activity-based assessments. Some of these are detailed in the following sections.

German adaptation of the Social Responsiveness Scale (SRS)

The Social Responsiveness Scale (SRS) has often been used as a quantitative measure of autistic traits in 4 to 18-year-olds. A cross-cultural validation of a German adaptation of the parent-report SRS was found to have internal consistency 0.91–0.97, test-retest reliability of 0.84–0.9, interrater reliability 0.76 and 0.95, and convergent validity with the Autism Diagnostic Observation Schedule (ADOS 2), as well as the Autism Diagnostic Interview-Revised, and the Social Communication Questionnaire (0.35–0.58). These ratings were described as "satisfactory to good".

The SRS total score was described as discriminating between autism spectrum disorder and other mental disorders and was sufficiently independent of general psychopathology. Construct validity was ensured by consistent correlations with the Vineland Adaptive Behavior Scales, the Child Behavior Checklist and the Junior Temperament and Character Inventory.

Taiwanese adaptation of the Social Responsiveness Scale (SRS)

A sample of 140 typically developing children and 167 with clinically diagnosed developmental disorders was undertaken using an adapted Mandarin version of the Social Responsiveness Scale (SRS). Total SRS scores, sensitivity and specificity of the scale for diagnosing developmental disorders were similar to those observed in Western studies, and SRS total and subscale scores distinguished significantly between autism spectrum disorder and other developmental disorders ($p < 0.01$).

Taiwanese adaptation of the Autism Diagnostic Observation Schedule 2 (ADOS-2)

Taiwan has also adapted the Autism Diagnostic Observation Schedule-2 (ADOS-2). The MC-ADOS 2 is adapted and validated for Mandarin Chinese and has been found to have sound statistical properties. Diagnostic specificity ranged between 0.71 and 1.00, and diagnostic sensitivity 0.83 and 0.96.

Autism Diagnostic Observation Schedule 2 (ADOS 2), Brazilian Portuguese adaptation

This project involved three stages:

- Translation and backtranslation of the ADOS 2 into Brazilian Portuguese.
- Semantic equivalence analysis.
- Pre-test to verify the agreement between mental health specialists and an ADOS 2 senior examiner regarding scoring procedure.

The translation and "back translation" involved an initial translation from English into Brazilian Portuguese conducted by two translators, followed by a "synthesis of translations", then a translation back into English, followed by review before the final Brazilian Portuguese version was adopted. The semantic equivalence phase of the project, based on specific guidelines, involved a comparison of the terms and expressions of the original version with the "back-translated" version for each of the questions, taking into account cross-cultural equivalence for use in Brazilian Portuguese. The quality of the translation according to the referential meanings of the words and phrases was used for the analysis of denotative equivalence.

Preliminary results suggested "good" equivalence between the original English version of the ADOS 2 and the Brazilian version. Some semantic differences were found between the original version and the back-translation into English, but they did not interfere with the first translation into Portuguese or into the final version. This study was of a small sample only but with "adequate" inter-rater reliability. This adapted assessment is not yet available commercially.

Afrikaans Autism Diagnostic Observation Schedule 2 (ADOS 2)

South Africa has 10 official languages, and Afrikaans was chosen for this translation project. A mixed-methods approach was used to evaluate three components associated with method bias in the Autism Diagnostic Observation Schedule-2:

- Language used.
- Social interactions and activities.
- Materials.

An ethnographic investigation of play, social interaction and social activities was conducted in a small community sample of 40, and the Afrikaans Autism Diagnostic Observation Schedule-2 was pre-piloted in a small clinical sample of 7. Results highlighted "unique" aspects of the language that need to be considered during Autism Diagnostic Observation Schedule-2 administration.

The social interaction requirements of the Autism Diagnostic Observation Schedule-2 appeared appropriate, and there was sufficient familiarity with the original test materials and activities to support the use of the adapted version.

Autism Diagnostic Observation Schedule 2 (ADOS 2) modified for use with children with visual impairment

The need for this adaptation of the ADOS 2 for children with impaired vision stems from the understanding that children with visual impairments are susceptible to developing autism spectrum disorder, one reason being that the lack of access to and experience of the "visuo-social environment" can delay or prevent the learning and understanding of mutual eye gaze, facial expressions, non-verbal imitations and gestures, social referencing and joint attention, including the ability to shift attention between objects and people. There are also "downstream" risk factors such as semantic and pragmatic language difficulties, affective reciprocal social relationships, and the development of "theory of mind". Many children with visual impairments learn and develop compensatory skills and strategies but some continue to manifest persistent social features of autism spectrum disorders. There can also be stereotypic self-stimulatory behaviours associated with visual impairment.

Autism spectrum disorder is reported as occurring more frequently in children with visual and/or hearing impairments than in the general population, with an incidence rate of 19% being suggested. But assessing and diagnosing autism spectrum disorder in young children with visual impairments is a challenging process due to the limitations of the current assessment tools.

To this end, Module 3 of the "gold standard" Autism Diagnostic Observation Schedule 2 was modified, trialled and validated on a selected sample of children with visual impairment, aged 4–7 years, as this Module is less reliant upon visual skills and object manipulation than are Modules 1 and 2. Tasks that required minimal visual involvement were retained in the modified test, and certain construction and manipulation tasks were adapted to make stimulus materials easier to see and handle. These toys and objects were introduced to the subject children through "multisensory" means.

Research findings suggested that one in three of the study cohorts could be considered "at risk" of autism spectrum disorder symptoms despite their average intellectual abilities and verbal fluency. Another finding was that the item changes and substitutions had in effect dictated a different algorithm from the original ADOS-2 Module 3, as despite the social motivation and interactional skills of some of the cohort, they were still considered at a "high risk" of autism spectrum disorder.

The Indian Scale For Assessment of ASD (ISAA), and the International Clinical Epidemiology Network Diagnostic Tool For Autism Spectrum Disorder (INTD-ASD)

These two scales have been developed in several Indian languages but do not accommodate all languages, verbal abilities and educational backgrounds. The Indian Scale for Assessment of ASD (ISAA) is a 40-item scale of six domains:

- Social relationship and reciprocity.
- Emotional responsiveness.
- Speech (language and communication).
- Behaviour patterns.
- Sensory aspects.
- A cognitive component.

Each of the 40 items are rated according to frequency, degree and intensity of behavioural characteristics observed. The range in which the final score lies is used to determine the degree of ASD (8). One concern is that this tool is not sufficiently "child-friendly" and lacks a visual component and a cohesive storyline.

The International NDT-ASD was a diagnostic tool originally developed using the fourth edition of the Diagnostic and Statistical Manual (DSM IV) but has been revised to accommodate the diagnostic criteria for autism spectrum disorder as defined by DSM-5-TR. It consists of two sections, one including questions related social interaction, communication and restricted interests.

The second section relates to scoring as well as arriving at diagnostic classification with reference to DSM-5-TR criteria for autism spectrum disorder. It is regarded a simple and structured instrument based on DSM-5-TR criteria, and can facilitate diagnoses of autism spectrum disorder with "acceptable" diagnostic accuracy.

To address the concern that these two measures were not sufficiently "child friendly" or orientated to a range of Indian languages and dialects, a home-based, audiovisual game app (Autest) suitable for autism spectrum disorder risk assessments in young Indian children was developed. It consists of five modules for specific age groups with specific peer interaction and play skill assessments. Each module follows a story from a popular Indian story series for children. Game play and behaviour are assessed to evaluate the risk of autism spectrum disorder. The Autest was rated by 30 psychologists to compare with other currently available tools.

It was noted that the game format reduced social inhibition and facilitated assessment by removing the language barrier and instead using emojis. This tool is described as particularly useful for minimally verbal, at-risk children.

Cultural adaptation and Northern Sotho translation of the Modified Checklist for Autism in Toddlers (M-Chat-R/FM)

To adapt the popular M-CHAT screening questionnaire for autism spectrum disorder, a qualitative design method was used so that perspectives, opinions and suggestions of various sources were reflected. Data was derived from self-completed questionnaires that included rating scales and structured review questions adapted from the International Test Commission (ITC 2016). Using both the ITC and World Health Organization (2019) adaptation guidelines, a test adaptation and double translation method were used, avoiding a literal translation and ensuring similarity of meaning of constructs across the two languages. The study was therefore undertaken in three consecutive phases: Adaptation, translation and reconciliation.

"Content equivalence" was reported as achieved between the "target translation", "back translation" and "source translation". A recommendation from this process was that the current Northern Sotho version of the M-CHAT-R/FTM should be formally evaluated to determine the feasibility, reliability and validity of the questionnaire.

Conducting assessments through interpreters and translators

It is highly improbable that psychologists will have ready access to any assessment tools that have been adapted for specific populations, ethnicities or language groups unless they are working with specific population groups. However, in today's climate of increasing migration and mobility, it is highly likely that many psychologists, particularly those working in government agencies and hospitals, will be required to interview families with languages other than their own, and in many instances to conduct assessments with their young children. Under these circumstances, the only practicable manner to conduct assessments and interviews is through interpreters or translators. This is a method which requires practice and skills development.

The Australian Psychological Society British Psychological Society, the American Psychological Association and other similar bodies, responding to the ethnic diversity of their populations, have all issued guidelines for the use of interpreter services by psychologists assessing and interviewing families and children from almost every corner of the globe. Amongst these recommendations are:

- Ascertaining whether a client family actually needs and wants an interpreter.
- Avoiding as far as possible the use of family members or friends when conducting clinical interviews or assessments, but instead using professional interpreters. Family and friends may not be able to translate unemotionally or accurately due to their links with client families and interpretations of their needs.
- Conducting a pre-session planning meeting with the interpreters.
- Remaining mindful of any possible shift in dynamics that interpreter might accidently cause to the psychologist-client relationship.
- Adjusting one's language and communication style to facilitate the presence and involvement of an interpreter.
- Clarifying the appropriate language and dialect to be used. It cannot be assumed that there is only one dialect for particular languages.
- Considering and clarifying a family's client's ethnicity and religion, as these may be important to some clients.
- Considering whether there is a family or cultural preference for an interpreter of a specific gender.

Additionally, there are important logistical processes and understandings to arrive at:

- Some interpreters translate one sentence or phrase at a time, whereas others are able to use "simultaneous translation", and it is important to clarify which method an interpreter will use.
- Whether an interpreter has any knowledge of disability issues in general, or neurodevelopmental disorders in particular.
- Whether an interpreter can translate accurately "beyond the words", for example relaying information about the specific cultural understandings and practices that might pertain to a family.
- In this respect, noting whether an interpreter may be imposing his or her own cultural values onto the circumstances which bring a family to assessment.

There are specific interview and assessment techniques which psychologists need to employ when working with interpreters:

- Interpreters should arrive earlier than the scheduled appointment so that the precise purpose and format of the interview or assessment can be explained.
- The interpreter is not the client; thus, the psychologists eye gaze and attention must be focused upon the child and family, not the interpreter.
- It is best to use short and concise sentences and wordings with an interpreter, particularly during the early phase of an assessment or interview when a collaborative working relationship is being developed.

- At regular intervals, it is beneficial to seek clarification as to the perceived effectiveness of the translation taking place.
- It cannot necessarily be assumed that because a family cannot speak the same language as the psychologist, they cannot likewise understand some or all of what is being said by the psychologist and interpreter. Caution and discretion must be exercised when speaking with the interpreter about the child or family.

Psychometric assessments by necessity involve the use of language. However, no two different languages align perfectly in terms of conceptualisation, vocabulary, grammar, intonation and expression, and communicative intent. Therefore, any interpretation of assessment results conducted through interpretation must be reported and analysed with considerable caution. There are many examples from intelligence and developmental assessments where even simple vocabulary differences might affect whether a test item is passed or failed. This means that scoring and report writing protocols may have to be phrased to allow for these variables. As with many other facets of psychological practice, the use of interpreter services is a subtle combination of experience, research, practice and learning.

Bibliography

Al Maskari, T. S., Melville, C. A., and Willis, D. S. (2018), "Systematic Review: Cultural Adaptation and Feasibility of Screening for Autism in Non-English Speaking Countries", International Journal of Mental Health Systems, 12, pp 1–19.

Bolte, S., Poustka, F., and Constantino, J. N. (2008), "Assessing Autistic Traits: Cross-Cultural Validation of the Social Responsiveness Scale (SRS)", Autism Research, 1(6) pp 354–363.

Brown, R., Hobson, R. P., Lee, A., and Stevenson, J. (1997), "Are there Autistic-Like Features in Congenitally Blind Children?", Journal of Child Psychology and Psychiatry, 38(6), pp 693–703.

Butchart, M., Long, J. J., Brown, M., McMillan, A., Bain, J., and Karatzias, T. (2017), "Autism and Visual Impairment: A Review of the Literature", Review Journal of Autism and Developmental Disorders, 4, 118–131, https://doi.org/10.1007/s40489-016-0101-1

Dale, N., Sakkalou, E., Erikkson, M. H., and Salt, A. (2024), "Modification and Validation of an Autism Observational Assessment Including ADOS-2 for Use with Children with Visual Impairment", Journal of Autism and Developmental Disorders, https://doi.org/10.1007/s10803-024-06514-z

Das, A., and Ray, A. (2021) "Culturally Adapted Assessment Tool for Autism Spectrum Disorder and its Clinical Significance", Journal of Emerging Investigators, 3, pp 1–6.

Fein, R. H., Mire, S., Umaña, I., Loria, E., and Duran, P. (2024), "Culturally Affirming Practices for Conducting Autism Assessments with Latine Children in the United States", APA PsycNet Practice Innovations, 9(4), pp 305–319.

Ferman, S., and Segal, O. (2024), "The Face of Autism in Israel", Neuropsychiatric Disease and Treatment, 20, pp 1677–1691.

Flood, L. N., Bulgrin, A., and Morgan, B. L. (2012), "Piecing Together the Puzzle: Development of the Societal Attitudes towards Autism (SATA) Scale", Journal of Research in Special Educational Needs, 13(2), pp 121–128.

Fonseca, H., Manao, A. A., Lemos, L., Cunha, M., and Carrieras, D. (2024), "The Portuguese Version of the Societal Attitudes Towards Autism (SATA) Scale: Psychometric Properties, Confirmatory Factor Analysis and Reliability", British Journal of Special Education, 51(3) pp 369–381.

Gulati, S., et al. (2019), "Development and Validation of DSM-5 Based Diagnostic Tool for Children with Autism Spectrum Disorder", PloS One, 14(3), p e0213242.

Harrison, A. J., Bradshaw, L. P., Naqvi, N. C., Paff, M. L., and Campbell, J. M. (2017), "Development and Psychometric Evaluation of the Autism Stigma and Knowledge Questionnaire (ASK-Q)", Journal of Autism and Developmental Disorders, 47, pp 3281–3295.

Harrison, A. J., Madison, M., and Campbell, J. (2024), "The Development of the Autism Stigma and Knowledge Questionnaire, Second edition (ASK-Q-2), through a Cross-Cultural Psychometric Investigation", Autism, 29(1), https://doi.org/10.1177/13623613241270916

Harrison, A. J., Naqvi, N. C., Smit, A. K., Kumar, P. N., Muhammad, N. A., Saade, S., Yu, L., Cappe, E., Low, H. M., Chan, S.-J., and de Bildt, A. (2023), "Assessing Autism Knowledge across the Global Landscape Using the ASK-Q", Journal of Autism and Developmental Disorders, 54, pp 1897–1911.

Harrison, A. J., Paff, M. L., and Kaff, M. S. (2019), "Examining the Psychometric Properties of the Autism Stigma and Knowledge Questionnaire (ASK-Q) in Multiple Contexts", Research in Autism Spectrum Disorders, 57, pp 28–34.

Kakooza, A. M., and Hansen, R. L. (2012), "Cross Cultural Issues in Tool Adaptation, Screening and Assessment of ASD Research Globally", Conference Paper given at 2012 International Meeting for Autism Research.

Memari, A. H., et al. (2013), "Cross-Cultural Adaptation, Reliability, and Validity of The Autism Treatment Evaluation Checklist in Persian", Iranian Journal of Pediatrics, 23(3), pp 269–275.

Pacifico, M. C., et al. (2019), "Preliminary Evidence of the Validity Process of the Autism Diagnostic Observation Schedule (ADOS): Translation, Crosscultural Adaptation and Semantic Equivalence of the Brazilian Portuguese Version)", Trends in Psychiatry Psychotherapy, 41(3), pp 218–226.

Papadopoulos, A., et al. (2024), "Evaluating the Psychometric Properties of the Autism Stigma and Knowledge Questionnaire (ASK-Q) among Greek Mental Health Professionals: An Exploratory Study", Neuroscience Research Notes, 7(3), pp 1–11.

Smith, J., et al. (2024), "'We Go through Trauma': South Asian Parents' Experiences of Autism Diagnosis and Early Supports for their Autistic Children in Australia", Research in Autism Spectrum Disorders, 114, pp 1–12.

Smith, L., Malcolm-Smith, S., and de Vries, P. J. (2016), "Translation and Cultural Appropriateness of the Autism Diagnostic Observation Schedule-2 in Afrikaans", The Counseling Psychologist, 21(5), 552–563.

Stickley, A., et al. (2017), "Assessment of Autistic Traits in Children Aged 2 to 4 and a Half Years With the Preschool Version of the Social Responsiveness Scale (SRS-P): Findings from Japan", Autism Research, 10, pp 852–865.

Wang, J., Lee, L. C., Cheng, Y. S., and Hsu, J. W. (2012), "Assessing Autistic Traits in a Taiwan Preschool Population: Cross-Cultural Validation of the Social Responsiveness Scale (SRS)", Journal of Autism and Developmental Disorders, 42(11), pp 2450–2459.

Zarokanellou, V., et al. (2023), "Societal Attitudes Towards Autism (SATA): Validation of the Greek Version in the General Population", Journal of Autism and Developmental Disorders, 54, pp 1582–1593.

Part IV

From theory to practice

How do we assess young children for possible neurodevelopmental disorders? How do psychologists plan for these assessments, accumulate relevant background information, select appropriate assessment tools and conduct assessments? What information do they derive from assessments and how is this information communicated to parents, referrers and other agencies?

Part IV explores the assessment process from referral through formal assessment, provision of feedback to parents, diagnostic considerations and formulations, and written reports. Reference is made to the use of specific developmental assessment tools and the manner in which these can be incorporated into the clinical armoury of psychologists.

18 From theory to clinical practice

Psychologists working with young children come from different academic and training backgrounds, professional and personal experiences. They work for different service providers, with different "charters" and clinical caseloads, eligibility criteria and service provision models. This variety overrides one "best way" to conduct assessment services for young children. Add to this the multicultural mix of young children, with their own personalities and temperaments, interests, levels of tolerance and obedience, strengths and weaknesses, to confirm the impossibility of a singular assessment "style".

Rather than attempting to provide explicitly prescriptive guidelines for the psychological assessment and diagnosis of young children, it is intended instead to highlight the many and varied ways assessment procedures can be offered and conducted. Psychologists and psychologists-to-be can reflect upon their own personal "styles", knowledge-base, preferences, strengths and "comfort zones". Every assessment of a child is a novel "learning experience", and Psychologists can always learn additional skills and insights. There are of course certain patterns and protocols which do occur frequently in early childhood assessments of the typical sequence of events that occur for developmental assessments of young children. Typically:

- A referral is made to a psychological service or practice.
- Background information is provided as part of that referral, although further information is generally sought.
- A family attends an assessment session, where referral information is clarified and discussed further.
- An assessment takes place, and formal assessment protocols used are scored.
- Feedback is given to the child's family.
- Sometimes further evaluation of a child occurs, through preschool observations, home visits or additional interviews.
- All information is consolidated and, where warranted, an appropriate diagnosis is either made or discounted.
- Reports are written and distributed.
- "Treatment" and management options are discussed, formulated and finalised.
- Follow-up assessments, observations or meetings are scheduled where necessary.

Within this framework, there are innumerable "variations on a theme", reflecting both the professional orientation of the psychological service involved, and the needs of individual families and their children. Hopefully, the following sections

DOI: 10.4324/9781003565338-23

will illustrate how this process can be applied to the maximum benefit of children and families.

Psychologists employed in government departments, or by non-government agencies, may feel they have limited influence over how diagnostic and assessment services are offered and provided but should always be encouraged to offer their opinions and suggestions in relevant forums, meetings and negotiations.

19 Pre-assessment preparation

Assessment contexts

Psychological assessments for young children with developmental delays and neurodevelopmental disorders take place in various settings, for example:

- Public hospitals such as a Children's Hospital, through a Child Development Unit or specific assessment and diagnostic service. Such services tend to be multi-disciplinary in composition, with perhaps a Consultant Paediatrician, Social Worker, Psychologist (sometimes Educational and Developmental, sometimes Clinical, and even Clinical Neuropsychologists), and even sometimes a Consultant Psychiatrist. One of these professionals may assume the role of Team Leader, who may assume responsibility for referral and intake procedures, oversight of assessments, and the ultimate formulation of diagnostic considerations.
- Non-government agencies with a specific "charter", for example treatment of cerebral palsy or autism spectrum disorder, may employ psychologists whose roles may include assessment and diagnosis, family support and counselling, staff education and development, and behavioural support programmes. Their level of direct supervision and "line management" may allow psychologists considerable autonomy, or even have them supervised by professionals other than psychologists.
- Private early intervention programmes, where a psychologist may be part of a small team, including speech pathologists, occupational therapists, and early intervention teachers. Psychologists in this situation may be entirely autonomous and reliant upon their own resources for ongoing professional development.
- Some psychologists work as "sole traders" and are entirely reliant upon their own skills and resources. They may align themselves to similarly focused professionals for mutual support and peer supervision.

Psychologists may therefore need to consider these factors in their career "journeys":

- Is the psychologist comfortable within the service or environment they are working?
- Do they have access to appropriate training, professional development and supervision? Are they given opportunities for responsibility and leadership, or expanded roles and responsibilities?
- Do psychologists have influence over such matters as: Case selection; choice of assessment tools; number of assessments to be conducted; diagnostic formulation; follow-up services?

Suggestions

a Psychologists may explore their professional development needs with line managers or supervisors. Needs should be made clear in the types of skills to develop, as well as clarification of an employer's staff development policy. This is particularly true for expensive training programmes for essential assessment tools such as Griffiths III, Bayley-4, ADOS-2, or ADI-R.
b Psychologists can arrange external professional development and training, for example through a peer supervision programme.
c Psychologists can investigate agency or departmental policies for study leave, personal and professional development time such as journal reading, or inter-agency visits.

Referral

All assessments begin with a referral, but different employment settings can impact upon how this occurs. For example, a Child Development Unit at a Children's Hospital may impose specific referral criteria relating to geographic boundaries, or prior evidence of "triage" and assessment. Sometimes only certain categories of children are eligible for assessment, for example within a certain age range or assumed level of developmental delay.

The referral process may occur through a formalised "intake" system such as regular meetings to consider the source and appropriateness of referrals. Individual "cases" may be allocated to team members either through general consensus, or by direct selection by the team leader. There may be an adherence to certain levels of background reporting prior to the intake process.

By contrast, non-government agencies may only accept referrals if there is clear evidence that the child is "at risk" of a particular disabling condition, for example autism spectrum disorder or cerebral palsy. These agencies may stipulate "payment for service", or sometimes any fees can be paid through government subsidy schemes. Such services may have a "priority-system" for acceptance. For example, precedence may be given to children for potential inclusion in the agency's programmes.

Psychologists who are sole traders in private practice are able to decide for themselves the make-up of their client intake. This may reflect their particular expertise and professional interests. They may conduct telephone intake or triage consultations, or referrals may be taken by a receptionist who then passes on the relevant information to the psychologist. There is also a growing trend for private psychologists to accept "online" referrals.

A psychological service may request the following:

- Background medical information such as reports from a consultant paediatrician.
- Where necessary, evidence of genetic assessment.
- Assessments of basic physical well-being such as vision and hearing.
- Reports from speech pathologists and occupational therapists if they are available.
- Previous assessment reports from other psychologists, particularly if a "second opinion" assessment has been sought.
- Reports, questionnaires, and checklists from childcare centres or preschools.
- Information from a child's parents about their concerns, and observations of their child's development and behaviour over time. Most assessment services require completed background questionnaires and checklists prior to assessment. There is also a

growing trend for mobile phone video vignettes to be requested to illustrate behaviours concerning parents.
- Most services request that background referral information be made available prior to scheduled assessments, for pre-reading, and scoring where necessary.
- Some services suggest or recommend that parents bring some of their child's favourite toys to help them feel comfortable and relaxed. Similarly, parents are also encouraged to bring snacks for their child, and even fresh nappies and a change of clothes.

Psychologists may therefore need to consider such issues as:

- What information does your service need to accept a referral? Does your employer use questionnaires or checklists which you feel are adequate for your needs? Does your service design and write its own background questionnaires, or commercially available examples?
- Are you permitted to purchase other questionnaires and checklists from your Team budget if you have a strong professional preference?
- Can you devise your own system of triage?
- How are cases allocated within your service?

Assessment room

It may be difficult to imagine, but not all early childhood assessments are conducted in purpose-built or allocated rooms. Psychologists may have little choice over the quality of office space given over to assessments and consultations. Rooms may need to be shared with other services, or pre-booked. Most dedicated assessment and diagnostic services do have specific assessment rooms, and this should always be the case for psychologists working in private practice, or small therapy services where they can influence their work environment more readily. In public and community health sectors, assessment rooms can vary greatly in size and format. Some are small and crowded, allowing a child little room or opportunity to move about. Some may be embedded in office buildings and have no external windows or views.

On the other hand, there are offices which are appropriately spacious, bright and airy, and allow for flexibility of use. They may include an internal bathroom (extremely important when assessing young children) (Figure 19.1). Assessment rooms may even have sufficient space for different "zones" to be established, for example:

- A separate interview area for parents and psychologist to sit prior to or after assessment, to prepare for assessments or discuss results and outcomes.
- A separate "free play" area for children to enjoy prior to assessment whilst they "settle in", and for post-assessment play. This room format is embedded in some assessment procedures, for example the psychoeducational profile (PEP).
- A formal assessment area, with an appropriately sized table and chair, room for equipment, and provision for parents to sit near or with their young child.
- Some assessment rooms include two-way observation mirrors, allowing parents to view the assessment process without being physically "present". Two-way observation rooms are also used for professional training and supervision sessions.
- Some assessment rooms are equipped for video recording, again for quality assurance and training purposes.

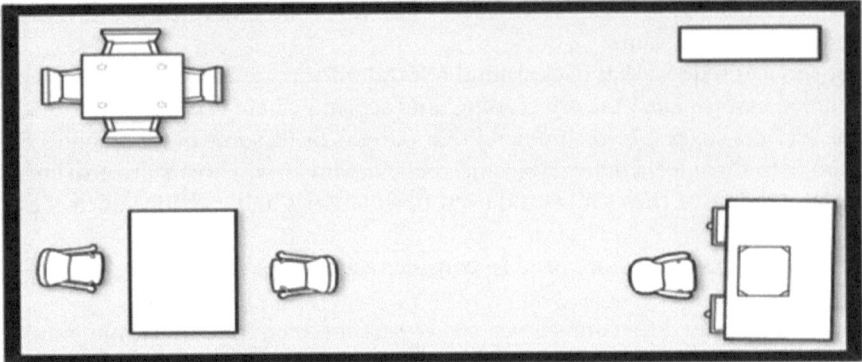

Figure 19.1 Suggested assessment room layout

- Some assessment rooms unfortunately are ill-equipped and unsuitable for assessing young children. They may have a clutter of desks, bookshelves, and filing cabinets. There may even be telephones and fax machines, which will invariably ring at an inopportune time during an assessment.
- Some assessment clinics include a formal reception area and waiting room, sometimes well-equipped with toys for little children and sometimes not.

Some issues to be considered include:

- Can a psychologist negotiate a more appropriate workspace for assessment if that provided is unacceptable?
- As a last resort, can assessments be conducted at a child's home or childcare centre?
- Can psychologists furnish their assessment room appropriately, from budgetary sources or "from home"?
- Is there a fair and equitable booking and priority system for any shared assessment space, for example a timetable?
- Is there sufficient storage space to temporarily relocate equipment needed only for assessments?

Equipment and toys

What toys and objects should be present in the assessment room over and above the equipment required for assessment? Young children are naturally drawn to toys to explore, manipulate, and play. This is to be encouraged provided they do not become a distraction to the formal developmental assessment. Letting a child play prior to formal assessment can give him/her time to acclimatise to the assessment room and become composed and happy. It also provides the psychologist the ideal opportunity to observe how a young child plays, both through their choice of toys and the way they use them.

Some young children like to help "pack away" when the time comes for formal assessment, and this can be an opportunity to observe a child's level of social cognition and maturity. Other children are less able to "help", and some may become fixated on certain toys or simply show age-appropriate reluctance to "give back". Developmental assessments are "social occasions", and every opportunity should be taken to observe social skills.

A skill for the psychologist to master is to divert children from such reluctance and "change the scene" for the formal assessment. Parents are usually skilled at "diversion", and a psychologist can learn from their strategies.

During formal assessment, some young children are more capable than others of ignoring extraneous toys and equipment and focusing on the formal assessment tasks. A psychologist needs to make instant judgements about these assessment variables and make appropriate arrangements. For example, some psychologists might store a range of toys in plastic containers or tubs, and bring these out or pack them away according to the "style" of the child at assessment.

Therefore:

- Selection of toys is developmentally important. Selections of toys can be stored in crates or tubs according to approximate developmental age levels and themes. One crate may, for example, contain simple cause-and-effect and exploratory toys such as pop-ups, blocks, Duplo materials, and other stacking or pushing toys. Another container may be for toys with more thematic and symbolic complexity, such as cars, trains, toy telephones, and animals. Yet another may have toys which require an understanding of thematic social role play, for example dolls, tea sets, and toy furniture. Young children have an innate ability to self-select toys according to developmental level and interest.
- Psychologists can note and record aspects of free play:
  - Functional play as opposed to stereotypic play.
  - Genuine "pretend" play rather than simple "modelled" play.
  - Social role play.
  - Thematic play, whether self-generated or imitated from sources such as cartoons or movies.
  - "Showing and sharing" play.
- As well as being a way to observe social maturity, helping to pack away also establishes a code of expected behaviour for the assessment. Packing away can be included in the "flow" of the assessment.

Scheduling

When is the optimum time to schedule an assessment? Some children are "at their best" early in the morning, some later. Some children can be slow to "get going", some others are easy. Some children have other morning commitments such as speech pathology. There are other family members to consider, such as another child who needs to be taken to school before the assessment.

Is there a young baby who is only minded by grandparents on certain days? Do parents need to negotiate certain days off? Are there days when only one parent can attend, even if both are eager to come?

Nowadays, both parents invariably work in order to pay the bills. They deal with traffic and transport delays, other family commitments to attend to or children to care for. It is sometimes impressive that families arrive at assessment at all! It is all the harder when a young child may have a developmental delay or disorder, anxiety or reluctance, or challenging behaviours. That they do arrive on time for assessment is testament to the value placed upon their child's well-being and their need for assessment. This commitment should be acknowledged, and assessments should be scheduled if possible for the parents' and child's benefit.

Psychologists may need to ponder:

- How flexibly can a service or Psychologist accommodate the needs of a family when scheduling an appointment? How early or late in the day can an assessment be scheduled?
- If there are only certain days when both parents can attend, can this be accommodated? Is there a rigid expectation that both parents will be present?
- If only one parent can attend, what arrangements can be made to meet with the other parent later to keep him/her fully informed of the assessment outcomes?
- Are childcare arrangements possible if a parent needs to bring a child's sibling?
- Can the service or psychologist provide a "letter of attendance" for parents if necessary for employers?
- Is the psychologist bound to a rigid "starting time" for assessments, or is there flexibility?
- Do families receive a reminder email or message prior to the assessment date?
- How many assessments per day or week is a psychologist scheduled to perform? Is this a reasonable expectation? Does it allow sufficient time for peer consultations, report writing, and parent follow-up meetings?
- If a service has a waiting room, is it well equipped with toys, reading material, or TV to keep the waiting period pleasant?
- How long do clients have to wait? Young children can easily become bored, anxious, or restless through prolonged waiting. They may also become tired or hungry. Such issues can adversely affect assessments. Minimum waiting periods should be the aim of any assessment service.

Bibliography

Aarons, M., and Gittens, T. (1992), The Autistic Continuum: An Assessment and Intervention Schedule for Investigating the Behaviours, Skills and Needs of Children with Autism or Autistic Spectrum Difficulties, NFR.

20 The assessment process

Let us imagine that a family and a young child have now arrived and are waiting. The psychologist has read all background material, read and scored psychometric background questionnaires, and the stage is set. When does an "assessment" actually commence? Is it when the child and family arrive, or the administration of the first subtest or test item? Is it in fact when referral information is received or returned? This will depend upon various factors, some of which relate directly to the original referral and background referral information, some to the psychologist's experience and clinical judgement, some to the immediate needs of parents, and a great deal to the initial demeanour of the child.

Background information

Background referral information informs psychologists about:

- Demographic information such as names, dates of birth, family members, contact details.
- Family "histories", for example the presence of developmental difficulties across generations.
- The child's birth and early developmental history, health concerns or serious illnesses, early developmental progression or regression, and early parental concerns.
- Early assessment history – hearing and vision, speech and language.
- Early or current paediatric assessments.
- Descriptions of behavioural, social and communication skills.

Such information should be received in advance to allow pre-reading and noting of "patterns of concerns". Background information informs the psychologist as to the type of assessment needed to be conducted, and the types of issues likely to be encountered. It also highlights any gaps in background information needing to be filled.

Questions and suggestions

- Does the psychologist or service request background information in a particular form? Do they use commercially available checklists, or do they collaborate and create "in-house" materials?
- Does background information include mobile phone video vignettes so that the psychologist can "meet" a young child in advance?
- When is background information used for formulating a "plan of action" for assessment?

DOI: 10.4324/9781003565338-25

Initial contact

Where does a psychologist first meet their family and young child? Is it in or near the carpark, or when they are in the waiting area and "checking in"? Does the family knock on the office door or ring the bell, or are they ushered into the assessment room by staff? "First impressions" are very important, and that applies both ways.

An assessment consultation can last 2 hours or more, and it is important to establish an appropriate relationship and rapport with families, so all involved can form an effective if temporary "team". This initial meeting phase is also an extremely valuable opportunity to observe the young child prior to formal assessment. Consider the following examples:

- **Child (a):** A family is in the waiting room. Their child happily and patiently sits, playing with the toys on offer. But the assessment does not start on time, as a team member is otherwise occupied, and the child becomes bored, irritated and fractious.
- **Child (b):** A family arrive and park their car, and the psychologist can observe that the child is anxious, clingy and reluctant to leave the car, let alone enter the assessment clinic. He/she is crying and holding close to his/her mother who is struggling to console the child.
- **Child (c):** Upon arrival, a child's parents are struggling to contain his/her behaviours. The child is continually breaking free from their grasp, running, climbing, exploring and hiding. Tubs of toys are noisily upended onto the floor in a random fashion, and no functional play is observed.
- **Child (d):** Upon arrival, a child immediately sits on the floor, and rocks backwards and forwards, making stereotypic sounds. Attempts to engage the child in play are unsuccessful, as the child shows no interest in these other than to mouth and bite them.

Each presentation is different but representative of the many and various scenarios which may confront a psychologist. There are an infinite variety of other "initial presentations", ranging from totally engaged and cooperative through to completely disengaged and disinterested, from happy and relaxed to distressed and highly anxious, from passive through to dangerously hyperactive. Knowing this in advance allows a psychologist to plan or replan their approach to assessment.

Questions

- How does the psychologist make use of these early observations? Are they, for example, informative for diagnostic purposes, or for test selection, or room preparation?
- How does the psychologist address these differing states of preparedness for assessment? Is there, for example, an urgency to commence assessment even when it is patently obvious that a child is not "ready"?
- How can a child's safety be ensured when he/she demonstrates a high degree of activity and disinhibited behaviour?
- How do a child's parents react when they realise their child is going to prove challenging to assess, and what can the psychologist do to ease any tensions and concerns?

Suggestions

Let us consider **child (a)**. How long should a family have to wait prior to an assessment commencing? How can assessments be scheduled and managed such that waiting times are at a minimum? It is appreciated that professionals can be extremely busy; however, young children do not respond well to long periods of inactivity such as waiting. Waiting periods should be as brief as possible, and suitable toys and stimulus material should be provided for the child whilst waiting. For example:

- It is almost universal nowadays that a parent will bring either an iPad or mobile phone for the entertainment of their child, but alternatively some waiting rooms include a TV monitor, which can run stimulus material such as cartoons.
- A range of suitable toys and equipment should be available in the waiting area.
- Perhaps the assessment should commence with those members of the assessment team who are ready and available, with any others entering the assessment room at a later stage. This is less than optimal, but is preferable to having a child wait for prolonged periods, become bored, anxious or distressed.

Child (b) is obviously very anxious, and children who are anxious do not simply "calm down" because they are asked to. Considerable patience is required whilst they work through their anxieties. Many young children presenting for assessment experience difficulties with "transitions" and entering the unfamiliar surroundings of a psychologist's office is an example. Helping such a child through a difficult transition period can be facilitated through:

- Giving the child as much space and time as necessary to settle in and regain composure. They may need to sit with their parents, but no immediate "performance pressure" needs to be placed upon them.
- This should include excessive "calming" by parents or psychologist. They can be left alone for a while, with one or two familiar or "easy" toys.
- The psychologist should observe signs of decreasing anxiety, for example reduced crying, voluntary separation from parents, and increased exploratory interest. Then, the psychologist might gradually introduce more toys and activities to the child and begin simple interactions and games.
- An intrinsic advantage of tests such as Griffiths III and Bayley-4 is their flexibility. Both have suggested starting points and order of item presentation, but they are not as pedantic as formal IQ tests can be. This inherent flexibility can be used to great advantage. For example, a psychologist may commence with tasks that are clearly too easy for the child, so that the child begins to engage, immediately experiences "success", and becomes increasingly confident and calm.
- It can often be best to start with non-verbal tasks requiring simple psychomotor abilities, for example stacking blocks, connecting Duplo materials, scribbling with a crayon or attempting simple puzzles. Children with speech and language delays do not appreciate excessive "language pressure" early in assessments. These tasks can be delayed until the child is ready to attempt these. Another approach can be to alternate verbal tasks and non-verbal tasks in quick rotation.

Child (c) raises the issues of safety and Duty of Care, and questions about the assessment process and setting.

- First and foremost, all psychologists have a "Duty of Care" over their clients. The safety and well-being of clients, particularly young children, is paramount in psychological practice. Duty of Care includes ensuring the physical safety of clients in assessment rooms.

- Assessment rooms should be lockable and safe during assessment, with no avenues to abscond. Furniture should be arranged to minimise dangerous climbing or jumping from heights.
- Psychologists working in private practice should hold public liability and malpractice insurance. Duty of Care considerations outweigh assessment completions.
- Parental involvement in challenging assessments takes on heightened significance. Parents and psychologist can "work as a team" to administer as many test items as possible, and to cross-reference parental knowledge of a child's skills. Parents may have specific behavioural support strategies for their children and may be called upon to administer test items under direction if necessary.

Child (d). This child clearly presents with significant developmental delays and even a developmental disorder. This assessment can be predicted to be complex, and again, a flexibility of approach will be necessary:

- If this child cannot be formally assessed, observations can still be made and "scored" through astute observations. This child will still demonstrate skills, even if these are at a basic level. They can be noted and scored from observation and reported accordingly as "observed".
- Both the Griffiths III and Bayley-4 provide normative data, which does not extend below the "moderate" range of developmental delay, and this child is more than likely to have a severe global developmental delay. "Downward-extrapolations" of developmental age equivalents are available for both tests but not recommended for use. It therefore becomes the responsibility of individual psychologists to make their own "clinical judgements" about whether a child may present with a "severe" or "profound" developmental disability.

These four examples reflect the varied scenarios and challenges a psychologist may encounter prior to or at the commencement of an assessment. Psychologists involved in early childhood assessments need to develop a flexible and adaptable approach to formal assessment, where pre-assessment expectations and plans can be changed or disrupted. Of course, there are children who present for assessment with no apparent behavioural or temperamental challenges, and who often enjoy the assessment experience because of its intrinsically motivating and rewarding nature and interesting tasks. But even when an assessment has started, things can change, the unexpected can occur and a presupposed assessment strategy will need to be re-evaluated "on the run".

During an assessment

An assessment has commenced. A young child and his/her parents are engaged, rapport has been established, base-level tasks have been attempted, and there is a clear plan ahead for completion of the assessment. What other issues can arise?

- A child may perform well on non-verbal and psychomotor tasks, particularly when they are easy and play-based. However, the child may react adversely when tasks become too difficult too quickly, for example when complex verbal expression tasks are introduced for a child with language delays.
- A child may fixate upon one particular activity, sometimes to the point of obsessionality. He/she may lack the ability to "move on" other tasks.

- A child may request parent help with various activities, particularly when they are too difficult to achieve easily.
- A child engaged in specific therapeutic programmes, such as applied behaviour analysis (ABA), may only complete tasks for a particular reward, or only if tasks are explained and demonstrated in a particular way.
- A child may fatigue quickly, lose concentration and interest, require food or a quick trip to the bathroom.
- A child who has thus far remained compliant, engaged and occupied, may become disengaged, leaving the table or desk and refusing to re-engage.
- A child who demonstrates signs of impulsivity and short attention may lose the ability to concentrate and become significantly distracted.
- Parents may wish to engage in the assessment tasks beyond a level deemed to be appropriate, perhaps attempting to help, re-explain and demonstrate "what to do", outside the allowable restrictions of test protocol.

Suggestions

Any suggestions made as to managing these issues are not intended to be prescriptive: They are to indicate that psychologists need to be creative, adaptable and resourceful when assessing young children. Some of the "solutions" to the issues raised hark back to the training and professional development psychologists have already undertaken, particularly on standardised assessments of child development such as the Griffiths III and the Bayley-4.

The Griffiths III and Bayley-4 tests require specific training, certification and guided usage immediately following this. Formal training magnifies what is already known about standardised tests and materials but emphasises additional "multi-tasking" skills required of test users. Reference is often made to the "75-25" theory of learning new tests: In the early phase of learning a new test, psychologists will give approximately 75% of their attention to the test protocol, materials and pass/fail criteria, but far less time to the child being assessed. Gradually over time, this ratio will change so that when "mastery" of the test is achieved, a psychologist will apply at least 75% of his/her concentration to the young child, as test administration becomes instinctive. The "probationary period" following formal training on either the Griffiths III, Bayley-4 or other "hands-on" tests comes with strong recommendations to facilitate this learning:

- There should be an initial focus upon engaging with and "enjoying" the child, rather than fixating too much upon "equipment and process".
- "Paired" assessments, with one psychologist conducting the assessment and the other assisting and recording responses, are strongly recommended. Initially, one psychologist should be experienced on the particular test, followed by paired assessments with two psychologists in "probation".
- Early assessment "practice" is recommended with children who perhaps do not need assessment, who are slightly older, and more likely to respond well to the assessment process.
- Filming or videoing test administrations and submitting these, along with scored protocols, for evaluation.
- Attending a follow-up evaluation day sometime after the formal training, to discuss any pertinent issues arising from the probationary period.

Griffiths III, Bayley-4 and ADOS-2 training is intense, and addresses some very important issues:

- The need to think flexibly and laterally during assessments, for example learning to "follow the lead" of the child and his/her behaviours and interests. This can mean deviating from any recommended "order of events" for item presentation, and instead "going with the flow".
- A thorough understanding of the toys and equipment from the tests, and an understanding that some equipment is used for more than one test item. Trainees from Griffiths and Bayley courses are often exposed to the "catchphrase: 'What else can I do with that?'", whilst particular toys and objects are in play. For example, blocks can be used to assess building towers, counting, making "trains" or packing away. If a child is interested in blocks, there are therefore a number of skills which can be assessed and observed in one sequence, rather than piecemeal.
- A central purpose of training on the Griffiths III or Bayley-4 is to educate psychologists about child development in general. Such knowledge can accelerate assessment through an understanding of "basal" and "ceiling" rules as applied to developmental assessments.
- For example, a psychologist may have a child attempt a task which is too easy for him/her just to establish a "basal" score, but if that item is too easy for the child because it represents an earlier stage of development, the child may technically "fail" that item. The skill being sought is no longer relevant to the child.
- Alternatively, knowing when a test item is inappropriate and unattainable by a young child because it is developmentally too advanced, can avoid pursuit of a meaningless test "ceiling", and frustrating the child by exposing them to "failure".

There are other issues to resolve along the road to "mastery" of developmental assessments:

- The decision needs to be made whether one parent or both remain present during assessments. Sometimes a parent will suggest that: "My child never performs as well at therapy when I am present". Often both can stay. Sometimes parents spontaneously organise a "division of labour" about "who should stay and who should go".
- Establishing a good working rapport with young children and their parents is vital. There is a clear benefit to having a well-organised room with a "meeting" area as well as the assessment area, so that issues such as parental involvement and explanation of the assessment process can be resolved.
- Parents like to reward their children for effort, and children enjoy rewards. There is more scope for rewarding and encouraging young children than with school-aged, and reward for early "success" can lead to sustained effort. Limits need to be drawn, however.
- For instance, parents may need to be dissuaded from excessively using food or unrealistically long-term rewards for motivation. It is generally best to work towards immediate social goals such as praise, particularly early in an assessment.
- Sometimes a child's ability to transition from a "free play" period to formal assessment is challenging. The child may wish to hold onto a particular toy, for example a car. A skilled practitioner may initially allow the toy to be near the child, perhaps on the desk, but to gradually "fade it out of the picture" by introducing other equipment and tasks.
- Not all children will be comfortable sitting at a child's desk or table, maybe due to age or reduced postural stability, or a desire to "move". A child may prefer to sit in a parent's lap or sit on the floor. It is important to judge whether sitting for long periods is a realistic expectation, or whether alternative solutions need to be found.

- Sometimes children will need a break for the toilet, or a quick snack or simply to move. Very young children may be unaware of their toileting needs or are not always reliable in their judgement. A short break is an opportunity for the psychologist to explore test items which require or allow parental response, such as self-help skills. A short break for any of these reasons is also an opportunity to judge whether a child can "reset" and return to table-and-task.
- Both the Griffiths III and Bayley-4 include gross motor tasks, which are traditionally administered towards the end of an assessment period. They involve many physical activities and are generally very enjoyable and exciting. If these tasks are attempted earlier in the assessment the young child may become too excited to settle to other tasks.
- The "75-25" theory is the basis for psychologists to note more than mere item "success". Passing an item provides only basic information. The "quality" of performance, whether successful or not, is equally important. Both the Griffiths III and Bayley-4 have clear scoring criteria and examples, but additional "qualitative information" can be derived from observing how skills were demonstrated and tasks attempted.
- For example, if assessing early drawing skills, did the child find it easy to grasp the crayon or pencil, or was the grip poorly formed and immature? Did the child exhibit any "associated movements" during the drawing task, such as restlessness or drooling?
- Parents, therapists and teachers appreciate "fine-grained" information of this nature for "benchmarking" current levels of skill and ongoing progress, particularly if this is subtle.
- Developmental assessments are often described as "social occasions" and include skills such as social greeting or farewelling. There is logic in attempting these items at the appropriate time during an assessment, for example waving "bye" when leaving, not on arrival or mid-assessment.
- A developmental assessment can be a long and tiring process for a young child, but also very exciting and unsettling. It is wise therefore to spend some time settling a young child down again before leaving the assessment room to go home.

Bibliography

American Psychological Association (2020), "Guidelines for Assessment of and Intervention with Persons with Disabilities", American Psychological Association, www.apa.org.

Australian Psychological Society (2018), "Australian Psychological Society Code of Ethics", Australian Psychological Society Website: www.psychology.org.au.

Bayley, N., and Aylward, G. P. (2020), Bayley-4: Bayley Scales of Infant and Toddler Development (4th Edition), Pearson Clinical.

British Psychological Society Code of Ethics and Conduct (2018), British Psychological Society Website, www.bps.org.uk.

British Psychological Society Division of Clinical Psychology, "Delivering Psychological Services for Children and Young People with Neurodevelopmental Difficulties and their Families".

Diemann, P., and Kasten-Koller, U. (2011), "Maternal Evaluations of Young Childrens' Developmental Status", Psychological Tests and Assessment Modelling, 53, pp 214–227.

Ellis, J., and Whaite, A. (1983), To Parents of Children with Disabilities, from Parents of Children with Disabilities, Social Evaluation and Research Ltd.

Stroud, L., Foxcroft, C., Green, E., Bloomfield, S., Cronje, J., Hurter, K., Lane, H., Marais, R., Marx, C., McAlinden, P., O'Connell, R., Paradice, R., and Venter, D. (2016), Griffiths III: Griffiths Scales of Child Development (3rd Edition), Technical Manual, Hogrefe Ltd.

21 "Driving" the test
The 75-25 rule and its application

The "75-25" rule generally pertains to the use of standardised assessment tools of child developmental milestones such as the Griffiths and Bayley Scales, where very young children are being assessed and there is a need for psychologists to allot as much of their attention to the child and his/her competency and engagement as possible (Figure 21.1). For new psychologists, this requires practice and increased competency as time passes. Young children cannot be left unsupported or disengaged for long periods, and thus, psychologists need to learn to expend most effort and concentration on the process of administering the assessment tasks:

- Knowing the materials and the protocol.
- Manipulating the test equipment, including stopwatch, and proformas.
- Remembering the precise or recommended order of tasks.
- Remembering basal and ceiling rules.
- Remembering and applying "pass/fail" criteria.

During this phase, the child receives less than optimal attention, which is why it is generally recommended that early practice be conducted on children who do not really need to be assessed, who are a little older or more mature, and who appreciate that in a sense they are "guinea pigs". As a practitioner's competence and confidence grows with a new test, less time needs to be devoted to the "mechanics" of the test, and more to the child involved. This facilitates increased opportunity for psychologists to focus upon other qualitative aspects of the assessment:

- The relationship with the child being assessed.
- The child's ability to concentrate and attend.

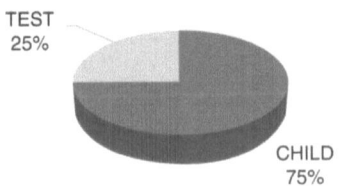

Figure 21.1 The "75%-25%" rule of assessment

DOI: 10.4324/9781003565338-26

- The child's demeanour.
- The child's ability to work to his/her best capacity for prolonged periods.
- The child's ability to learn, generalise and apply different problem-solving strategies across different types of tasks.
- The quality of a child's performance on tasks, whether passed or failed.

Understanding this "75-25" rule is most important for mastering the art of assessing very young children through a rapid period of development, from "toddler" age through to late preschool. Young children are less able to maintain concentration and task orientation skills. They need more support, prompting, encouragement and rewarding to remain on-task.

This is very difficult to achieve when assessing the psychologist's attention is predominantly focused on the test. They will not necessarily "wait" for the psychologist to sort out the test logistics. It is for this reason that Griffiths III, Bayley-4 and ADOS-2 training courses strongly recommend "paired" practice for as long is required to gain sufficient competency to assess alone. Griffiths III, Bayley-4 and ASOS-2 training procedures stipulate evidence of such competencies, including where appropriate video evidence of skills acquisition and mastery. From then on, the psychologist is "licenced" and can genuinely begin to "drive the test".

What information do developmental assessments derive?

Standardised developmental tests provide considerable statistical information:

- Developmental quotients.
- Developmental age equivalents.
- Standard scores and Z scores.
- Percentile ranks.
- Stanines.

Some of these can be reported as "absolutes" and others in "confidence intervals" based on standard deviations and standard errors of measurement. These metrics can be presented through various histograms: Bar graphs, line graphs, pie charts, coloured or monochrome. Some of this data is necessary for "systemic" purposes such as bureaucratic needs, or for research purposes. But there is another dimension of analysis to be elicited, and this is dependent upon the psychologist's ability to observe what the child actually did during an assessment.

Developmental tests are predicated upon a child "climbing the developmental ladder": Trying, failing, learning, practising, mastering, consolidating and applying new skills. Having achieved mastery of one particular skill, he/she moves on to conquering the next, often abandoning or "casting off" acquired skills that are no longer required. And this process occurs across the five subscales inherent in both the Griffiths III and Bayley-4 tests.

Child development is not linear. There are rapid phases of development in some areas followed by periods of consolidation and refinement. There are skills which are only required for a short time, such as "reflex" skills in early infancy, which then become purposeful action. There are transitions from core skills to applied skills, for example "grasp and release" skills, which children learn and then eventually apply to meaningful and productive activity with toys, utensils, clothes and academic tools.

There are early learning skills which shift from "concrete" tasks to abstract and conceptual thinking. There is the development of social cognition from expressing basic needs to developing friendships, theory of mind and social responsibility. Developmental tests are carefully crafted to organise these sequences of development into a coherent hierarchy of item classification and order.

Both Doctor Ruth Griffiths and Doctor Nancy Bayley achieved impressive "item placement" accuracy without technological aids such as computers or calculators. Both were diligent observers of play and development. They both judged with remarkable accuracy the timing, acquisition and mastery of skills, using strict "pass/fail" criteria, which has proven valid over decades. Observation was the key to this achievement.

That developmental tests such as Griffiths III and Bayley-4 do not possess a high degree of predictive validity is not a failure but a function of the reality of child development – it is not a uniform or linear process. A common experience for psychologists conducting developmental assessments is to hear that an item "failed" on the day of assessment was suddenly "mastered" only a few days or weeks later. There are also occasions when a child demonstrates skills at assessment which parents have never previously seen. This brings into focus two very important issues:

- How a child achieves a "pass" or a "fail" on an assessment task is best described as a "qualitative" issue".
- Children frequently demonstrate "emerging skills" at assessment. A skill may not be quite within their reach at assessment but may soon appear.

This is germane to "driving" a test: Looking beyond "passing" or "failing" and considering what is actually happening as a function of development.

Emerging skills

Let us consider some. For both Griffiths III and Bayley-4, there are gross motor tasks such as observing whether children can jump at floor level, deliberately coordinating their movements to facilitate a brief "airborne phase", often accompanied by associated arm movements. Prior to "success" on this item, parents and psychologists will observe a child's strenuous efforts to jump-squatting, puffing up chest, springing on legs and feet, but never quite attaining "flight".

The child's intention is very clear-he/she wants to jump but lacks the strength and co-ordination to achieve "take-off". The skill is "emerging" and will probably be mastered soon after the assessment. There are many similar examples:

- Being "almost ready" to rise from kneeling to standing, without using hands on the floor for assistance.
- Imitating circular scribble, but not quite a "round and stop" circle.
- Holding a cube in each hand, dropping one in order to accept a third, but not holding all three at once.
- Imitating one's first name, but not yet stating it in response to a question.
- Indicating some awareness of toileting needs through physical movements, but not being able to state what is needed.
- Naming toys and pictures when shown, but not consistently defining these by use.
- Placing different sized circles into a circle board, but only if the pieces are next to the appropriate holes.

- Tracing over a letter or number, but not imitating it.
- Counting orally, but not coordinated with finger pointing.
- Self-calming skills evident, but not being able to prevent a tantrum when thwarted.
- Using personal pronouns such as "he/she", but not always appropriately.
- Attempting to hold scissors and cut, but eventually tearing the paper in frustration.
- Trying to self-dress with a T shirt but becoming "stuck".
- Trying to pedal a tricycle but moving "backwards".

It is gratifying to note that the Bayley-4 includes codings for "emerging skills", rather than applying a simple "pass/fail" criterion to tasks. The significance of "emergence" lies in how a psychologist conceptualises "pass or fail" events and report them to parents, medical practitioners and therapists. Developmental tests are hierarchical in structure. Test items are "age and stage"-related and become increasingly more difficult. A "failure" is not necessarily an indication of a "problem". Psychologists need to differentiate between a child's chronic inability to perform certain developmental tasks rather than simply not being "ready".

"Benchmarking" emerging skills serves other functions, for example reviewing children after a time lapse, it is easier to determine the best "starting levels" for re-assessment. Developmental tests allow for test-retest interval as short as 6 months, and progress noted to occur during that interval should be positively reported. A lack of progress is a point for clinical consideration and discussion. Parents can nowadays keep psychologists updated as to progress through on-line media or mobile phone vignettes for instant feedback and discussion.

Qualitative aspects of developmental skills

The "75%-25%" formula is at its most relevant when psychologists consider through observation how a child achieves "success" or "pass/fail" on test items. This is a skill which develops over time with practice and illustrates the advantage of "paired" assessments in the early phase of test usage. One psychologist may be tasked with undertaking the assessment, but the second may be very useful in making and recording qualitative observations for later discussion. Some assessment clinics are equipped with recording and playback facilities, which provide excellent training and professional development opportunities.

A young child may "pass" certain test items, but the manner in which they do so may be more important to the understanding of their medical or therapeutic needs, programme selection, or concern for other as yet undiagnosed difficulties. "Passing" or "failing" test items is only one way to elicit information about possible developmental delays and difficulties. Below, two hypothetical children of the same age are compared on a number of developmental tasks. Each child in fact "passes" the relevant test items, but there are obvious differences in the ease and quality by which they do so (Table 21.1):

What are the implications of the qualitative aspects to child 2's performance for:

- Item scoring.
- Feedback to parents.
- Diagnostic considerations.
- Reporting.
- Recommendation for possible further assessment.
- Coordination with therapists, teaching/learning programmes.

Table 21.1 Qualitative descriptions of test items passed

Task	Child 1	Child 2
DRAWS A CIRCLE	Sits still, good posture, draws neat circle, good "tripod" pencil grip	Restless. Unable to maintain posture. Immature grip, excessive downward pressure, "associated movements" such as tongue thrust, but draws a circle
INSERTS PUZZLE PIECES	Places pieces quickly and accurately, works methodically, uses good pincer grip, responds positively to "time challenge"	Attempt to push pieces with palm of hand, finds it difficult to orientate pieces, struggles to develop learning schema such as matching, but inserts pieces
THREADS BEADS	Calmly and methodically threads beads onto string. Adapts strategies "on the run". No associated movements. Enjoys pretend nature of task	Fails to find alternate strategies as task becomes complex. Restless and reluctant, needs parental assistance. But threads beads. Laboured breathing and effort required
MOVEMENT SKILLS	Engages well in coordinated physical movements such as throwing and catching. Minimal clumsiness	Loses balance and falls over. Trips over furniture. Attempts tasks but clumsy. Becomes overactive
SPEAKS IN 5-WORD SENTENCES	Speaks in clear and lucid five-word sentences with correct grammar	Speaks in five-word sentences, but dysfluency and difficulty with words order evident
GREETS, ENGAGES SOCIALLY, AND FAREWELLS	States first name spontaneously, responds to simple questions, waves goodbye at conclusion, all without prompting	Requires prompting and modelling to greet and farewell. Little response to questions, requests and social overtures
EATS SEMI-INDEPENDENTLY	Clearly understands eating utensils and uses these appropriately	Finger-feeds and requires assistance with cups, spoons and general cleanliness. Messy eater
COUNTS BLOCKS	Counts with coordinated verbal and finger-pointing skills. Conserves quantity	Finger-counts and speaks numbers, but not coordinated. Omits individual numbers. Unable to conserve value

These relatively straightforward examples raise another key issue related to item placement in developmental tests. It is the notion that a child can "fall between" test items. Try as they might to be "fine-grained", developmental assessments can only include a finite number of test items, and that can mean that progression from one level of skills to the next might not be achievable during the test-retest interval. But this does not necessarily mean that "progress" has not been made. For example, at a subsequent re-assessment, "child 2" may not have made sufficient gains to pass the next test item in a particular sequence but may find it easier to reach the same level of performance. He/she may for example still have limited verbal expression, but there is more fluency, clarity, spontaneity and accuracy than previously. In short, "passing" or "failing" test items is only a part of the purpose of developmental assessment. Qualitative aspects of a child's efforts on test items are equally important. Below is an example of how this quantitative/qualitative dichotomy may be described in a subsequent report (Table 21.2):

Table 21.2 Pass/fail and qualitative descriptions of item attempts

Pass/fail:
"Jill successfully completed a three piece and a six piece insert puzzle within the requisite time limits. She was unable to complete an 11-piece puzzle. These were at an approximate three year developmental age level."

Qualitative:
"Jill tried a number of insert puzzles. Although she was able to insert circles, triangles and square shapes into the appropriate holes when these pieces were aligned to the holes, she found it difficult to generalise a problem-solving strategy. She looked to her mother and suggest that she help her. With smaller puzzle pieces such as those associated with a six-piece puzzle, she found it difficult to insert pieces with irregular shapes, particularly triangles, diamonds and squares. It was also noted during this task that Jill did not consistently use a mature pincer grip to grasp and release the puzzle pieces. Instead, she tended to push the pieces in with the palm of her hand, and the resultant difficulty caused her obvious frustration."

Achieving a "75%-25%" ratio comes with repeated and either paired or supervised practice, and teamwork is required for maximum benefit. A colleague or supervisor may ask: "What else can you do with that equipment now the child is engaged with it"? This can help the "flow" of an assessment, avoiding the need to search for the next piece of equipment. The "paired Psychologist" may act as "hander upper" of equipment or may time relevant timed tasks. He/she may distract and amuse a child whilst the assessing psychologist gathers his/her thoughts and equipment for the next task. A trained and experienced "helper" may suggest alternative strategies to help maintain a child's engagement and reassure the parents present that "all is well".

This "paired" learning process should also extend to scoring the test upon completion, to clarify specific item "pass/fail" criteria, to indicate if any items were accidentally omitted or forgotten, and to confirm mathematical accuracy. There is a great deal to learn and practise before mastery is achieved. It is no disgrace to have to serve an apprenticeship!

Special circumstances and adaptations

Developmental assessments already assume the need for flexibility and adaptability of administration by virtue of their applicability to very young children, particularly with developmental delays and disorders. But even within that framework, there are other "special circumstances", which need to be addressed so that children can be assessed. These relate to two sets of circumstances:

- Language and communication differences, for example the use of interpreters when families speak a language other than English.
- Service access difficulties, for example rural and remote families who cannot physically access assessment and diagnostic services.

The one agency which clarifies "what to do" under such circumstances is the American Psychological Association, through its **"Guidelines for assessing individuals with disabilities"**. Three specific guidelines are relevant to these considerations (Table 21.3):

How can these guidelines be applied in clinical settings? Let us take the following examples.

Table 21.3 American Psychological Association test adaptation guidelines

- **Guideline 14:** Depending on the context and goals of assessment and testing, psychologists strive to apply the assessment approach that is most psychometrically sound, fair, comprehensive and appropriate for clients with disabilities.
- **Guideline 15:** Psychologists strive to determine whether accommodations are appropriate for clients to yield a valid test score.
- **Guideline 16:** Consistent with the goals of the assessment and disability-related barriers to assessment, psychologists in clinical settings strive to appropriately balance quantitative, qualitative and ecological perspectives, and articulate both the strengths and limitations of assessment.

The use of interpreters

Countries across the world are becoming increasingly multicultural in makeup, with people from many different cultural and linguistic backgrounds, and it is inevitable that some assessments will be made more complex by the lack of commonality of language between child, family and psychologist:

- A family may indicate that their child does not speak English but does possess vocabulary from another language.
- Or, although the child may not speak much at all, he/she may comprehend better in one language or another.
- Or, a family may feel their own familiarity with English is still developing and they would be more comfortable if interpreter services were available.

There are solutions to these situations:

- Some government-provided assessment services such as children's hospitals or assessment clinics can arrange for interpreter services to be made available.
- Some parents may bring a friend or relative who can act as interpreter.
- Interpreters can be hired, but this can be expensive for psychologists in small private practices.
- There is a difference between using interpreter services for communicating with parents and assessing the abilities of young children.

Let us consider some examples:

Scenario 1: A young child is described as being able to name toys and pictures in a language other than English. This child is so young that only single-word responses are to be expected at best. If the child is shown a toy and utters a word in his/her home language, can we ask the parents: "What did he/she say?"

- Different languages do not necessarily "line up" as simply as that. Different languages may describe and categorise objects and pictures differently. What appears to be a "label word" (e.g., car) may in fact be an action word, for example "drive". Does this invalidate the test item and its response?
- Questions posed in one language may not have exactly the same imperative as they would in English. "What is this?" when asked in English may translate as "say car for me" in another language.

- Different languages can have different grammatical structures, so a language task requiring the correct use of pronouns or grammatical terms may be hard to assess as there may not be an exact equivalent in another language.
- Speech pathologists often refer to language development through "mean length of utterance", meaning how many syllables are strung together. A string of five syllables may not equate to five words in English, but perhaps in another language it does.

Scenario 2: At a post-assessment feedback discussion, important diagnostic information needs to be communicated to a family, but one parent has greater facility with English than the other. Does the psychologist use that parent as the "interpreter", assuming an accurate translation of information? If it is a family friend or relation who is translating, can the psychologist be sure of accurate and literal interpretation of what is being conveyed?

Scenario 3: A professional interpreter is assisting an assessment service. After the assessment, the psychologist indicates the need to discuss and explain findings to the child's family. The interpreter indicates that the parents have only restricted understanding of the assessment process, and that the psychologist's language and terminology is inconsistent with and perhaps absent from the dialect of the family in question. For example:

- There is not an equivalent concept to autism spectrum disorder in the family's language background.
- Or, in describing a developmental delay, the family interpret this as if it is a "disease" which will need a specific "cure".

Working through interpreter services can be challenging but satisfying. Some suggestions to maximise the effectiveness of professional interpreter services or other "third party" translators include:

- Meeting with the interpreter prior to the assessment or interview to discuss and agree upon the most appropriate "modus operandi". For example:
  - Explaining in detail the reason for the assessment or interview, the types of assessments to be undertaken and the possible issues to be discussed.
  - Whether the translator translates one sentence or phrase at a time or can translate simultaneously.
  - Confirming whether the interpreter can clearly phrase the intent of the assessment in the family's home language, or if particular idioms need to be utilised or avoided.
  - Whether the interpreter is aware of any cultural beliefs or attitudes, which may need to be addressed during assessment to facilitate effective communication.

Assessing and interviewing through interpreter services is a reality that many psychologists face frequently. It is a skill which improves through practice, care and attention. Skills such as maintaining eye contact with the family, speaking directly with them and listening directly to them even when the interpreter is speaking, may feel counterintuitive at first, but the family are there to communicate with the Psychologist and not the interpreter. When parents translate the words of their children, this fact should be highlighted in subsequent reports to provide accurate commentary as to the conditions of the assessment.

The use of signing and communication devices

Non-verbal children can access communication devices to substitute for the spoken word. This frequently occurs when speech pathologists consider the use of augmentative non-verbal communication systems essential to a young child's therapeutic programme.

Some children may be taught signing language such as (in Australia) Auslan so that they can communicate basic needs such as "more", "drink", "finished" or "toilet". For some children, signing becomes their primary language, for example children with significant hearing and speech impairments.

For other children, augmentative communication devices and programmes are more suitable, for example Boardmaker, Proloqo2go or Lamp Words for Life. These programmes allow children to indicate their needs and engage in communication through use of pictures or icons. Children with autism spectrum disorder are often assisted through these methods, sometimes as an intermediary step towards the development of spoken language, and sometimes as their "primary" language. Intervention programmes for children with autism spectrum disorder often have as their primary objective the development of a "portable" augmentative communication system, with an increasing emphasis upon technology as "signing" per se can be restrictive in its utility because the broader community is not familiar with its "vocabulary".

As with language translated through interpreters, psychologists need to judge whether communication from a child through devices or signing carries the same "communicative intent" as the spoken word. Examples such as whether a sign or computer-generated symbol represents the name of a toy, or its action, are the most common clinical decisions to be made in assessments. Clinical judgement is the preserve and responsibility of the psychologist "in the room". Reference to the American Psychological guidelines listed above should help assuage concern about such professional and ethical decisions.

Observing children "off-site"

How naturalistic is an assessment clinic or a psychologist's office? Is it always the best place to observe young children and undertake assessments? Certainly, an assessment clinic is a "controlled environment" and most ideal for standardised assessments. There are few distractions, and the psychologist can manage their assessment setting to suit their clients. But sometimes, it is advantageous to leave one's office and observe young children in more naturalistic circumstances.

Young children invariably attend childcare centres, long day care centres, nursery schools or preschools. Here, they interact with other children, follow the dictates of adults in authority and adapt to environments and routines not replicable in clinical settings. Questionnaire-based assessments of adaptive behaviour skills attempt to quantify these experiences, but discrepant information can result. Observational visits to preschool and childcare centres can unearth a wealth of information about a child's "real world" adaptive behaviours and skills. Maximising the time spent in such observations is not complex:

- Arriving early at a preschool allows observation of a child's ability to separate from parents, and how "drop-off" is best managed.
- Young children generally enjoy free play upon arrival, inside or outside. This is an opportunity to observe their choices:
  - Does the child spontaneously follow organisational routines such as unpacking his/her bag and placing it in the relevant place?
  - Is the child able to self-direct towards chosen activities, or is he/she dependent upon adult guidance?
  - Does the child have a favourite place to go, for example the sandpit?
  - Is there evidence of functional or symbolic play, or a notable absence of these?
  - Does the child engage with other children, or remain isolated?

- Preschools and childcare centres provide many examples of "transitions". For example, there is the move to "morning circle", where songs are sung, names called out and the role marked. This provides opportunity to observe:
  - The ease with which a child makes transitions.
  - A child's ability to sit within a group without adult support.
  - Social response such as responding to the call of name in roll call.
  - Engage in early morning "settling" activities such as singing songs, particularly when these involve "actions".
  - Further transition to specific activities or free play.
- Preschools provide a rich variety of activities, toys and games for children:
  - Does the child engage in play with other children, imitating, turn-taking, cooperating and jointly problem-solving?
  - Does he/she retreat to one specific activity or toy? Do preschool teachers confirm a limited repertoire of play and interest?
  - Does the child merely self-stimulate with certain objects or pieces of equipment?
  - Does the child "sample" various activities?
- Preschool routines often include formal sit-down morning tea:
  - Does a child follow known and practised rules for this?
  - Can the child eat with simple utensils, or finger-feed?
  - Does social interaction and communication occur during this morning tea?
  - After morning tea, is the child independent in toileting and self-care?
- Activities such as "big book" are part and parcel of preschool programmes:
  - Can the child able sit and remain transfixed by stories, or does his/her attention wander?
  - Does he/she comment upon stories and pictures, or does he/she appear bemused by the content?
- There may be examples of developing relationships and friendships in preschool:
  - Is the child beginning to make social connections and relationships, or is he/she remote from other children?
  - Does the child demonstrate emerging social communication skills, such as sharing, negotiating and cooperating? How does the child negotiate having a toy taken from him/her, or how does he/she request one from another child?
  - Is the child developing emotional regulation and self-calming skills when things do not go his/her way?
  - Does the child possess awareness of personal space?

Childcare and preschool visits also afford the opportunity to discuss young children with teachers and caregivers. These personnel are intimately involved with the daily lives of their children. The quality and depth of their observations of their young children is extremely valuable. Childcare centres and preschools can photograph and video events that occurred during the day to keep parents informed of their child's daily activities. This can be another source of invaluable information.

Visits to childcare centres and preschools also facilitate discussion about the types of support services available, and whether these can be provided on the basis of a psychologist's report. Some preschools have close professional relationships with speech pathologists and occupational therapists, even allowing them to work on-site. This is another opportunity for psychologists to liaise with relevant professionals. Preschool and childcare visits are not mandatory for psychologists, but it is important to stress the benefits which can flow from them.

Observing children on mobile phone video

Psychologists increasingly request mobile phone video vignettes of young children prior to assessment. Parents are usually happy to provide such footage, and many do so as a matter of course. Useful information can be gleaned from such footage:

- Evidence of behaviours causing concern, for example stereotypic movement patterns, or behavioural tantrums.
- A young child in play, demonstrating the toys, equipment and interests a child may have, and the "quality" of play.
- Social interactions, often those occurring with a child's siblings or cousins.
- Behaviours associated with change of or interruption to routines and activities.
- Language and communication samples.
- Evidence of maladaptive behaviours such as possible convulsive activity or self-harm.
- Response to call of name, requests and social overtures from parents.

Parents often collate "libraries" of these behaviours and skills over time, recording on-going progress or areas of concern. Parents can also video therapy sessions with permission, both as a learning strategy to apply therapeutic techniques at home and as a marker of progress or difficulty. Videos of behavioural sequences at preschools and childcare centres can be hard to obtain due to privacy concerns and restrictions.

In recent years, mobile phone videos have also aided the medical professions. Whereas paediatricians and neurologists may have been traditionally "evidenced-based" about certain behaviours, they are now more amenable to considering video examples of concerning behaviours, rather than relying solely upon parental report or "direct evidence" of issues, which may or may not occur in a Doctor's surgery. Video examples of the "lead-up" to behavioural outbursts can be enlightening by highlighting the antecedents of such episodes, the course of the outburst, and the possible intended or unintended consequences. Even possible epileptic convulsions can be evidenced in this matter. This helps bring the "real-world" to a professional's office.

Bibliography

American Psychological Association (2020), "Guidelines for Assessment of and Intervention with Persons with Disabilities", https://www.apa.org/pi/disability/resources/assessment-disabilities.

Bayley, N., and Aylward, G. P. (2020), Bayley-4: Bayley Scales of Infant and Toddler Development (4th Edition), Pearson Clinical.

British Psychological Society (2018), Code of Ethics and Conduct, https://www.bps.org.uk/.

British Psychological Society Division of Clinical Psychology, "Delivering Psychological Services for Children and Young People with Neurodevelopmental Difficulties and their Families", https://www.bps.org.uk/.

Ellis, J., and Whaite, A. (1983), To Parents of Children with Disabilities, from Parents of Children with Disabilities, Social Evaluation and Research Ltd.

22 Remote and online assessments

Not all client families have immediate access to specialist developmental clinics or assessment services. They may reside in rural and remote locations in small towns or villages, farms or mining sites. The nearest available services may be great distances away, with extended waiting lists and little by way of immediate follow-up or feedback. Visits from these services are often sporadic. Much is made of the "tyranny of distance" in countries such as Australia, but as romantic as this can be portrayed, remote families are placed at a considerable disadvantage.

In the "commercial" world and in politics, online video and streaming services such as Skype, Teams and Zoom play an increasingly important role in allowing communication and contact, and this is extending to online medical services. Video and live streaming are used more often to observe young children, interview their families and come to diagnostic decisions where appropriate. These procedures became increasingly important and advantageous during the COVID-19 epidemic which started in 2020, changing the world irrevocably.

Countries went into "lockdown", and "social distancing" became the new norm. Suddenly, "working from home" became the only feasible way to conduct one's employment, profession or trade. Amongst the hardest hit by the various restrictions were professionals working with young children's teachers, childcare personnel, doctors and nurses, and of course psychologists and other allied health workers and therapists engaged in young children requiring assessment and treatment.

How did they meet these unforeseen challenges and continue their professional responsibilities in these unforeseen and "unprecedented" changes of circumstances? Firstly, "telehealth" systems were created to facilitate online mental health consultations with doctors and psychologists, and the success of these methods was soon selectively transferred to the field of developmental and diagnostic assessments of young children such as assessments and diagnoses of conditions such as autism spectrum disorder and global developmental delay.

New protocols and adapted methodologies were developed to maximise the efficacy of online assessments, and these were, in the main, found to be satisfactory and successful. One well-documented example was the Australian Psychological Society guidelines for conducting clinical neuropsychological assessments:

1 Determine your reason for referral and to what extent the referral is "high stakes".
2 Determine your comfort level with the limitations associated with using telehealth for neuropsychological assessment (versus alternatives).
3 Determine the suitability of a telehealth assessment in terms of practicality.
4 Determine your response for referrers and clients.
5 Consider broader professional issues.

Secondly and very much at odds with the tightly controlled protection of copyright of published products, some assessment tools were modified to allow for materials such as checklists, and even toys and puzzles, to be sent to parents in order that they could administer certain subtests and tasks under the online supervision of psychologists. For example, the Association for Research in Infant and Child Development (ARICD), the custodians of the Griffiths III, released new resources and stated the following:

> The ARICD wishes to support practitioners in their professional roles during the Covid-19 pandemic and are putting together a Griffiths III telepractice assessment format to ensure that practitioners do not infringe the copyright. Meanwhile, these points may be helpful for practitioners to consider: Practitioners should follow the advice of the country where they work and of their professional bodies in regard to social distancing and alternative methods of consultation, assessment, and treatment.
>
> If assessment using Griffiths III cannot be completed in the normal standardised procedure, the scales may be used as a tool to obtain qualitative and/or quantitative information about the child's developmental strengths and weaknesses.

These modifications and adaptations were consistent with the guidelines of the American Psychological Association (APA) in reference to assessments of children with disabilities:

> **APA Guideline 14**: *Depending on the context and goals of assessment and testing, strive to apply the assessment approach that is most psychometrically sound, fair, comprehensive, and appropriate.*
> **APA Guideline 15**: *Strive to determine whether accommodations are appropriate to yield a valid test score.*
> **APA Guideline 16**: *Strive to appropriately balance quantitative, qualitative and ecological perspectives, and articulate both the strengths and limitations of assessment.*

Psychologists who utilised these assessment protocols and strategies quickly learned that some assessment tools were more readily adapted to these techniques than others, and traditional allegiances to some tests were challenged in favour of others. They found it surprisingly easy to provide ongoing feedback around the nature of behaviours observed online and to comment upon behaviours they were noting in the child, sometimes not noted by parents. This allowed the exploration of behaviours possibly associated with global developmental delay or autism spectrum disorder.

Nothing emphasised this new-found sense of flexibility and creativity in the normally "rigid" psychometric world than an ARICD Educational Meeting in October 2020 with the theme "Innovative Ways of Using the Griffiths III", including a review of the "Experience of Using Remote Developmental Assessment."

It is not easy to "assess" a child remotely, but creative adaptations can be made and already exist in some circumstances. Working online with families to demonstrate a child's skills or difficulties is merely an extension of procedures from, for example, the ASQ-3. Specific skills and behaviours can be explained, demonstrated and taught remotely to families so that observations of a young child can be made. In-depth interviews such as adaptive behaviour assessments can be conducted online.

Reporting results from these "adapted" assessments may need to be more carefully worded to allow for these accommodations, and diagnostic decisions may need to be more cautious or conditional, but these restrictions far outweigh the consequences of "no service". Living in rural or remote locations should not impose an unfair "barrier" upon families in such need. A core philosophical aim of any disability-related service is to remove such barriers. It is not suggested that technology-based assessments of young children should become "the new norm", as they are not as accurate or effective as face-to-face interactive assessments. But it should never be too early, too late or too hard to learn and adapt new methods.

Bibliography

American Psychological Association (2020), "Guidelines for Assessment of and Intervention with Persons with Disabilities", American Psychological Association, Association for Research in Infant and Child Development, www.aricd.ac.uk.

Association for Infant and Child Development (ARICD Statements, Use of Griffiths III by means of Zoom, Skype or other means of telehealth services during COVID-19, including Parental Questionnaire and Guidelines, June and July 2020, and Education Meeting Agenda for 9 October 2020. Association for Research in Infant and Child Development, www.aricd.ac.uk

Australian Psychological Society (2007), "Australian Psychological Society Code of Ethics" www.psychology.org.au.

Australian Psychological Society (2020), Guidelines for the Use of Telehealth for Clinical Neuropsychological Services, https://psychology.org.au/.

Katakis, P., et al. (2023), "Diagnostic Assessment of Autism in Children using Telehealth in a Global Context: A Systematic Review", Journal of Autism and Developmental Disorders.

23 Scoring developmental tests

Scoring developmental tests is not as simple as with other assessments. Developmental assessments using measures such as Bayley-4, Griffiths III and Autism Diagnostic Observation Schedule 2 (particularly Modules 1 and 2) are very "busy" occasions. They are for young children with differing degrees of engagement, compliance, activity levels, language and concentration. There are many toys and objects involved, and the order of item presentation is not necessarily as preordained as would be the case in a standardised assessment of intellectual abilities with an older, school-aged child. Developmental assessments can be fun, taxing, organised or frenetic, depending upon circumstances.

In the "post-training" period when a psychologist is just starting out with such tests, it is therefore difficult to keep track of all the items administered, and some may be inadvertently omitted. This is when "tandem" post-training assessments are of immense benefit, working as a team to ensure that all relevant items are in fact attempted or a record of those missed is kept. Then there is the process of checking task completion against what can be complex scoring criteria to ensure accuracy, followed by double-checking basal and ceiling requirements. This shared process is also an opportunity for "debriefing" about the assessment process. Scoring and debriefing should take place without parents, perhaps after a short break. Scoring should be conducted slowly and carefully:

Questions and suggestions

- Check and cross-check all the items attempted and completed. Were any items accidentally omitted? If so, be aware of the scoring and reporting conventions for such omissions.
- Refer to the user's manual for specific item administration instructions, scoring and "pass/fail" criteria and basal and ceiling rules. This particularly applies when pass criteria relate to different "stages" of mastery which may apply, for example, to early drawing skills.
- Clarify item administration protocols. Any doubtful administrations or interpretations can be set aside for discussion and review.
- If two psychologists are working "in tandem", discuss scoring criteria and reach a consensus about the final interpretation and scoring.
- Check demographic details, particularly dates of birth and chronological ages. Chronological age conventions are detailed in developmental tests, particularly the process of "rounding up", and allowing for cases of premature birth.
- Calculate all relevant scores: Raw scores, scale scores, developmental quotients and developmental age equivalents. Use a calculator to ensure accuracy.

- Determine appropriate "scoring ranges", for example, a developmental age range of ±3 months depending on chronological age.
- Notate any specific issues for immediate feedback to parents. Complete relevant graphic representations of scores, for example, histograms.
- Compile notes describing qualitative performance observations such as the child's behaviour at assessment, approach to tasks, and levels of concentration.
- Flag-specific recommendations and courses of action to be taken, so they will not be accidentally omitted from feedback discussions and final reports.

Care and maintenance of test equipment

As scoring a developmental assessment generally takes place soon after completing an assessment, it is a convenient time to also "pack away" the equipment. It is also an opportunity to do "scheduled maintenance". Developmental assessment test kits for very young children, by definition, comprise toys and items of interest to young children. They are played with (sometimes gently, sometimes not), hit against each other, thrown, sucked, licked and mouthed. Sometimes toys break, and sometimes they mysteriously vanish and escape the assessment room or are hidden in the most unlikely places. It is prudent therefore to maintain a stock of spare toys and objects as near as possible to equivalence with those supplied with specific tests such as Griffiths III or Bayley-4. Cars, dolls, trains, blocks, toy animals, toy scissors and the like are easily sourced and relatively cheap.

A matter of serious concern however is the maintenance of cleanliness with test materials. Cytomegalovirus (CMV) is a common virus. Once infected, the body retains the virus for life. Most people do not even know they have the virus because it rarely causes problems in healthy people. CMV spreads from person to person through body fluids, such as blood, saliva, urine, semen and breast milk. There is no cure, but there are medications that can help treat the symptoms. Babies and young children are inclined to mouth, lick and suck toys such as those in test kits, and it is a wise practice to clean all test materials regularly with disinfectant.

This precaution is particularly important for pregnant women or people with compromised immune systems. Women who develop an active CMV infection during pregnancy can pass the virus to their babies, who might then experience symptoms. CMV is a known contributing factor in the causation of disabilities such as cerebral palsy. For people who have weakened immune systems, for example, after an organ, stem cell or bone marrow transplant, CMV infection can be fatal.

Teachers who work in day care centres, nurseries, preschools and kindergartens are specifically cautioned about CMV due to the sheer number of young children in their care and their propensity to transmit illnesses in their young, formative years.

Bibliography

Centers for Disease Control and Prevention (2000), "Cytomegalovirus (CMV) and Congenital CMV Infection", https/www.cde.cde.gov/cmv/index.html

24 Giving feedback

After a child has been assessed and where appropriate a diagnosis made, how is information relayed to a child's parents? How is the issue of "feedback" managed, and how does this relate to the ongoing support for the child and family? Are results and diagnoses simply relayed and reports written and then cases simply filed away as "finished"?

Feedback in essence is another example of communication, a combination of content, form and context, but with the addition of extra layers of complexity. Assessments of young children are often conducted with one or both parents present, or perhaps watching through a two-way mirror. Parents have observed a psychologist interact with and develop a degree of rapport with their child, and in so doing, a degree of trust and credibility has hopefully developed. This may be based on parental perceptions of the following:

- The psychologist's competence.
- The feeling of empathy imparted to parents and child.
- The quality of the psychologist-child relationship.
- The "customised" nature of the assessment to suit circumstances.

This "closeness" can influence the manner in which information is relayed to a family and even the substance of that information. If psychological practice is the art of developing a professional and caring relationship with clients, it is often in the process of "feedback" that is most important. And even when rapport, trust and confidence have been achieved between parents and psychologist, the "language" of feedback is very important, particularly when complex, technical information needs to be discussed (Figure 24.1).

This cartoon illustrates the point that the trust and rapport developed between psychologist and parents during an assessment needs to extend into the process of later feedback discussions. It is the role of the psychologist to make judgements not just about what to feed back but also about the most appropriate "form" and "content" so as not to distance the family from the assessment process and outcomes through any unintended disenfranchisement. Practitioners can risk lapsing into excessive technical terminology and jargon during feedback at a time when parents simply want to know what is happening and what to do about it.

Parents of young children will vary in what they do and do not want to hear about their child. Some will desire an instance "answer" as to possible diagnoses and courses of action; others will want to hold on to hope that in fact, nothing is wrong, that their

DOI: 10.4324/9781003565338-29

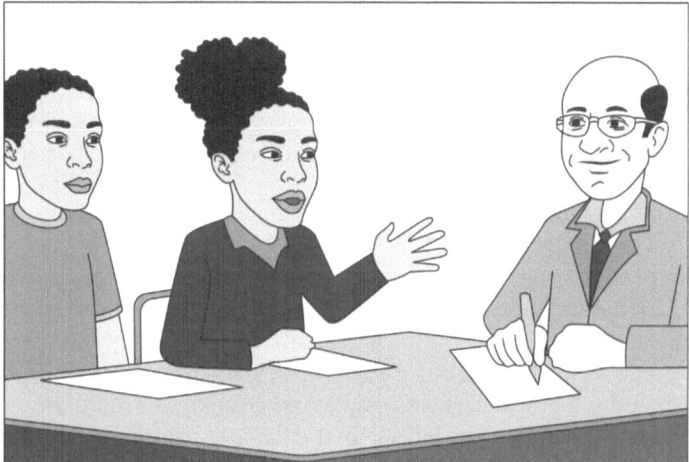

Figure 24.1 Providing feedback to families
"Thanks for explaining our child has a disorder we've never heard of in words we don't understand".

worst fears have not been realised or that the diagnostic outcomes are incorrect and a further opinion should be sought. All of these are justifiable responses to the trust families have placed in a psychologist who had been up until their appointment a complete stranger.

When should feedback occur?

Whichever way individual psychologists function in their assessment setting, it is the confidence and trust that parents have developed with that professional which initially impacts the nature of feedback given. Often, a determining factor in how individual psychologists "feed back" their findings is the specific employment contexts in which they work and the conditions which influence their post-assessment roles:

- Follow-up is sometimes immediate or soon after assessment and diagnosis has occurred, or may be after a period of time in which families have had the chance to process the information given, to make specific enquiries and arrangements regarding service provision, or to simply attend to other matters.
- A psychologist may judge that a family may require time to process information and observations and return later for more comprehensive discussions. Or it may simply be the case that families need to leave an assessment immediately after its completion to tend to other duties and responsibilities.
- If a "team" assessment has been conducted, formal feedback may be delayed until all team members have had the opportunity to compile, compare and discuss their individual findings.
- In the case of young children attending preschools, a psychologist may decide to visit and observe the young child in that setting to garner further "contextual" information and schedule follow-up discussions for a later date.
- Or perhaps a diagnostic assessment can only be completed after further assessment by medical practitioners or therapists has been undertaken.

What to feed back

What does a family want to know, and how can this information be best imparted? What does a psychologist feel is necessary to relay to parents? In some instances, there is a perfect alignment between these two dimensions of feedback. Standard psychological practice dictates that the following should be discussed and explored after assessment:

- A review of the original referral question and background information provided by parents, specialists and other caregivers.
- A restatement of the parents' concerns and their expectations of the assessment process.
- An appraisal by the family as to whether their child's observed behaviours and skills were what they expected. Were they representative of his/her typical presentation?
- A review of the assessment process, for example, the name of the tests and what they assess. This includes helping parents understand complex terminology such as standard scores or age equivalents, developmental delays or disorders.
- Explanation of results obtained, using the most appropriate modality, for example, age equivalent scores presented graphically. It is sometimes useful to reflect upon a family's previous experience with young children, particularly if they have an older child to compare with. Some parents will express, for example, "we still find that he/she speaks like a 2-year-old".
- An explanation of the "basics" of psychometric assessments, particularly the meaning of age equivalent scores, "ranges of confidence" and that assessments are a "snapshot" of today's level of skill, and not predictive of the future.
- Salient features and highlights from the assessment, emphasising strengths and weaknesses, and behaviours of note. These should be related to the original referral "question". For example, "that constant arm flapping can be a sign of Autism Spectrum Disorder" or "your child's delays are not just in the area of speech and language—they are more global than that".
- Feedback sessions should allow for as much "question and answer" discussion as possible, and parents should be encouraged to take notes or even record discussions on their phones. They should be reassured that further clarifications are always available and a full report provided.
- There should be a discussion of further observation or assessment outside of the assessment clinic, if applicable, for example, through preschool observations.
- Parents should be encouraged to attend assessments and feedback sessions with an independent "third party", perhaps a friend or relation, if they so wish, for support, accuracy and clarification of detail.

Feedback often involves the discussion of diagnostic outcomes which may not be favourable. Bartolo discusses the "giving of news" to a family as being a dipolar paradigm: "Realism versus hopefulness". Three "frameworks" are described to express and explain "bad news":

- **Parent-friendly frame:** This incorporates an empathic relationship with parents and child, reassuring a family that they were doing all they could to meet their child's needs but suggesting additional strategies or services, if appropriate. Time should be allowed for parents to seek clarification of important or unfamiliar issues. For multidisciplinary teams, there is a need to have clarified any professional differences of opinion before the feedback session so that "one story" can be presented to a family.

- **Hopeful formulation frame:** This approach emphasises the positive aspects and achievements of the child, with a focus on "what to do next" to further this progress.
- **Defocusing frame:** This approach avoids "labelling" a child with any particular diagnosis but instead focuses upon a child's progress and needs. The obvious difficulty with this approach is the nexus between "diagnostic precision" and service delivery/programme access.

Practitioners eventually formulate their own individual "style" of news-breaking and explanation, often a combination of all three of the above. They adapt their processes according to the needs of their client families and their understanding of assessment processes. They need to ask the following questions:

- Why did they come for assessment?
- What information did they provide?
- What pre-assessment understanding did they bring to the assessment?
- How well "did" they understand the "story" unfolding during the assessment and feedback session?
- Did the assessment process unearth or raise new insights and understandings of their child? Did it provide additional strategies for interaction, communication, play and management of difficult situations?
- Does a family need "time and space" to read subsequent reports, consider the information provided, ask further questions or seek further opinions about the child's diagnosis?
- Does a formal diagnostic need to be made immediately? Is there further information needed to be considered, for example, preschool observations, further information from other professionals or a later review of the child following therapeutic intervention?
- Feedback sessions invariably raise questions about "diagnosis", and it may or may not be appropriate to determine diagnosis at this point. It is also important to consider:
  - Is a family "ready" to consider a diagnosis of a neurodevelopmental disorder?
  - Is the psychologist ready to make a clear diagnosis?

An essential aspect of any feedback to families, before, during or after assessments, is the need to hold discussions in a manner which is respectful to families and their cultural and linguistic backgrounds and appropriate to their level of understanding and experience. This is termed a "common language" of communicating information, whereby medical and psychological terminology are phrased in a manner facilitative of easy and unambiguous discussion and comprehension. This will be expanded upon in a later section concerning report writing.

Bibliography

Aschieri, F., Cera, G., Fiorelli, A., and Brasil S. (2024), "A Retrospective Study Exploring Parents' Perceptions of their Child's Assessment", Frontiers of Psychology.

Bartolo, P. A. (2002), "Communicating a Diagnosis of Developmental Disability to Parents: Multi-professional Negotiation Framework", Child: Care, Health and Development, 28(1), pp 65–71.

Bowen, C., and Snow, P. (2017), Making Sense of Interventions for Children with Developmental Disorders, J&R Press.

Caithness, T., and Moore, E. (2011), "A Common Language for understanding disability, development, emotions, and behaviour", In Dossetor, D., White, D., and Whatson, L. (Eds.),

Mental Health of Children and Adolescents with Intellectual and Developmental Disabilities, IP Communications.

Ellis, J., and Whaite, A. (1983), "To Parents of Children with Disabilities, from Parents of Children with Disabilities", Social Evaluation and Research Ltd.

Gilmore, L. (2018), "Supporting Families of Children with Rare and Unique Chromosome Disorders", Research and Practice in Intellectual and Developmental Disabilities, 5(1), pp 8–16.

Snoyman, P., and Veddovi, M. (2001), "Changes to Parents Expectations of their Child's Behaviour following Assessment", Unpublished Paper.

Tharinger, D. J., Finn, S. E., Hersh, B., and Wilkinson, A. (2008), "Assessment Feedback with Parents of Pre-Adolescent Children: A Collegiate Approach", Professional Psychology Research and Practice, 39(6), pp 600–609.

25 Intervention strategies

Some questions inevitably raised by families at assessment, during "feedback' and even at later follow-up meetings include: "What do we have to do now? How do we help our child? What therapies and treatments work? Are there any medications that will help? Can he/she be cured? What will our child's future be like?"

These questions are clearly too numerous and a child and family's circumstances too varied and individual for a psychologist to answer all of these queries. Nowadays, there are a plethora of programmes and resources, medications and service providers, too many for any one psychologist to know. These various programmes, resources, treatments and "cures" range from thoroughly researched and "evidence-based", peer-reviewed and government-sanctioned to discredited and baseless shamanism. Many offer realistic explanations about efficacy and treatment outcomes, and some make wild and outlandish claims about "cures". Some are advertised in a variety of media, including online forums, books and magazines, TV content, as well as "word of mouth" through service providers, doctors, schools and other psychologists. There are:

- Individual and group therapy programmes and educational programmes.
- Medical and biomedical "treatments".
- Books and resources, including online "apps".
- Support groups and societies.
- Claimed "cures" and "miracle workers".
- Special preschools and early intervention programmes.

Parents are far more able to access information today in the "connected" world, but this does not mean they possess the requisite critical evaluation skills to decide whether treatment options are validated and therapeutically sound or simply unproven fads or trends. Psychologists by virtue of their education and training should possess a good working knowledge of "scientific method", critical thinking and evidence-based veracity. Although psychologists cannot make decisions on behalf of their client families, they can use these skills to help their clients navigate the complex, confusing and often contradictory maize of "treatment options". This may include directing families towards useful information about support and treatment options, how to better "evaluate" the claims that may be made and how to consider "for and against" evidence for contentious programmes.

An understanding that psychologists need to hold is the stressors that families will be experiencing at this time:

- Shock, grief and anxiety at the realisation that their child needs help.
- Guilt through feelings of "complicity" in causation.

DOI: 10.4324/9781003565338-30

- "Expectation pressure" from other family members.
- Time and financial pressure at the prospect of paying for expensive programmes and finding time in their already busy lives to undertake treatments.
- Confusion and trepidation at the prospect of navigating through the bureaucratic labyrinth of applications, phone calls, application forms and letters, appointments and further referrals.

This early post-assessment phase can be when families most need a psychologist's support but also a time when they can least afford the time and emotional "space" to engage. A theme sometimes encountered by psychologists at this time is that a family may feel "too busy to grieve", but this can be mistaken as resiliency. Families need to know that their psychologist is available when as a family they are "ready".

Psychologists cannot "know" each and every therapy option, programme, or treatment. There should always be literature available pertaining to these, and psychologists should make their own evaluations and judgements as to their scientific efficacy. But it is also important for psychologists to appreciate that families will make their own decisions about treatments and programmes and accept their right to do so. Families might concede later that they made the "wrong decision", and a phrase often used is that parents should be allowed "the dignity of failure". Similarly, families in these situations may experience "decision regret" when they do decide to change their minds. Again, a psychologist's role is to support and not to judge.

Specific treatment modalities: Therapists

Speech pathology, occupational therapy and physiotherapy are often "frontline" interventions for neurodevelopmental disorders, but this does not mean that all therapists will assist in the same manner. There can be:

- Individual therapy sessions are to enhance communication skills, fine and gross motor coordination skills, emotional regulation and play skills.
- Some programmes are tailored specifically to the individual child, or some may be particularly "designed" programmes.
- Some therapists may offer home-based services, others at their clinics, and some are mobile and visit preschools and schools.
- Some may only offer advice and recommendations rather than "hands-on" treatment.
- There can be group sessions where a small number of children are treated together.
- Particularly with speech, language and communication skills, some therapists may make use of device "apps" and other technologies to facilitate "augmentative communication." Others may make their own augmentative communication materials depending on a child's specific needs.

Examples of specific and researched therapeutic programmes and modalities include various autism spectrum disorder–specific programmes, where treatment options have grown considerably:

- Applied behaviour analysis (ABA), described as "the process of applying principles of behaviour to the improvement of specific behaviours" through systematic instruction

and repetition of learning sequences. Originally pioneered by Ivar Lovaas in the 1970s in the United States, it has been adapted over the decades into a variety of similar approaches but all based on the "discrete trial training" (DTT) method.
- "Relational-based", for example, "Floortime" (Developmental, Individual-Difference, Relationship-based model) and Relationship Developmental Intervention (RDI), both of which are very child-centred.
- Communication-based programmes such as Hanen's "More Than Words", where language use is encouraged and developed through using everyday activities as the vehicle for learning.
- Sensory integration therapies (SRIs), based on sensory integration theory whereby sensory stimulation received from the environment is integrated and interpreted.

Specific treatment modalities: Early childhood centres including early intervention programmes

These are usually offered through government services although there are an increasing number of private centres. Early intervention centres and preschools are often an ideal mix of both individual therapy where skills can be learned and developed and a social milieu where they can be applied to "real-life" interactions, play and learning. There are also mainstream preschools and childcare centres which can carry a specific "loading" of children with special needs, for example, a formulaic decrease in overall enrolment numbers if a child with "special needs" is enrolled.

Specific treatment modalities: Medications

Psychologists are not doctors. They have no medical training or prescribing rights. Parents often raise questions about the usefulness of medications for their children, and these questions should be immediately referred to an appropriate medical practitioner for expert advice. Psychologists do not possess these areas of knowledge or skill.

However, it is of benefit for psychologists to have at least a background knowledge of the medications often prescribed to children with neurodevelopmental disorders, the reasons for such usage, the potential benefits or side effects and the role that psychologists may play in supporting families or monitoring progress.

Firstly, however, there are no medications which "cure" neurodevelopmental disorders. Medications, when prescribed, are used to reduce if possible the impact of specific symptoms which may be impinging upon a child's daily functioning:

- Maladaptive behaviours.
- Excessive emotional reactivity.
- Short attention or impulsivity.
- Sleep disturbance.
- Obsessiveness.
- Anxiety.
- Aggression.

At early ages such as under 6 years, they are generally prescribed as a "last resort" when other behavioural or therapeutic processes have not resolved specific issues or

Table 25.1 Selected medications used with neurodevelopmental disorders

Drug Class	Example	Usage
Antipsychotics	Risperidone Aripiprazole	Aggression, self-injury, tantrums, withdrawal, tics, rituals
Antidepressants	Fluoxetine Sertraline	Repetitive and stereotypic behaviour
Anticonvulsants	Valproic acid (Epilim) Clonazepam	Epilepsies, bipolar disorders, externalising behaviour problems
Stimulants	Dexamphetamine (e.g. Ritalin) Concerta	Attentional problems
Supplements	Melatonin	Sleep disturbance

when a child's behaviour may be placing himself/herself, or others, at risk (Table 25.1). To this end, the following classes of medication may be prescribed by medical specialists:

- Medications for overactivity, impulsivity or short attention. These are generally of the same class of medications prescribed to children with attention deficit hyperactivity disorder. These are frequently "stimulant" medications. Examples of their usage include young children whose behaviours are so impulsive or erratic as to place them in danger of unsafe absconding, road crossing or other issues associated with community access.
- Medications or naturally occurring agents to improve the quality of sleep experienced by a young child, for example, melatonin.
- Medications to reduce underlying levels of anxiety, particularly when this is causing significant behavioural disturbance or interruption of daily activities. Such medications can also be used to help reduce obsessive behavioural traits if these are excessively problematic.
- Antipsychotic medications. These are generally prescribed to older children with neurodevelopmental disorders when they are demonstrating extremely aggressive behaviours or early prodromal signs of possible psychosis.
- Anticonvulsant medications. As is implied by this very description, anticonvulsant medications are used to treat and manage epileptic conditions in young children, but it is known that some such medications can have other beneficial effects, for example, mood stabilisation.

All such medications can be efficacious, but all drugs can also cause side effects. Even though psychologists will have no direct role in recommending and prescribing medications, they can assist prescribing medical specialists and of course families in monitoring the impacts, both positive and negative, of any medications used. Medical specialists, in particular, rarely have the opportunity to escape their busy caseloads at hospitals or their own clinics to observe young children at home, at school or in the community. They will sometimes therefore request information from parents, therapists or psychologists involved for information and observations about a child's progress during a medication regime. "Charting" of progress is a relatively simple and effective means of giving useful information to medical specialists. An example of a simple chart is included in Table 25.2.

Every medication, despite its intended medicinal benefit, is capable of causing unwanted side effects, and referring specialists are very conscious of the need to monitor

Table 25.2 Sample medication side effect chart

Code	0 = No problem 1 = Slight problem 2 = Major problem			
Symptom	Week 1	Week 2	Week 3	Week 4
Sleep trouble				
Appetite loss				
Headaches				
Anxiety				
Irritability				
Withdrawn				
Digestion				
Drowsiness				
Teariness				
Nail biting				
Euphoria				
Facial tics				
Aggression				
Restless				
Self-harm				
Negative thoughts				

a child's progress and demeanour when medications are prescribed. They are generally receptive to objective and detailed feedback from other professionals such as psychologists who may have better opportunities to observe young children.

Psychologists employed in multidisciplinary teams and services which include paediatricians are often called upon to be part of any review of a child's response, either positive or negative, to specific medication regimes, and the methodical and objective data derived from such checklists or sampling techniques can be incorporated into the clinical decision-making processes of treating specialists or may indicate other hypotheses to be considered about treatment modalities.

Most psychological registration and licencing organisations offer ongoing education and training programmes for their members, and a common theme in at least some jurisdictions is awareness programmes around medication and the ethical requirements inherent in the psychologist's role in such matters. There are many and varied textbooks and other sources of useful information to inform psychologists about matters of medication, but it is imperative that correct clinical judgement be applied to any discussions with parents about medication issues.

Psychologists cannot be expected to have intimate or in-depth knowledge of every type of treatment modality available for young children; however, they can access objective reviews of these programmes and remedies through relevant literature which provides reviews of the many treatment options and support methodologies for young children, ranging from the scientifically based and researched to the specious and unsupported.

"Treatments" can be categorised according to whether there is clear evidence of research and efficacy or whether they simply tap into the hopes and aspirations of families at their most vulnerable as they search for "answers" for their children's difficulties.

Bibliography

Bowen, C., and Snow, P. (2017), Making Sense of Interventions for Children with Developmental Disorders, J&R Press.

Keen, D., and Rodger, S. (2012), Working with Parents of a Newly Diagnosed Child with an Autism Spectrum Disorder, Jessica Kingsley Publishers.

Popow, C., Ohmann, S., and Plener, P. (2021), "Practitioner's Review: Medication for Children and Adolescents with Autism Spectrum Disorder (ASD) and Comorbid Conditions", Neuropsychiatry, 35(3), pp 113–134.

Zehetner, A. A. (2011), "Psychopharmacology: The Use of Medication to treat Challenging Behaviours in Children and Adolescents", In Dossetor, D., White, D., and Whatson, L. (Eds.), Mental Health of Children and Adolescents with Intellectual and Developmental Disabilities, IP Communications.

26 Diagnostic considerations and formulation

What is a "diagnosis", and why are they so important? How does a psychologist formulate an appropriate diagnosis on the basis of assessments they have undertaken, observations they have made and information they have received, collated and considered? Is the "end product" of an assessment always a "diagnosis"?

What is a diagnosis?

A diagnosis is defined as *"the identification of the nature of an illness or other problem by examination of the symptoms"*, and although this is a medically orientated description, it can equally apply to psychological and developmental disorders. A key difference is in the nature of "symptoms", which for childhood conditions can be contextually and culturally based and subjective in their interpretation. The diagnostic process for neurodevelopmental disorders can be slow and multifaceted. Information from various sources needs to be collated, compared and verified against specific criteria. There is a different "evidence base" to medical conditions where "hard science" and physical evidence are germane. There is the perception of "subjectivity" around psychological disorders of children: "It's just your opinion", "where is the evidence supporting this diagnosis?" or "all children are different, aren't they?" can be the responses to diagnostic decisions.

Parents more accustomed to receiving definitive medical diagnoses may worry about the lack of "precision" in psychological assessments. Receiving "bad news" is never enjoyable, and parents of young children will react in ways reflecting their levels of understanding, grief, anger or anxiety. Psychologists need to be aware of these background issues during their assessment and diagnostic processes.

Is the "diagnostic process" like following a recipe? Do psychologists simply follow a templated order of events, for example:

- Collate background information.
- Conduct tests.
- Combine results.
- Compare with diagnostic criteria.
- Formulate diagnostic result.

Some researchers have produced "decision tree" models of assessment and diagnosis that would suggest that this is simply the case in models predicated upon "test-diagnose-treat-retest", but although a "diagnosis" may appear to be the final step in a linear

DOI: 10.4324/9781003565338-31

228 *Diagnosing Young Children with Neurodevelopmental Disorders*

process, it is not that simple. Assessment is multifaceted. Information and "evidence" come from many sources to inform the assessment process:

- Medical reports.
- Parental reports and descriptions.
- Therapeutic information.
- Formal test results from other practitioners.
- Psychological assessments such as developmental tests.
- Preschool observations.
- Video vignettes.
- Questionnaires and checklists.

This information will vary in specificity, veracity, orientation and possibly "agenda". Parents will vary in their understanding and interpretation of this input and likely be unfamiliar with the actual "act" of assessing their child. The dynamic process of assessment-testing hypotheses from disparate information sources, followed by a simple diagnosis, is not necessarily the "end product". The stylised representation of assessment in Figure 26.1 highlights that information is always "present and active" during the assessment. It will churn through the assessment process from beginning to end, through "forward and backward referencing" with additional information arising *de noveau* during assessment through questions and observations. There are new hypotheses to test, all occurring simultaneously. There are cultural issues, language differences, beliefs and feelings to accommodate. There are child-centric factors such as age and behaviour. Families have background histories to divulge. This treasure trove of information needs to "align" with observed "symptoms" to warrant a "diagnosis".

Some diagnoses are easy to make. A child arrives at a psychologist's office and "on cue" demonstrates the core symptoms of a diagnostic category. Other children are difficult to diagnose as their presentations do not readily align with specific criteria, or it is difficult to accurately appraise the child for "operational" reasons. Some children should not be diagnosed as their presentations are at odds with known diagnostic criteria.

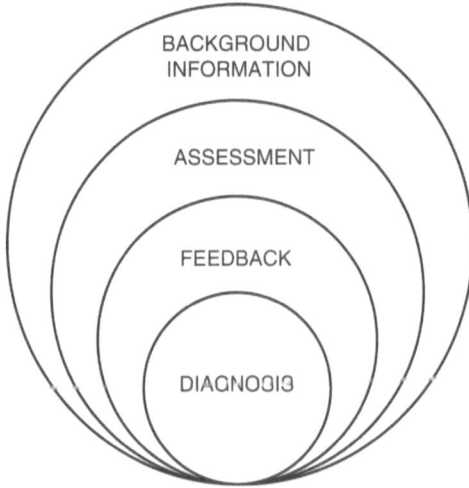

Figure 26.1 "From referral to diagnosis to action" flow chart

Diagnosis can be the "end product" of information and evidence provided, refined and then compared with relevant diagnostic criteria. It can be akin to a "sorting" task where different symptomatic "proofs" are placed into the appropriate "slots". Whichever way "diagnosis" is characterised, it is predicated upon a number of considerations:

- An understanding of diagnostic criteria from DSM-5-TR or ICD-11, which should be readily available to the psychologist.
- An understanding of the "condition" under consideration for assessment. If a clear but less well-known condition has been referred for assessment, pre-reading can lay the foundations for the assessment.
- Salient background information about the child from multiple, credible sources.
- "Face-to-face" interaction with the child, possibly in multiple contexts.
- Training, qualification and experience with specific testing procedures.
- Awareness of advantages and disadvantages associated with diagnosis, including "systems-related" factors and family perspectives.

Which disorders do psychologists commonly diagnose?

Psychologists have no medical training or qualifications; thus, their expertise will be required for the assessment and diagnosis of conditions observable through "behaviours". They will not be involved in diagnosing genetic disorders in children but may be involved in assessing their developmental skills, behavioural attributes, strengths and weaknesses and progress through intervention. A "most likely" list of diagnostic conditions for psychological/developmental assessment is likely to include:

- Global developmental delay.
- Specific delays in development, for example, language delay.
- Autism spectrum disorder.
- Developmental coordination disorder.
- Stereotypic movement disorder.
- Attention deficit hyperactivity disorder.

These categories can constitute a "primary diagnosis" when there is no genetic "underlay"; however, children with genetic disorders can also present with symptoms from those listed above. This is referred to as "comorbidity" and is not uncommon. Many genetic disorders will have issues with inappropriate development of milestones as an artefact.

Some present with an increased likelihood of autism spectrum disorder. Down syndrome, for example, is associated with a 5–10% chance of autism spectrum disorder. Some genetic conditions, for example, Smith–Magenis syndrome, are characterised by behavioural "phenotypes" such as stereotypic movements, and these can cause diagnostic confusion. Global developmental delay is common in genetic disorders. Therefore, psychologists undertaking early childhood assessments need to develop expertise and experience in:

- Collating relevant background information.
- Observing and interacting with young children.
- Undertaking a psychometric assessment of developmental skills.
- Formulating diagnostic outcomes.
- Relaying information to parents, caregivers, and other professionals.

- Liaising with other professionals.
- Understanding support agencies and services.

Examples of diagnosis

Scenario 1: A hypothetical assessment for a child with possible global developmental delay. The child has been assessed by a developmental paediatrician, and there is no evidence of underlying genetic disorders or neurological conditions. How might this referral and assessment progress?

Background information

- Is there a comprehensive report from the developmental paediatrician, indicating possible causative factors?
- Did the child experience normal early development of milestones?
- Is there a family history of developmental delay or disorder?
- Is there a history of chronic health conditions such as glue ear?
- Has the child's hearing been assessed, and if so, is it within normal limits?
- Has the child been assessed by professionals such as speech pathologists or occupational therapists? If so, what were their findings?
- Did the child present with consistent skills development in some areas but delayed development in others, or were concerns expressed about all areas of development?
- Does the child attend a playgroup, childcare or preschool? If so, how is this child's progress rated by carers? Is he/she achieving the outcomes expected for children of his/her age?
- Does the child come from a stable home environment, or is it characterised by disruption, neglect or abuse? Does the child receive adequate environmental stimulation and opportunity at home?
- What is the family language background? Is the child exposed significantly to languages other than English?

Pre-assessment questionnaires

- Which questionnaires are sent to parents, childcare centres or preschools? For example, questionnaire-based assessments of adaptive behaviour, autism spectrum disorder or milestone development?
- Are questionnaires returned prior to assessment for scoring and interpretation?
- Do parents provide written accounts of their observations of their child or mobile phone video of behaviours or issues of concern?
- What early hypotheses and "lines of enquiry" are apparent to the psychologist?
- Does background information indicate assessment procedures to be undertaken?

Assessment procedure

- Do the parents understand the assessment procedure, or is there a need for further discussion, explanation and development of professional rapport?
- If a formal psychometric assessment such as Griffiths III or Bayley-4 is necessary, is there a "back-up plan" if it proves unworkable? How else can skills be recorded and benchmarked?
- After assessment, is there sufficient time for test scoring, notetaking, and reporting back to parents?

Feedback to and from parents

- Which of the following information is relayed to parents at this stage?

  - Psychometric test results.
  - Qualitative observations.
  - Reference to specific diagnostic conditions and labels.

- What other information is sought from parents at this stage?

  - Did the assessment represent an accurate picture of their child?
  - Did the parents observe familiar skills and behaviours, or were there tasks which they felt under- or overestimated his/her ability?
  - Were the parents surprised by any skills revealed by this assessment?
  - Did the parents feel their child was developing appropriately? Did they compare their child to a younger family member?
  - Did the parents note any issues of concern which they had not encountered before?

Diagnostic consideration

- What psychometric information did this assessment provide, and did the psychologist's observations correlate with these results? Did they tally with pre-assessment adaptive behaviour questionnaires?
- How did these psychometric results and observations align with diagnostic criteria from either DSM-5-TR or ICD-11?
- How does a family prefer diagnostic information to be used? Is a diagnosis what they perceive as the best outcome from assessment, or do they have concerns about "labelling" their child?
- What "systems" issues emanate from a diagnosis of this child? What information needs to be provided to service providers?

Consider at this point DSM-5-TR criteria for global developmental delay (Table 26.1).
It is a psychological convention that a "global developmental delay" can be diagnosed when there are significant delays and deficits in at least three of the five developmental areas assessed. Both the Griffiths III and Bayley-4 tests provide:

- Age equivalent scores and developmental quotient scores for each of the five areas, as well as overall scores.
- Standard scores and confidence intervals, again by subscale and overall scores.
- Developmental quotients that do not extend below 50, so more "weight" is often applied to developmental age scores when considering diagnosis.

If our hypothetical child was 4 years of age but functioning at approximately a two-year-old level or younger, with such delays in at least three subscales, he/she would be considered as having a global developmental delay as defined by DSM-5-TR. A developmental age of less than 50% of the child's chronological age is generally viewed as being a "moderate" global developmental delay. If our child was achieving developmental scores of approximately 3 years, a "mild" global developmental delay would be a more likely diagnostic outcome.

Questionnaire-based assessments of adaptive behaviour such as Applied Behavior Assessment System 3 and Vineland-3 also focus on early developmental skills, and

Table 26.1 DSM-5-TR criteria, global developmental delay

"This diagnosis is reserved for individuals under the age of five years when the clinical severity level cannot be reliably assessed during early childhood. This category is diagnosed when an individual fails to meet expected milestones in several areas of intellectual functioning, and applies to individuals who are unable to undergo systematic assessments of intellectual functioning, including children who are too young to participate in standardised testing. This category requires reassessment after a period of time."

corroborating evidence is an important "check" when considering assessment results, particularly if information is derived from parents or preschools. Assessment results from speech pathologists or occupational therapists also provide corroborating evidence, particularly if their assessments make reference to age levels or degree of severity.

What if this hypothetical child was found to have only one or two areas of delayed development? Would this be a "global developmental delay"? DSM-5-TR and ICD-11 refer to specific developmental delays and disorders affecting speech, language and movement skills. If our hypothesised child presented only with delays in speech and language, reference would made to DSM-5-TR or ICD-ICD-11 criteria for communication disorders such as language disorder. Both DSM-5-TR and ICD-I1 refer to "developmental coordination disorder" with its focus upon "activities of daily living" such as dressing and undressing and eating and feeding. These mirror the skills assessed by Griffiths III, Bayley-4 and adaptive behaviour tests, adding validity to such a diagnosis. Developmental assessments such as Griffiths III and Bayley-4 do not substitute for formal speech pathology or occupational therapy assessments. However, they can augment existing information about a child and add strength to diagnostic certainty.

Scenario 2: Not all referrals for early childhood assessments relate to disability concerns. What if the parents of a 4.5-year-old child with mildly delayed speech and language were concerned about their child's school readiness—should they enrol him/her straight away or delay for a further 12 months? The child presents as charming and bright, clearly able to perform most age-appropriate preschool activities. Background information from preschool includes an adaptive behaviour assessment, which indicates overall "below average" functioning, accompanied by written reports expressing their concerns about the child's ability to separate from parents and to cope with a full school day. Developmental assessment indicates age equivalent scores a few months below the child's chronological age but with greater delay in speech, language and social, emotional and self-help skills:

- Would a diagnosis of mild global developmental delay be appropriate, in fact, should any diagnosis be made?
- What other assessments could be undertaken with this child? Are there more detailed assessments of social-emotional readiness for school entry?
- How else could information about this child be derived? Would it be advantageous to observe this child at preschool to gain further insights into his/her "readiness"?
- Would a preschool observational visit allow for discussions not only about their concerns but also the assistance they would provide should he/she "stay on" for another 12 months?
- What additional programmes might be put in place to extend the child's maturity? Are there obvious or potential disadvantages to repetition at preschool?

- Are there alternative options to those proposed? Might the child undertake "orientation visits" to the proposed school to see whether he/she is in fact "ready"? Could school personnel visit and observe the child at preschool and offer their appraisal of the child's readiness?

School systems have their own guidelines regarding "readiness" skills. However, they are "guidelines" and not "policies". This scenario occurs often, and although not truly "diagnostic," the recommendations discussed are important to parents. A potential assessment tool for these situations is the Vineland Social-Emotional Early Childhood Scales (Sparrow, Balla and Cicchetti), conducted by interview with parents and yielding standard scores, bands of error and confidence intervals in these areas:

- Interpersonal relationships.
- Play and leisure time.
- Coping skills.
- Social-emotional composite scale.

This assessment protocol of course emanates from the United States of America, and it is therefore necessary to consider whether there are universal standards around the concept of "school readiness". Entry ages vary from country to country, and even jurisdiction to jurisdiction, so school readiness is very much a localised issue around which psychometric assessment would be only one of a number of "proofs" in any decision-making process.

Diagnostic formulation of autism spectrum disorder

Reference is made to Chapter 1 and the changes in understanding, classification and diagnostic criteria for autism spectrum disorder over the decades. There was a time of scepticism when "autism" was not acknowledged or was under-diagnosed. Sustained educational and training programmes, publicity campaigns and community activism have all played their part in bringing about changes in attitude and awareness, along with an explosion of research, literature and personal accounts.

Autism spectrum disorder is now supported through financial schemes and allowances, special schools and classes and therapeutic programmes for communication, behavioural support, social skills development and sensory processing help. Accurate assessment and diagnosis of autism spectrum disorder is imperative to access such services. All countries have some kind of inclusion criteria.

As with Griffiths III and Bayley-4 tests, specialised training programmes are required to become licenced to use "gold standard" assessments such as the Autism Diagnostic Observation Schedule-2 or the Autism Diagnostic Interview. These assessments require a similar process and skill set to other assessments of neurodevelopmental disorders and delays:

- Collation of background referral information from multiple sources.
- Use of appropriate tests. Autism spectrum disorder should be assessed and diagnosed using "autism-specific" tests. Paired or supervised assessments are recommended for psychologists in the post-training period.
- Detailed observational skills, preferably in more than one context.

234 *Diagnosing Young Children with Neurodevelopmental Disorders*

- Detailed record keeping and scoring.
- Aligning of observations and assessment results with diagnostic criteria.
- Collegial discussion and consideration of diagnostic hypotheses and findings.

In some assessment clinics, it is mandatory for screening of possible autism spectrum disorder. Screening questionnaires such as the Autism Spectrum Rating Scales are often used for this purpose, as are "in-house" questionnaires and checklists. Information from these is used as part of referral "triage."

Psychologists who administer developmental tests such as Griffiths III or Bayley-4 are already engaged in interaction and observation with young children, and some question the need to complete an autism-specific assessment as well. Both Griffiths III and Bayley-4 are excellent "vehicles" for observing a child's social, emotional, communication, play and problem-solving skills, but they are not "autism-specific".

The "gold standard" autism assessments arose from the need for reliable research instruments into the condition. Griffiths III and Bayley-4 allow a "window" into autism assessments, and some practitioners feel confident in administering developmental tests and autism spectrum disorder tests concurrently. This is a matter of professional and ethical judgement.

Scenario 3:

Background information

- A three-year-old child is referred by a paediatrician for assessment of possible autism spectrum disorder. No genetic testing has been considered necessary as the child does not present with dysmorphic features.
- The child developed minimal spoken language, perhaps two single words, by 12 months of age, but these ceased to be heard at approximately 15 months.
- Non-verbal gestural communication such as pointing has not developed, nor has clapping, waving or other communicative gestures.
- Despite apparently normal hearing, there is no social response to the call of the child's name.
- The child is described as not seeking comfort or as engaging with other children at childcare.

Pre-assessment questionnaires

- Autism Spectrum Rating Scale questionnaires completed by parents and childcare centre both indicated "Very Elevated" scores for social communication problems, unusual behaviours, total scores and DSM-5 scores.
- Parent-completed questionnaires indicate ongoing concerns about the child's lack of eye contact and social engagement, empathy for others and lack of anticipatory social reactions.
- Mobile phone video vignettes include examples of the child lining up toys on the floor, but not engaging in meaningful play. Also noted are repeated arm flapping when excited and a tendency for the child to "run and dart" and to walk on toes for no particular reason.
- Observations are made of the child's immediate response to certain sounds such as TV themes, in contrast to the lack of social response to the call of his/her name.

Assessment procedure

- The psychologist at this stage of their career has no training in either the Autism Diagnostic Observation Schedule or Autism Diagnostic Interview but is familiar with a range of autism spectrum disorder assessments such as Gilliam and CARS 2.
- An attempt to engage the child in formal psychometric assessment using Griffiths III or Bayley-4 is unsuccessful as the child is unable to follow instructions, imitate play or procedures or settle to any particular activity. Instead, the assessment period becomes one of observed play and attempts at engagement without reference to strict assessment protocol or scoring guidelines.
- The child is observed to repeatedly line up toys, as well as engage in a non-purposeful exploration of the "parts" of toys.
- Stereotypic babble is repeatedly heard, for example, "digadigadiga", with no apparent communicative intent.
- Stereotypic hand and arm flapping are both noted, sometimes in excitement and sometimes through anxiety at "change."
- No non-verbal communication strategies are noted, other than the child taking his/her parents' hand and placing it on chosen toys or objects.
- The child engages in covering his/her ears when loud noises occur.

Feedback to and from parents

- The child's parents confirm that observations made at the assessment are consistent with their own experiences of their child at home. They are familiar with autism spectrum disorder through conversations they have had with their paediatrician and friends and through their own internet searches.
- The alignment of observed symptoms from autism spectrum disorder is discussed and indicates that the child's parents are not surprised or disturbed by this reference.

Diagnostic consideration

From all background information received and observations made, could this psychologist validly make a diagnosis of autism spectrum disorder? What other information would be seen as useful or necessary, and how would this be obtained?

- If the psychologist has not used an autism spectrum disorder–specific test, would a diagnosis of autism spectrum disorder be "system-acceptable"? How should this diagnosis be ethically reported under those circumstances?
- How would the psychologist determine the appropriate level of support required for this child? Would additional information be necessary?

Scenario 4: An infant of 2 years of age is referred for assessment due to observable features of autism spectrum disorder such as delayed language, restricted social response, immaturely formed and repetitive play. He/she has not attended preschool and has not commenced therapies such as speech pathology. Paediatric reports indicate chronic glue ear, and grommets have recently been inserted. Hearing appears to be normal. The young child has been cared for by loving grandparents, whilst the mother and father work, but the grandparents have only limited English skills and the ability to engage with the child.

Is this presentation best described by reference to global developmental delay or autism spectrum disorder as defined by DSM-5-TR? Let us consider the factors:

- This is a very young child, who has not had the opportunity to engage in childcare programmes or social engagement with other young children.
- Language modelling and development has been restricted by two factors: Glue ear and subsequent early hearing difficulty and lack of stimulation of language and communication.
- Speech pathology assistance is yet to commence for this child.
- The child is about to commence a dynamic phase of development where change can be rapid and significant. This can include the diminution of early symptoms or the appearance of new symptoms.
- But it can also herald significant progress, particularly when therapeutic, health and environmental factors are remediated.

Imagine that developmental assessment of this child produced psychometric results consistent with mild global developmental delay, with the child functioning at approximately a 16-month level but with severely delayed speech and language scores at approximately a 12-month level.

Observations made by the psychologist highlighted the impression that the child lacked experience with many of the toys from the test but was enthralled by them. Imitative play was noted through psychologist demonstration, and increasing social engagement was achieved over time.

- Would a psychologist diagnose "mild developmental delay" as defined by DSM-5-TR or a specific language delay?
- Would a psychologist also diagnose autism spectrum disorder as defined by DSM-5-TR?
- What would be the relative advantages and disadvantages of this diagnosis?
    - Does it accurately reflect the child's current status?
    - Does it address the child's present and future needs?
    - Does it allow access to funding and support programmes?
    - Would the psychologist recommend a review assessment following a period of sustained therapeutic assistance?

Scenario 5: Not all children can be successfully psychometrically assessed, but that does not mean "assessment and diagnosis" are impossible. This hypothesised child was referred for psychometric assessment to facilitate school enrolment. He/she is approaching 5 years of age; has no meaningful language, play or object use; and suffers significant epileptic seizures. There is no known genetic or chromosomal condition and no family history of developmental disorders.

At assessment, he/she does not relate to the psychologist at all, makes continuous non-speech sounds with no communicative intent and chaotically explores the assessment room in an unsafe manner, necessitating the locking of the office door to prevent absconding. Toys and objects are either mouthed or thrown randomly, and maladaptive behaviours such as self-biting and hitting occur. There are instances of stereotypic hand movements. Any attempt to engage the child in developmental tests is unsuccessful. How would a psychologist "assess" this child, and what would he/she diagnose given the following?

- Scores from adaptive behaviour questionnaires are in the "Extremely Low" range, with no variation by subscale. The child is entirely dependent upon caregivers for all daily needs.

Diagnostic considerations and formulation 237

- Little discernible progress has been reported through either speech pathology or occupational therapy services.
- Enrolment in a special school for children with moderate-to-severe intellectual disability is sought, but that requires psychometric test results and a "diagnosis" to satisfy eligibility and funding criteria.
- When given free access to standardised test materials, observing the child confirms the behavioural presentation, and "scores" using developmental test norms are consistent with an approximately 12 months developmental age. Noted are:
  - "Grasp and release" behaviours such as dropping and throwing.
  - Some variation in vocal tone, pitch and volume and occasional use of vocal consonants.
  - Some ability to make eye contact.
  - The ability to run, climb and jump.
  - Some exploratory play such as tipping objects from containers.
  - Occasional close "visual stimulation" with toys and objects.

The psychologist needs to make a "clinical" decision about diagnosis on the basis of the evidence available:

- Will the psychologist report the psychometric assessment results even though they were based only on observation?
- Is it likely that the child will be diagnosed with a severe developmental delay or severe intellectual disability, regardless of psychometric results?
- Will the psychologist indicate that formal psychometric assessment was not possible and report only the results of adaptive behaviour assessments?

The process of assessment and diagnosis can be quite straightforward, but it can also be a complex process where a psychologist needs to apply common sense, clinical knowledge and judgement, to the various challenges that occur when young children and their families are faced with complex interactions with government departments and services, agencies, schools and other bodies.

Who decides to diagnostically "label" a young child?

Is this for the parents to decide or the psychologist? Is it by mutual agreement? Psychologists do not "own the child." Should parents have the final say? There will be occasions when psychologists will know "what is best" for a child for service access, therapeutic needs and the particular idiosyncratic rules of service providers. They may feel that a "diagnosis" is:

a Warranted on the basis of all clinical assessments undertaken.
b Necessary for entry into specific therapies, educational programmes or funding and support arrangements.

But parents are not required to agree. They are entitled to their own opinions, choices and decisions. They may have some suspicion and scepticism about government departments and agencies. They may feel that a "diagnosis" or "label" will remain with their child for life and affect his/her future reputation and opportunities. Parents may have personal and philosophical views about treatments, including those which may be "unorthodox" or lesser known.

Parents may not yet "believe" or accept the underlying story about their child, even when comprehensively assessed and diagnosed. They may not be "ready" to hear the story. This is not irrational—it is a phase of the grieving process. Emotions may drive a family's ability to accept diagnoses and recommendations. There may be wounded pride—they do not need help and will proceed "their own way". There may be cultural beliefs and traditions preventing even close family assistance. There might be feelings of guilt, embarrassment or shame.

Families in these situations are sometimes described as "in denial", but that is not to apportion blame. Families in denial sometimes appreciate all too keenly the underlying "truth" of their situations but are just not ready to deal with it. Families have rights as well as responsibilities, and one "right" is to the "dignity of failure", where they may choose to believe certain "truths but not others.

Psychologists, social workers and other allied health workers have an important role to support families when disabilities and disorders have been diagnosed. They need to "be there" with and for families as their "stories" unfold and change, and their actions and decisions adjust accordingly. It is important to "work with" families as they come to terms with the news imparted to them. This can be long and complex.

Bibliography

American Psychiatric Association (2013), Diagnostic and Statistical Manual 5 TR, American Psychiatric Association.

Ellis, J., and Whaite, A. (1983), To Parents of Children with Disabilities, from Parents of Children with Disabilities, Social Evaluation and Research Ltd.

Gilmore, L. (2018), "Supporting Families of Children with Rare and Unique Chromosome Disorders", Research and Practice in Intellectual and Developmental Disabilities, 5(1), pp 8–16.

Reed, G. M., et al. (2019), "Innovations and Changes in the ICD-11 Classification of Mental, Behavioural and Neurodevelopmental Disorders", World Psychiatry, 18(1), pp 3–19.

Part V
Report writing and case studies

For some psychologists, written reports are a chore to be endured; for others, they are an enjoyable creative process. Regardless of preference, psychological reports are a vital and mandatory part of developmental and diagnostic assessments of young children. Access to funding and services, information to parents, therapists, medical practitioners, government services and agencies generally depend upon timely, accurate, informative and helpful information.

What information should be included in reports? How much technical information and psychometric data should they contain? Are there different report writing styles depending on the recipients of reports? What in fact is the overriding function of written reports?

This chapter tackles the process of writing reports emanating from developmental assessments. Various report writing structures and templates are discussed, and examples provided in the context are case examples. These cases are drawn from "real-life" clinical practice over many years and have been appropriately anonymised and redacted to ensure that none of the children and scenarios presented can be associated with actual cases.

The essential role of reports—a means of "telling the story"—is central to this chapter, as is the need for psychologists to experiment and develop their own report writing style. The different case examples demonstrate the variety of purposes reports can serve and the range of issues which may come to psychologists for assessment, review, advice, intervention and advocacy.

DOI: 10.4324/9781003565338-32

27 Report writing

Reports! Some psychologists love writing them; others find them the bane of their existence. Some love to express their thoughts and opinions through words, to tell the stories of their clients; others merely report psychometric and diagnostic results. Report writing is integral to the role of psychologists involved in assessments as other parties need to have results, information and diagnoses. Often there are deadlines for completion, and different formats are required.

Why do we write reports?

Reports from assessments serve many purposes and many masters. Reports can:

- Record the details of a child's assessment for parents.
- Inform other professionals about a child's assessment and diagnosis.
- "Benchmark" a child's current skills and weaknesses.
- Help plan for future needs.
- Assist in advocating for children and families.
- Secure funding and services and access to specific schools and programmes.
- Offer programming and support suggestions.
- Provide support and encouragement for families.
- Educate parents and professionals about neurodevelopmental disorders.
- Address legal proceedings associated with diagnoses and support needs.

To whom do psychologists write reports?

A psychological report can have many "audiences", depending upon circumstances:

- Parents and caregivers.
- Medical practitioners.
- Therapists such as speech pathologists and occupational therapists.
- Government departments and agencies and non-government organisations.
- Early intervention teachers and personnel.
- Government and non-government schools and educational bodies.
- Lawyers and solicitors.

Do different "audiences" require different reports?

Let us consider the differing needs of report recipients and how these perspectives may be encapsulated in reports.

DOI: 10.4324/9781003565338-33

Families

Parents need to know in succinct terms about their child's diagnosis: What it means, how it may have occurred and what should be done immediately to begin remediation. They need to know what to do immediately to secure support and funding and where to find appropriate therapeutic, medical or educational services. They need to know which programmes and resources are "the best" for their child and who to contact. They need to know as much as they can about the future for their child. They need to know how and what to tell family and friends. As much as these issues should and can be discussed at the time of assessment, a written report "secures" the information for later use and consideration.

Written reports allow families to make informed and appropriate choices about therapies, medical treatments and intervention, and educational options. A written report also serves as a "passport" for a family and their child, confirming "eligibility" and "right of entry" to the complex world of services. Without a written report, they may be "ineligible." A poorly written report can cause delay, refusal and "denial of service".

Medical practitioners

Most young children who come for psychological and developmental assessments are already under the care of paediatricians, neurologists, general practitioners or geneticists. The medical profession requires the circulation of information through referrals and reports. Psychological reports provide the additional information that specialists need to clarify their ongoing services for a child. For example, a psychological report may confirm a diagnosis of autism spectrum disorder, allowing the paediatrician to engage with the child's family at a different level. There may be supporting evidence required for a paediatrician to secure specific services or funding support. There may be implications for the paediatrician to consider such interventions as medications.

Medical specialists are inordinately busy and rarely have the opportunity to speak to psychologists by phone or in person but will liaise through reports and emails. A temporary "team" may come about with psychologist, medical practitioner and family working towards common goals. Reports become the "common language" shared by those involved and can serve as the "handshake" by which a professional relationship of trust and respect can develop.

Therapists

Speech pathologists, occupational therapists, physiotherapists, other psychologists, behavioural therapists and early intervention teachers will invariably read psychological reports about young children. They rely upon this information to alert them to specific issues prior to their own assessments and interventions. Reports provide qualitative information which serves as "benchmarks" and starting points for therapists and early intervention professionals. Reports from psychologists can serve an educational purpose for other professionals, clarifying diagnostic criteria for neurodevelopmental disorders and illustrating a child's observed behaviours in that context.

Therapists and early intervention services often contact psychologists to discuss details of behaviour, performance, progress and achievement. Their relationships with young children and their families can be very close and sustained, and they can bring insights into other family issues to psychologists. These professionals will know when to refer families for additional assessment, support or information. They may even become aware of concerns regarding a child's sibling. Again, written reports are the "common language" and medium of communication for therapists.

Government departments and other agencies

Nations worldwide provide funding for early intervention, therapeutic and educational support programmes for children with neurodevelopmental disorders through a complex array of service providers; some funded directly through state agencies while others through government-funded organisations such as religious bodies, charities and private service providers. Each may have its own eligibility criteria, similar no doubt from context to context, but with subtle variations which can inadvertently prevent service access if not understood. Psychologists should be as far as possible *au fait* with these criteria and procedures and structure their reports accordingly to service provision. There should be:

- Clear and accurate demographic information.
- Clear reports of assessments undertaken, including relevant psychometric results and diagnostic terminology.
- A clear statement of a particular child or family's needs.
- Completion of relevant application forms and checklists.
- Reference to supporting evidence such as confirming medical reports.
- Evidentiary proof of the psychologist's credentials.

Government departments and agencies are perhaps less interested in fine-grained qualitative assessment information, but non-government agencies and services may require information of that kind. Writing reports for government departments and agencies can be pedantic and repetitive, but it is an "essential service" for young children with neurodevelopmental disorders.

Lawyers, solicitors and court proceedings

From time to time, a psychologist may be requested by lawyers to provide information for upcoming legal proceedings, for example, separation or divorce cases where there are disputes about the costs of care of a child with a disability. Sometimes this is a voluntary process; at others, reports and client notes may be subpoenaed. These cases may involve requests for highly specific and sometimes unanswerable questions such as the likely duration and course of a disabling condition, the costs of treatment and the availability of alternate courses of action. Where possible, psychologists should avail themselves of any opportunity to attend seminars on the responsibilities they have in relation to such matters.

How can a single report accommodate these needs?

Report writing may be considered by some as an "art," and there are as many report writing "styles" as there are psychologists. Report writing is a developmental process. Change in style can occur over time through experience and practice. There is one core issue to consider—reports are a form of "communication".

Writing as "communication"

Speech pathologists describe "communication" as the intersection of three factors (Figure 27.1):

- **Content:** What is being spoken about?
- **Form:** The language, vocabulary, idioms, syntax and terminology in use.
- **Context:** Where, why and with whom the communication is occurring.

Communication around disability challenges parents with labels, diagnoses, clinical terminology, medical and psychological nomenclature. Technical terminology is of course essential to all professions. It is a set of "abbreviations" to be used "in-house" for those who share and understand the content. But what is being discussed is a child, not a collection of psychological or medical terms. These discussions often take place in doctor's surgeries or hospitals, psychologists' offices or schools, which for families may be alien territory. The "context" is generally about assistance, but this can be rendered meaningless if the "form" and "content" are not appropriate for that context. Under those circumstances, effective communication may not occur. This also applies to written reports.

Written communication also needs to be "fit for purpose". Given the complex nature of information and terminology inherent in developmental assessments, it is often discussed that there needs to be a "common language" for understanding disability and developmental disorders, whereby information can be effectively communicated across all parties involved—parents, clinicians, agencies and government departments (Figure 27.2):

Under this model, interdisciplinary communication would endeavour to ensure that all parties would share information in its most accessible and coherent form, whether written or spoken. There would be minimal use of confusing jargon or terminology and statistics and avoidance of language which may inadvertently be "offensive" or derogatory to children or families. A simple example is of a child with "bizarre" language and another a child with "primitive" facial features. Reaching a common language consensus may be easier in multidisciplinary settings where teams can discuss and clarify these issues, but psychologists working independently can help by clarifying and simplifying information from other professionals.

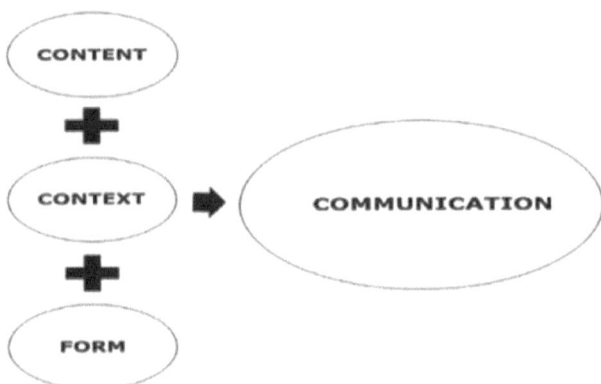

Figure 27.1 The components of communication

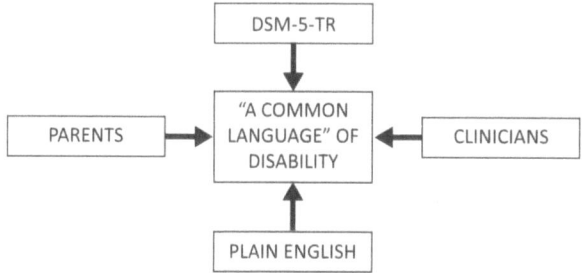

Figure 27.2 A "common language" for discussing and reporting

The following is an actual case example of medical terminology associated with chromosome 9p deletion syndrome presented to a family by written report, with no explanatory notes as to the meaning of the symptoms:

- **Trigonocephaly**: This relates to the premature fusion of skull bones giving the forehead a triangular shape.
- **Brachycephaly**: This refers to the condition where the head is disproportionately wide.
- **Metopic Ridges**: This refers to an abnormal shape of the skull. The ridge can be seen on the forehead.
- **Frontal Bossing**: This describes an unusually prominent forehead, sometimes associated with a heavier than normal brow ridge.
- **Camptodactyly**: This is a rare disorder characterised mainly by permanently flexed fingers, deafness and hair and teeth abnormalities.

It is unlikely that families will be able to decipher such complex terminology, and the net effect may be anxiety or confusion on their part as they struggle to understand what is wrong with their child and what courses of action, if any, can be taken to remediate the situation. The symptoms described above essentially relate to the physical appearance of a child and not to life-threatening illnesses. A simplified, "plain English" version of such a report created by the psychologist involved helped clarify parental concerns.

Can a psychological report successfully convey all requisite information to all "stakeholders"? There will be times when different reports will be needed for different "audiences". Sometimes a "template" report can be written, but two or more different "endings" are used, depending upon "audience" and purpose. The following section provides examples of these various methods and formats, but firstly, it is important to address the modern trend towards automatic generation of scoring profiles and results through artificial intelligence.

A note on computer-generated scoring, reporting and artificial intelligence

The "art" or craft of report writing in psychology continues to evolve through advances in technology. Psychologists who have been practising for a long time will remember writing reports by hand and then passing them on to typists or other clerical staff for transformation into official copies. It was a significant change for many when desktop computers were introduced at workplaces, as it meant "thinking" and writing through a keyboard instead of the human hand. Nowadays, one can dictate directly by voice-translating software text on screen, another skill to learn in the processing and expressing of thoughts and ideas.

Technology continues to permeate almost every facet of our lives, including our professions, and work practices. Psychometric tests can now be administered "online" rather than through pen and paper pro formas. Results can be instantaneously scored, tabled, graphed, compared and interpreted through sophisticated software packages. For some but not all psychometric test instruments, reports can be generated automatically from these results, including interpretation of results and subsequent recommendations. And the development and growth of "artificial intelligence" (AI) and readily available programmes for computers such as "ChatGPT" pose many questions for the role of psychologists in their professional practice. At the time of writing, only one psychological society (the New Zealand Psychological Society) has published a set of coherent guidelines as to the use of AI in the writing of reports, but it is expected that others will follow suit. The guidelines reflect the following points of concern:

- **Variable depth of knowledge:** The effectiveness of AI is contingent on the quality and breadth of the data it processes.
- **Bias and inaccuracy:** Identifying biases within AI algorithms can be challenging.
- **Subtle biases:** The subtlety of biases in AI-generated content can complicate their identification, especially in areas unfamiliar to the practitioner.
- **Misinformation and ethical misuse:** The deliberate use of AI to fabricate or distort information is ethically indefensible.
- **Plagiarism and intellectual honesty:** Particularly in research.
- **Accountability:** Again, particularly in relation to research.

The associated guidelines include some which relate directly to New Zealand Maori culture and are paraphrased below:

- Psychologists need to consider the unique cultural context of "Aotearoa" (Mauri name for New Zealand) when using AI in their practice.
- Psychologists are encouraged to view their obligations in understanding an AI tool as similar to those when using psychometric measures.
- Psychologists need to consider their obligations under Te Tiriti (the Treaty of Waitangi) and the principles of Māori Data Sovereignty when using AI tools.
- Psychologists need to consider the potential biases in results from an AI tool and avoid perpetuating any form of discrimination based on biased data sets.
- Psychological services and opinions that a registered psychologist offers should not be exclusively delegated to AI.
- Psychologists should only use AI tools that they have assessed as being ethically robust and transparent about the parameters of data sharing.
- Psychologists should consider the principles of the Privacy Act 2020 (New Zealand) and a privacy impact assessment when using AI tools in their work.
- Psychologists should be transparent about the use of AI and inform colleagues and clients that they are using AI.
- The onus is on the psychologist to ensure the person(s) with whom they are working understands the role of any AI, to facilitate an informed choice about its use.
- Person(s) working with a psychologist should not be disadvantaged if they do not wish to have AI tools used in their care, particularly in relation to stored data.

It is a matter of individual professional choice and judgement as to whether reports generated in part or whole using AI adequately "tell the story" of a clinical assessment of a young child, where a great deal of the perception and understanding about a child comes from the clinical but personal interaction with that child and family "in the room".

The concern expressed by many practitioners, including the author, is that there can be no substitute for clinical experience in describing a child's presentation and that reports generated purely from psychometric algorithms are significantly limited in their ability to accurately or adequately narrate the experience of such clinical interactions and observations. A previous chapter has highlighted the need to incorporate information about the qualitative aspects of test performance as well as the purely psychometric. Report writing is, as has been expressed, a "communication" and resides perhaps in a space between an "art" and a "craft". Practitioners will need to determine for themselves whether the convenience of software-generated reports is compromised by a lack of direct "expression" of what has been assessed or whether there is justification in implicitly trusting the metric information produced electronically to be sufficient.

Typical psychology report layouts

Section 1: Identifying demographic information

- File or reference number (if applicable).
- Name of child.
- Date of birth.
- Date of assessment.
- Chronological age (years and months or just months).
- Parental details—names, addressed and contact details.
- Name of assessing psychologist.
- Referring doctor (where applicable).

NB: Developmental tests such as Griffiths III and Bayley-4 are predicated upon birth date for accurate calculation of chronological age, including. "rounding up" rules when calculating chronological age "to the months."

Section 2: Executive Summary (optional)

- Generally, a dot-point precis of main points for specific "audiences." An executive summary can be useful for agencies only requiring the report to validate a child's eligibility for a programme. The remainder of the report is more appropriate to other professionals involved.

Section 3: Background information

- Referral purpose or referrer.
- Summary of medical assessments if relevant.
- Summary of other reports of relevance.
- Family history.
- Parental account of child's developmental history and presenting issues.
- Information from other involved parties, for example, preschools.
- Summary of information obtained through checklists and questionnaires.

NB: Section 3 "sets the scene" and context for the assessment report, facilitating the "reframing" of information from various sources into a coherent story. Finally, Section 3 validates various opinions about a child.

Section 4: Psychometric tests used and results obtained

For example:

- Griffiths 3 and Bayley-4, with results tabulated appropriately.
- Adaptive behaviour assessments with results tabulated appropriately.
- Diagnostic assessment outcomes, for example, autism spectrum disorder assessments.
- Any other relevant psychometric assessment results, for example, executive functioning assessments.

NB: It needs to be considered how much psychometric and diagnostic information is sufficient, who will be reading this information and whether it will be understood and how such information should be presented, for example, tables, graphs and histograms.

Section 5: Child's observed behaviour and assessment performance

For example:

- Behaviour on arrival and observed behaviours during assessment.
- Free-play observations.
- Levels of concentration, anxiety, compliance and engagement.
- Qualitative aspects of task attempts, completions and failures.
- Specific behaviours of concern noted during assessment.

NB: This section allows psychologists to relate as accurately as possible the observations made during assessment. Psychologists are trained to observe and report on "behaviours", such as how children attempt tasks, whether successfully or not. Such observations should go beyond simple "pass/fail" criteria for test items, also commenting upon the "quality" of attempts made.

Section 6: Test findings and diagnostic considerations

For example:

- Global developmental delay.
- Autism spectrum disorder, including degree and support levels.
- Other neurodevelopmental disorders.

NB: Background information, observations, assessment results, hypotheses and theories can be condensed into a coherent summation. Not all assessments culminate in a diagnosis, and if a psychologist is undecided about a clear diagnosis, he/she should state this and make recommendations, for example, for:

- Further assessments and observations.
- Reassessment at a future date, particularly after therapies and remediation programmes have subsequently been put in place.

When diagnoses are made, DSM-5-TR coding should be used when applicable. A psychologist needs to "argue his/her case". It is the professional role of psychologists to present independent and objective findings and not merely opinions. Diagnosis follows analysis of accumulated evidence aligned to internationally recognised diagnostic criteria.

Section 7: Recommended courses of action

For example:

- Referral to therapists or programmes.
- Applications to funding or support agencies and services.
- Follow-up observations at (for example) preschools.
- Follow-up meetings with parents and other involved parties.
- Recommendations for further assessments, for example, hearing.

NB: It is general psychological practice that "generic" recommendations can be made about intervention programmes and therapeutic options, but specific programmes or individuals should not be recommended. Conflicts of interest need to be declared. For example, the Australian Psychological Society Code of Ethics states the following:

C.3.4. Psychologists declare to clients any vested interests they have in the psychological services they deliver, including all relevant funding, licensing and royalty interests.

- Brief restatement of referral purpose and outcomes.
- Commitment to follow-up actions.
- Salutations, for example, gratitude for information provided to assist assessment.

Section 9: Score summary page (optional)

For example:

- Standard scores.
- Stanines.
- Percentiles.
- Developmental age equivalents.
- Any other specific information.
- Graphing and charting (optional).

NB: Section 9 is specifically for reports when another psychologist will be reading the assessment details (Figure 27.3).

Psychometric results are generally presented "visually" on test protocols, variously as tables, charts and graphs. These graphs, tables, charts and diagrams can be useful in representing psychometric data in differing ways. It is a matter for psychologists to determine which format is most appropriate for specific assessments, target audiences and report purposes (Figure 27.4).

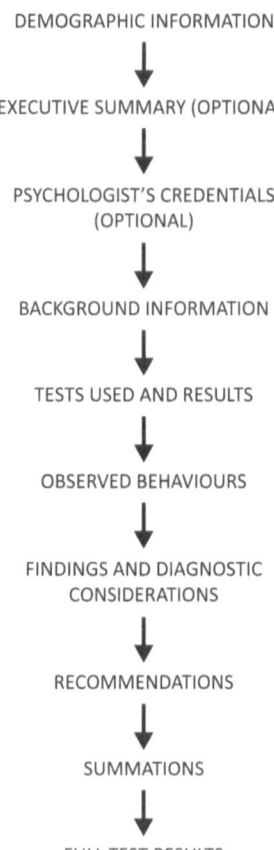

Figure 27.3 Summary of suggested report structure

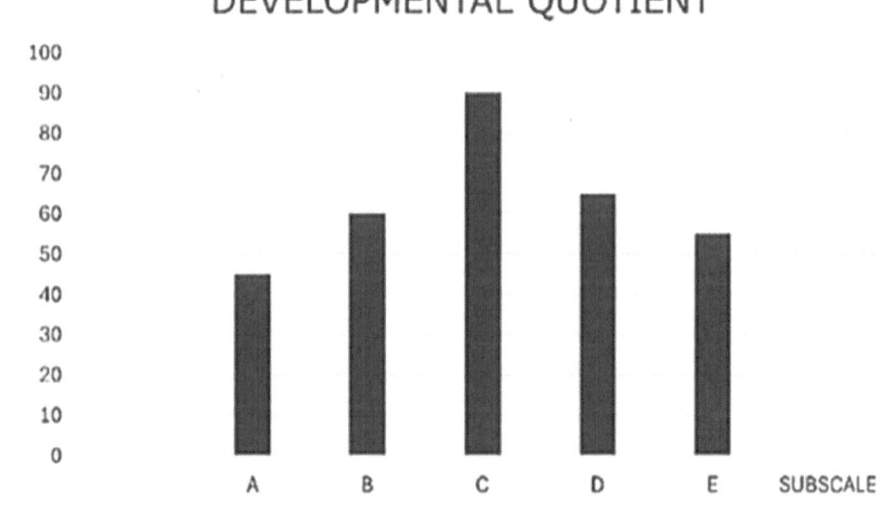

Figure 27.4 Sample graphic representations of psychometric data

Final points

Reports are invariably time-consuming but are best when written immediately or as soon as possible after an assessment. Firstly, the detail and "immediacy" of an assessment may be forgotten or lost if there is a significant time delay between assessment and report. Many things will intervene in that time. Secondly, reports for applications for funding, service access or school enrolment are often "driven" by urgency. There are deadlines and "cut-off" dates. The sooner a report is completed, the faster it can be sent or lodged to secure the support and services required for a child and family.

On the other hand, reports need to be written carefully and checked for accuracy. Trivial mistakes can occur, such as spelling errors or even wrong names. Dates of birth can be erroneous; test results may be reported incorrectly. "Save-as" reports need to be carefully checked to ensure no residual information from a previous report is inadvertently left behind in the new version. It is always better to complete a report "once" accurately even if some extra time and effort is required.

Finally, but perhaps most importantly, psychological reports are a means of "telling the story" of children with disabilities, neurodevelopmental disorders and other compromising conditions. These are young children and cannot speak or advocate for themselves. Families of course do advocate for their own children but rely upon "expert" evidence to bolster their claims for legitimate help. As much as psychologists' reports must detail and present such evidence, it must never lose sight of the subject of their reporting. "Telling the story" of the child should be at the heart of every report.

Bibliography

Australian Psychological Society (2007), Australian Psychological Society Code of Ethics, https://psychology.org.au/.

Australian Psychological Society Information Sheet 2, www.psychology.org.au, "Writing reports for court"

Caithness, T., and Moore, E. (2011), "A Common Language for Understanding Disability, Development, Emotions, and Behaviour", In Dossetor, D., White, D., and Whatson, L. (Eds.), Mental Health of Children and Adolescents with Intellectual and Developmental Disabilities, IP Communications, pp 36–50.

Goldfinger, K., and Pomerantz, A. M. (2013), Psychological Assessment and Report Writing (2nd Edition), Sage Publications.

Huff, C. (2020), How to Write More Useful Assessment Reports, American Psychological Association.

Pelling, N. J., and Burton, L. J. (2017), The Elements of Psychological Case Report Writing in Australia, Routledge Publishing.

Wiener, J., and Costaris, L. (2012), "Teaching Psychological Report Writing: Content and Process", Canadian Journal of School Psychology, 27(2), pp 119–135.

28 Case studies and reports

The following reports are derived from clinical assessments of global developmental delay as defined by DSM-5-TR, autism spectrum disorder as defined by DSM-5-TR, other specific diagnoses or dual diagnoses. Some are derived from unusual requests, subpoenas and submissions from specific situations and referrals. The names and demographic information of the children involved have been changed to ensure anonymity and specific details such as children's dates of birth, names of doctors, therapists, preschools and childcare centres and have also been redacted. These extracted samples also indicate the range of diagnostic questions posed prior to assessment and the range of diagnostic outcomes which can eventuate or be considered.

Case Study 1:   Autism Spectrum Disorder and Global Developmental Delay

Child's Name: Mario
Chronological Age: 2 years 9 months

Referral information

Mario is a 2-year-9-month-old male child, who was referred by his neurologist for a neurodevelopmental evaluation due to concerns with his attention, socio-emotional and language development. This evaluation is being completed to gather a better understanding of his current functioning, consider a diagnosis of autism spectrum disorder, as well as provide recommendations for services not already in place.

Background and history

Information about Mario's history was obtained through a semi-structured clinical interview with his mother and through review of data provided by his mother. The clinical interview was completed in English.

Mario's parents first became concerned with his development at the age of eighteen months due to a regression in his overall language skills. He was saying single words and some two-word phrases, but he lost this ability and other social communication skills (such as spontaneously greeting others). He was recommended to undergo a neurology consultation, as well as being connected to the relevant early medical screening services.

DOI: 10.4324/9781003565338-34

Mario completed a developmental screening assessment with the relevant service provider and was noted to have delays across most of his areas of development. He was recommended to receive in-home early education services twice per week. He also received occupational therapy services earlier this year (6–7 sessions) to address sensory difficulties. However, sessions were discontinued for reasons unknown.

Mario recently completed a neurology consultation in July 2020. Results of the evaluation indicated learning, social and language delays which ruled out diagnoses of attention deficit hyperactivity disorder (ADHD), obsessive compulsive disorder (OCD) and generalised anxiety disorder (GAD). His neurologist recommended that he obtain a speech and language evaluation, occupational therapy evaluation, neurodevelopmental evaluation, continuation of early intervention services as well as being connected to the local school district at the age of three.

Currently, Mario is demonstrating delays in his communication skills. He is exposed primarily to English at home. He can produce several word approximations with consistency, but they are not used functionally. However, his mother noted that he has recently started saying "No" and "Mum". Mario mostly speaks in jargon speech and open vowel/nasal sounds to communicate his needs. He also engages in hand leading, using others' hands as a tool and whining to communicate with others. He is not yet consistently imitating simple words but can imitate play sounds such as "choo" with a train and howling like a wolf. Several speech abnormalities were reported: Grunting sounds, repetitive vocalisations and heavy breathing. He occasionally makes high pitched sounds when he is excited and playing with his sister.

In terms of his receptive and nonverbal communication skills, Mario is not consistently responding to his name or to simple commands. His mother believes he understands some simple instructions but chooses not to respond. Mario is able to use some communicative gestures to compliment his speech, such as using a communicative reach, pointing, facing away to indicate no and clapping to himself when he is happy. He is not yet waving to greet, pointing to show or nodding his head for yes. He uses well-developed facial expressions, but he is described to occasionally laugh to himself without purpose. Mario demonstrates inconsistent use of eye contact when he is initiating a social interaction. He is not yet engaging in flexible joint attention, but he consistently socially references others while playing on his own.

Mario offers affection to his loved ones. However, he does not consistently tolerate unexpected touch and affection from anyone other than his mother. In terms of social skills, Mario prefers to engage in solitary activities. He demonstrates a limited interest in his peers. Most of his interactions are object oriented and physical in nature. He will tolerate playing next to his peers and adults. He can engage in some simple reciprocal interactions. He is not yet sharing and showing his interests with consistency. He occasionally has difficulty tolerating transitions and unexpected changes during his day, but he is easy to redirect.

In regard to his play skills, he is engaging in functional play, but he often engages in cause-and-effect play actions. He is demonstrating a restricted interest in playing with toy vehicles, playing with sand and dirt and playing with water, but he enjoys exploring all toys. He also demonstrates a restricted interest/behaviour in placing toys on tabletops and windowsills. Most of his play is one-sided and follows his own train of thought.

Atypical and other repetitive behaviours were reported to occur occasionally: Pacing, flapping, squinting, finger play, grimacing, jumping, placing his arm on his eyes and peering out of the corner of his eyes. He also enjoys climbing on others (particularly his mother), receiving squeezes and hanging on people. Additional concerns include Mario's sensory processing difficulties. He has an aversive reaction to haircuts, water over his head and touching sticky or slimy objects. He prefers to be naked and barefoot. He enjoys playing in darker lit spaces such as under tables. He also has a history of engaging in staring spells. He also engages in repetitive sensory-seeking behaviours; licking, mouthing and biting toys; visually inspecting toys; staring at bright and blinking lights; and rubbing his face on others' legs. Although he is not described as a picky eater, he is noted to have some difficulties with certain textures, such as gooey and tacky textures in his food. He also engages in some repetitive routines with his food such as dumping his food before eating it. He is also demonstrating a heightened threshold to pain.

In regard to his motor skills, no concerns were reported regarding his early developmental milestones. He walked at 12 months and ran at 13 months. Currently, he is able to run and jump, and he enjoys being outside. However, he is described as clumsy and uncoordinated, and he also walks on his toes throughout his day.

No fine motor delays were reported, but he is not yet efficiently using feeding utensils and prefers to use his hands. He is not yet toilet-trained, and he is not showing signs of being ready. No sleep difficulties were reported.

In terms of his emotional regulation skills, Mario is described to have some difficulty adapting to changes in his schedule, transitions and when his needs are not immediately met. In times of stress, he engages in tantrum behaviours: Screaming, crying, falling to the floor, running away. He can become aggressive such as throwing toys, pushing and hitting (however, this has decreased over time). A history of self-injurious behaviours was denied. His tantrums are frequent and occur a few times per day, but he is easy to soothe and redirect. There are also some mild safety concerns, eloping in the community, wandering away, climbing on furniture and demonstrating little sense of danger.

Psychosocial/Family history

Mario lives with his mother, father and his sister (age 5). His mother denied being impacted by any recent significant psychosocial stressors, and a history of trauma was denied. There is a family history of autistic spectrum disorder in a paternal first cousin. There is a history of anxiety and depression in his father, paternal grandmother and paternal uncles and aunts. No other family history of mental, psychiatric, neurological or genetic problems was reported.

Birth/Medical history

Mario's mother had an uneventful pregnancy. His mother had appropriate prenatal care, and Mario was not exposed to any teratogens in utero. He was born 7 pounds 9 ounces by normal spontaneous vaginal delivery and term gestation without any complications. He was born with jaundice and was discharged after two days with a "biliblanket", and symptoms were quickly resolved. Currently, Mario is in good general health and is not taking any medications. A history of seizures and head trauma was not noted. Vision was not described as of concern. Previous audiology evaluation showed no concerns. A history of allergies was not noted.

Behavioural observations

Mario's grooming was neat and appropriate. Mario easily transitioned into the testing area. When prompted by his mother to greet the examiner, he ignored her request and quickly began playing with the toys in the room. The examiner attempted to wave at him, but he did not respond. He was noted to babble and jargon to himself during the clinical interview. He was not observed to show toys but often brought his mother toys and placed them on the table in front of her, placed them in her lap or placed toys in her hand and then walked away. He mostly spoke in open vowel and nasal sounds, with occasional jargon speech. He was observed to say a few words during the clinical interview, but they were not directed at others (i.e., no, "choo choo" for a train). He often used hand leading and used his mother's hands as a tool to get his needs met.

No gross motor concerns were noted. He was observed to walk on his toes. He was observed to engage in cause-and-effect and explorative play and occasional functional play. He enjoyed playing with toy animals and a farm. He played on his own, rarely asking either his mother or the examiner to join in. He came to others for help by placing toys in their hands or by hand leading. Mario played on his own without guidance for over 30 minutes. He engaged in some repetitive mannerisms: Grimacing, peering out of the corner of his eyes, flapping, squinting. He was not observed to share his enjoyment while he played on his own.

Mario was able to transition from playing to engaging in structured activities, particularly while sitting on his mother's lap. He often wiggled, asked to get down and threw items off the desk but was easily redirected with the presentation of new tasks. He rarely responded to any social praise during the cognitive/language testing but enjoyed the presentation of novel stimuli. Mario was able to complete all parts of the cognitive and language testing. Some caution was taken while interpreting the results on the Bayley-4 due to behavioural interference and modification to the presentation of instructions, for example, the examiner wearing a mask due to COVID-19 regulations).

Scores on the ADOS-2 were not provided at this time, due to modifications during testing (the examiner and mother wearing face masks due to COVID-19 restrictions), but testing was completed for qualitative purposes.

Tests administered

- Autism Diagnostic Observation Schedule, Second Edition (ADOS-2), module 1.
- Bayley Scales of Infant and Toddler Development, Fourth Edition (BAYLEY-4), Cognitive and Language Subtests.
- Bayley Scales of Infant and Toddler Development, Fourth Edition (BAYLEY-4), Social-Emotional and adaptive Behaviour Scales, parent report.
- Behaviour Assessment System for Children, Third Edition (BASC-3), parent report.
- Ages and Stages Questionnaires, Social Emotional, Second Edition (ASQ:SE-2), parent report.

Bayley Scales of Infant and Toddler Development, Fourth Edition (BAYLEY-4)

Area	Standard Score	Percentile	Interpretation	
Bayley-4 Cognitive Composite	55	0.1	Extremely low	
Bayley-4 Language Composite	45	Below 0.1	Extremely low	
Domain	Scaled Score	Percentile	Age equivalent	Interpretation
Bayley-4 Cognitive Scale	1	0.1	19 months	Extremely low
Bayley-4 Receptive Language Scale	1	0.1	7 months	Extremely low
Adaptive Behaviour Scale and Social-Emotional				

(Continued)

Area	Standard Score	Percentile	Interpretation	
Bayley-4 Communication Composite	50	Below 0.1	Extremely low	
Bayley-4 Daily living skills composite	75	5	Borderline	
Bayley-4 Socialisation	59	0.3	Extremely low	
Bayley-4 Adaptive Behaviour	55	0.1	Extremely low	
Bayley-4 Social Emotional scale	55	0.1	Extremely low	
Domain	Scaled score	Percentile	Age equivalent	Interpretation
Bayley-4 Receptive	1	0.1	8 months 15 days	Extremely low
Bayley-4 Expressive	2	0.4	10 months 15 days	Extremely low
Bayley-4 Personal	5	5	18 months 5 days	Borderline
Bayley-4 Interpersonal relationships	1	0.1	1 month 15 days	Extremely low
Bayley-4 Play and leisure	4	2	9 months 15 days	Borderline
Sensory Supplementary analysis Bayley-4	Raw score		Interpretation	
Bayley-4 Sensory processing	25		Possible challenges	

Test results

Social and emotional development

Asq-se-2

Area	Raw score/cut-off score	Interpretation
Asq-se-2	170/105	Elevated

Socio-emotional perception

Basc-3 preschool aged 2–5 years

Area	Raw score	Interpretation
Validity scales		
F	0	Acceptable
Response pattern	98	Acceptable
Consistency	6	Acceptable
Clinical scales	T-score	Interpretation
Hyperactivity	59	Within normal limits
Aggression	58	Within normal limits
Anxiety	44	Within normal limits
Depression	48	Within normal limits
Somatisation	57	Within normal limits
Attention problems	61	At risk
Atypicality	70	Clinically significant
Withdrawal	88	Clinically significant
Externalising problems composite	59	Within normal limits
Internalising problems composite	50	Within normal limits
Behavioural symptoms index	68	At risk

(*Continued*)

Adaptive scales

Adaptability	48	Within normal limits
Social skills	28	Clinically significant
Functional communication	31	At risk
Activities of daily living	32	At risk
Adaptive skills composite	31	At risk

Content scales

Anger control	54	Within normal limits
Bullying	43	Within normal limits
Developmental social disorders	83	Clinically significant
Emotional self-control	52	Within normal limits
Executive functioning	60	At risk
Negative emotionality	56	Within normal limits
Resiliency	42	Within normal limits

Clinical Diagnosis: Global developmental delay. On this basis, he is eligible for consideration of attendance at an early intervention centre conducted through his local school district, and his family entitled to apply for the Supplemental Security Income (SSI) programme to help with the costs of additional therapeutic assistance such as applied behaviour analysis.

Case Study 2: Autism Spectrum Disorder and Global Developmental Delay

Child's Name: Ethan
Chronological Age: 3 years 8 months

Background

Ethan is aged 3 years 8 months and was referred by his consultant paediatrician for formal assessment of possible autism spectrum disorder. The paediatrician refers to Ethan's poor social interaction and language skills, his tendency to be totally involved in his own world, excellent memory skills, restricted diet and his tendency to vocalise by singing and reciting songs and poems.

Ethan attends a childcare centre. He is under the care of a speech pathologist, and a summary report indicates social communication difficulty, severe receptive language delay and severe expressive language delay. This report highlights Ethan's inconsistent social engagement skills, with instances of solo play but at other times being responsive to games and activities. He was described as being a pleasure to play with, but difficulties were noted in maintaining eye contact, turn taking, expressing needs, asking and responding. It was particularly noted that there were times during the assessment when Ethan remains non-verbal. It has been suggested that Ethan also should be assessed by an occupational therapist.

Diagnostic assessment outcomes

Autism Diagnostic Observation Schedule 2, Module 1

DSM-5-TR Diagnosis: Autism Spectrum Disorder
Level of Support: Level 2 "Substantial"

258   *Diagnosing Young Children with Neurodevelopmental Disorders*

Background

Ethan attended assessment with his mother, and it was a pleasure to meet them. He presented as a child with considerable variation in his ability to interact and respond socially, communicate and play. Initially, he was left to play as he saw fit whilst a background case history was taken. This is summarised below:

- Ethan's mother described a family history on the male side of significant learning difficulties and rigidity of behaviour patterns.
- In relation to Ethan, she described that there were few early concerns about his development until somewhere between 18 months and 2 years of age. At this point, there was stoppage and regression in relation to his spoken language and a distinct change in his ability to tolerate various foods. Subsequent assessment of hearing indicated no difficulty, but Ethan is now extremely fussy about what he will and will not eat.
- It was described that Ethan had become fixated upon a particular colour for his drink bottle and as possessing a most impressive memory as to where toys and objects were located or hidden.
- Some early toe walking was reported, but not stereotypic hand or arm flapping. Ethan was described as having engaged in close visual inspection with his toys, namely, putting his head on the floor when pushing cars. Some instances of turning toy cars over and spinning the wheels were reported.
- Ethan was described as being inconsistent with his social and communication skills. On the one hand, he was described as at times showing empathy and concern for his parents, by sitting in their lap and cuddling. On the other hand, he was described as being disengaged and inconsistent in terms of turning to the call of his name unless he was "motivated".
- Ethan was described as singing and reciting rhymes on a frequent basis. He was described as not engaging in immediate echolalia but as having some instances where spoken words did not appear to connect to any immediate context.
- Ethan was described as being particularly sound-sensitive, perhaps more so when younger. This included instances of Ethan having to cover his ears to loud noises. Although he was not described as "sniffing and sampling" foods, it was clear from description that he was extremely sensitive to certain foods and even food brands of essentially the same product.
- At his childcare centre, Ethan's interaction with other children was described as being inconsistent in terms of frequency and quality. He was described as taking part in some of the routines but again mostly when he was motivated or interested to do so.
- Ethan was described as already developing and expertise with early reading and letter naming and recognition. He was also described as having an interest in car number plates.

Behavioural observations

Following this case history, Ethan was assessed through direct interaction and play, using a variety of toys and materials from Griffiths III and activities from the Autism Diagnostic Observation Schedule 2, and scoring of this process is tabled above.

After 2 hours of assessment in this manner, it was my decision that Ethan did meet DSM-5-TR criteria for a diagnosis of autism spectrum disorder.

Most of his symptoms were mild, with some "classic" signs of autism spectrum disorder not noted at all. However, sufficient symptomatology was noted for a clear diagnosis to be made. Given his age, it is imperative that early therapeutic intervention be continued and extended. For this reason, Ethan meets DSM-5-TR criteria for level II "substantial support needed" in relation to his diagnosis of autism spectrum disorder. The following specific points were noted:

- There were considerable periods of time throughout the assessment when Ethan essentially remained non-verbal. When he did speak or vocalise, it was often in the context of singing or "jargoning". Some of the sounds made were distinctly stereotypic in quality. On other occasions, Ethan was heard to vocalise clear words and phrases although not necessarily related to the immediate context of interaction or communication. One such instance was when for no reason he pronounced "word". Ethan also made a small number of non-speech sounds which may have been self-stimulatory. He was also described as having a tendency to teeth-grind.
- Ethan's social engagement was very variable. At times, he responded quite well to verbal redirection, particularly when it was related to stopping him from attempting to leave the room, to climb onto high bookshelves or to engage with office equipment.
- On other occasions, he remained non-responsive to social cues, the call of his name or specific instructions. At other times, he was capable of making good eye contact and displaying warm and engaging social smiles and some variation in facial expression. He particularly enjoyed anticipating simple physical games such as tickling. There were also times when Ethan was able to demonstrate anticipatory language, such as finishing someone else's phrase.
- Ethan was affectionate with his mother, but it was noted that this often consisted of him sitting on her lap for a cuddle but then nuzzling his nose against her face or her clothing. On one occasion, he displayed a distinctly concerned facial expression, but it was not possible to gauge any particular context for this. Ethan was noted on at least one occasion to give his mother something for her to help him with, but social showing and sharing was not noted.
- It was noted that Ethan was usually quite negotiable in terms of giving toys and equipment back, but his mother did note that temper tantrums were possible when routines were interrupted.
- In terms of words spoken, Ethan spontaneously named shapes and colours which were being used in play. He did not necessarily repeat these words when requested. Throughout assessment, Ethan was not heard to say his name or to use any personal pronouns although he was described as being able to say "mine" on occasions.
- In terms of non-verbal communication, Ethan was described as having previously made considerable use of pushing his mother towards what he wanted or leading her by the hand and placing her hand on what he wanted.
- These non-verbal communication strategies were described as decreasing over time and were rarely noted at assessment.
- On the other hand, Ethan did not spontaneously engage in non-verbal communication skills of a symbolic nature, for example, pointing, clapping or waving, gesturing or demonstrating. It was possible to engage him in high-fives if this was initiated by the adults present.
- Ethan's play also presented as being inconsistent and mixed in quality. He was at times able to push toy cars, and the previously mentioned spinning of the car wheels was not noted. He demonstrated some early symbolic play interest with cups which he held to his mouth. Stereotypic lining up was not noted, but Ethan did display some interest in sorting objects by colour.
- It was noted during assessment that Ethan clearly possessed some ability to imitate toy use and basic play themes. This "foundation skill" was very important in the context

of future learning and therapeutic processes, as many children with autism spectrum disorder do not learned through imitation.
- On the other hand, Ethan's play was somewhat chaotic at times, with little development of play themes.
- Ethan did not display the sound sensitivity behaviours described by his mother, but it must be noted that my assessment room is quiet and devoid of such distractions.
- As well as nuzzling his nose against his mother's face and clothing, Ethan was noted to place other objects against his nose, for example, a ball of Play-Dough. However, it was not immediately clear whether this was a sensory processing behaviour or an attempt to play with this material. Ethan was also described as being very sensitive to various parts of clothing, for example, the labels and tags on shirts. This was not noted at assessment. Ethan is not yet toilet-trained, but he did appear to be aware of his needs by clutching at his body.
- Ethan certainly presented as being strong-willed and possessed of an acute understanding of what he wanted, but when denied this, he did not respond with temper tantrums. He was quite negotiable for most of the morning.
- Of concern was the fact that Ethan enjoyed attempting to open my office door in order to get out and also enjoyed moving furniture closer to cupboards and bookshelves so as to be able to climb higher. Ethan's mother related that he was not safety-aware at all in terms of cars and traffic and that he needed a considerable amount of supervision at home in relation to safety. Ethan was described as having previously been sensitive to various lights, and at assessment, it was noted on one occasion that he turned off my ceiling lights.

Psychometric assessment

Test Used: Griffiths III

The Griffiths III scales are a series of standardised activities to provide a comprehensive screening assessment of milestone development. They are not intended to substitute for comprehensive physiotherapy, occupational therapy or speech pathology assessments. It proved to be difficult to assess Ethan completely on these scales due to his inconsistent social engagement and ability to follow tasks set by others.

However, sufficient tasks were completed to note that his overall development was mildly delayed. His age-equivalent results are tabulated below, and it will be noted that they are recorded in a range of ages to allow for the fact that there was some difficulty in concluding whether he could do certain things or simply would not.

Overall Developmental Age: 21–24 months

Ethan was found to be functioning at approximately a 2-year-old level. This overall result is consistent with a mild developmental delay. Ethan scored similar results or slightly higher in the various subscales and areas of functioning and lower in others. This was consistent with a DSM-5-TR diagnosis of mild global developmental delay.

Subscale A: Foundations of Learning
Developmental Age: 24–30 months
- Ethan was already developing excellent skills with highly structured tasks such as inserting shapes into puzzles. He particularly enjoyed naming the various shapes.

His approach to solving these puzzles was quite methodical, and he was clearly learning methods from which he could develop further skills.

- Ethan demonstrated the ability to unpack boxes of blocks and play with them and to imitate simple play themes such as making trains and tunnels. He repacked these materials by colour-matching, but as indicated previously, there was another instance where he sorted the materials out by colour for no particular reason.
- Ethan was beginning to be able to use coloured blocks to imitate simple patterns demonstrated to him on a demonstration cards. He had a tendency to need to put the blocks on the cards rather than making the pattern on the table, but the impression was gained that he would learn further symbolic skills quite quickly. An attempt was made to have Ethan draw a human face or basic figure, but his drawing skills (which will be described later) did not allow for this.
- An attempt was made to assess whether Ethan could demonstrate understanding of verbal learning concepts such as big and little, but this was unsuccessful. It also appeared that Ethan did not yet understand the instruction or concept of "matching" or "making the same".

Subscale B: Language and Communication
Developmental Age: 20–26 months

- Ethan has been expertly assessed by a speech pathologist, and a diagnosis of severe receptive and expressive language delay has been made.
- At assessment, Ethan was at his most verbal in a purposeful manner when naming shapes and colours. His other vocalisations were generally not related to the particular tasks taking place, but on one occasion, he did very clearly say "No!" when he was losing patience and becoming fatigued.
- Ethan was described as being able to place his finger upon pictures in books and identify some of these pictures. He certainly presented as having the technical ability to name toys and objects, but Ethan's mother felt that he had not yet been able to do so at his speech pathology sessions. This presented in my experience as being more related to his willingness to undertake certain tasks when requested.

Subscale C: Eye and Hand Coordination
Developmental Age: 25–31 months

- Ethan did not present as being clumsy. He manipulated toys and objects with ease and was not noted to use heavy breathing sounds, dribble or excessive noise when doing so.
- With a pen, he was able to scribble on paper and begin to imitate circular scribble and straight lines scribble. This did not occur spontaneously, nor was it sustained for long.
- Ethan experienced no difficulty inserting small pegs into a pegboard, connecting Duplo-type materials, putting foam puzzle pieces together and opening a screw toy. He was impressive in his ability to manage scissors and cut paper and also to fold paper in half.

Subscale D: Personal-Social-Emotional Scale
Developmental Age: 15–21 months

- Ethan was clearly delayed socially and emotionally but at this assessment presented with a relatively calm disposition. His inconsistent and somewhat disengaged social skills were clearly delayed, but another "foundation skill" was the fact that at times, he would engage socially with good eye contact and social smile.

- Ethan's current limited diet was noted, as this would impact upon his need to learn to use eating utensils appropriately. Ethan is not yet toilet-trained, and it has been my experience with children with autism spectrum disorder that some delays to be expected. It was encouraging in my view that he was aware to a degree of his needs as demonstrated by his clutching at himself.

Subscale E: Gross Motor Scale
Developmental Age: 25–31 months

- Ethan did not present with any coordinational difficulties. His score on this scale tends to reflect the skills that he would demonstrate as opposed to those that he could.
- Ethan is clearly capable of running, climbing, sitting, jumping and kneeling. He is described as having difficulties "stopping" some of these actions when they would be unsafe, and particular caution was taken at assessment not to place him in such danger, particularly outside of my rooms.
- At no stage during the morning did Ethan present as being clumsy or prone to falling off chairs or having other accidents. He enjoyed climbing and descending stairs, but an attempt to have him jump from a low step did not eventuate as he was not in the mood to do so. Ethan was also described as being able to kick a ball and as beginning to engage in some weekend activities of this nature.

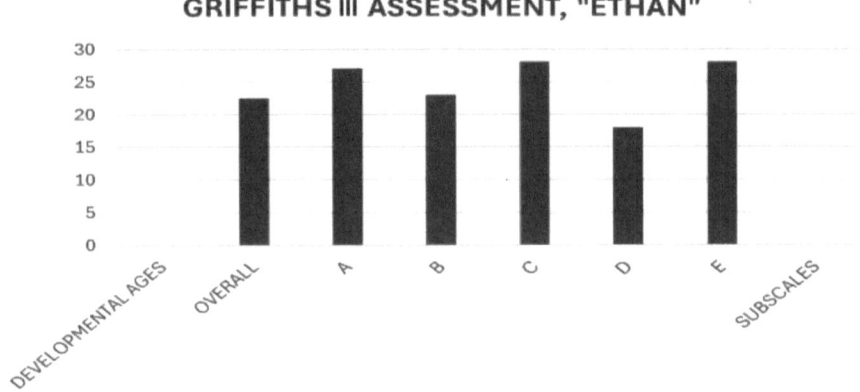

Discussion

This assessment confirmed that Ethan continued to present with symptomatology consistent with a DSM-5-TR diagnosis of autism spectrum disorder, with level II "substantial" support needs. This assessment also confirmed that Ethan presented with mild global developmental delay as defined by DSM-5-TR criteria.

Recommendations

Several specific recommendations arose from this assessment and diagnosis:

- This report should be added to any current application for support funding, as well as applications for further support.
- Ethan presents with a clear need for ongoing speech pathology with Ethan but also other avenues of therapeutic assistance such as occupational therapy, for assistance

with sensory processing difficulties such as food sensitivities and reluctance, improving Ethan's ability to play and interact socially.
- There are also combined programs which incorporate teaching and learning opportunities, social skills training, speech pathology and occupational therapy services, and these should also be investigated and considered to assist with Ethan's progress.
- Ethan's progress should be reviewed through formal assessment in approximately 9 months' time to monitor the impact of his therapeutic intervention programs.

Case Study 3:   Global Developmental Delay

Child's Name: Charlie
Chronological Age: 27 Months

Background

Charlie was referred at 27 months of age by his consultant paediatrician for comprehensive developmental assessment following early developmental difficulties. These included concern about head size at approximately the 97th percentile, dilated ventricles, a history of glue ear and bilateral Eustachian tube dysfunction and a familial chromosomal microduplication thought to be of no significance. His adenoids were removed and grommets inserted in relation to early hearing difficulties and snoring. Charlie also experienced acute pneumonia but is now of good health. There is a family history of sensorineural hearing loss with no particular aetiology. Brain scans and other neurological assessments have indicated no specific diagnostic conditions.

Charlie has been diagnosed by his consultant paediatrician as having a developmental delay on the basis of informal observations and receives government financial support which is used to access speech pathology assistance for delayed speech and language skills. Occupational therapy and physiotherapy have also been considered but hindered by poor service access.

Charlie lives in a remote rural location where access to early intervention services is limited; however, there is strong community involvement in family day care, and Charlie will eventually attend preschool locally. There are early intervention services available in a nearby major town, but this is some distance from the family farm. Formal developmental assessment was requested to quantify Charlie's level of developmental delay for future funding reviews and ongoing service provision. Charlie was shy upon arrival, having woken up from a sleep in the car, but he acclimatised quickly to the assessment room and proved to be a delightful little child.

Behaviour at assessment

An initial decision was made not to place Charlie under undue "task performance pressure", as he has not had much experience in table-top activities. Instead, he was allowed to move about and play with toys. Specific toys and equipment were gradually introduced into his play repertoire. In this way, Charlie completed all relevant tasks from Griffiths III for his age group.

Test used 1: Griffiths III

Developmental assessments such as Griffiths III are designed to be a "snapshot" of a child's developmental skills on the day of assessment. They therefore have strong concurrent validity but weaker predictive validity. In Charlie's case, there were a number of instances of his performing "in-between" levels of achievement on certain tasks, and it was felt that it would not be long before he fully achieved mastery of these skills. Charlie's approximate age equivalent scores reflect his performance on the day and are tabulated and discussed below.

Subscales →	A	B	C	D	E	Overall
Age equivalent →	15 months	14 months	18 months	21 months	22 months	18 months

Outcomes

Charlie's overall developmental age equivalent of 18 months was consistent with a mild global developmental delay. Charlie scored significantly differently on language-based tasks than "performance" tasks, consistent with his history of glue ear, delayed speech and language skills.

In subscale A, **Foundations of Learning,** Charlie was clearly more able in non-verbal tasks than verbal and was at a developmental stage where fine motor skills such as grasp and release could be used for problem-solving. For example, he was beginning to understand how to place a circle or a square piece in a puzzle board although not at the same time. This was a clear example of an emerging skill for the future.

Charlie engaged in the typical play of younger children, for example, exploratory play with boxes of blocks. He took them out and returned some, rattled the box and placed a block upon a lid. Charlie enjoyed exploring and playing with a toy handbell, ringing it and following its sound when played for him. He was able to grasp and hold two blocks at a time, and consistent with his age, he needed to drop one of these blocks in order to accept a third one. He used both hands in play and manipulation and was able to pass items from one hand to the other and swap hands when necessary.

In subscale B, **Language and Communication,** there was opportunity to observe both Charlie's expressive and receptive language skills. Charlie's parents estimated his verbal expression skills as being approximately consistent with a one-year-old child, and this proved to be accurate. One clear word and one-word approximation ("mama" and "dada") were heard often during the assessment and in context. They were not merely play sounds. No other clear words were heard, but Charlie engaged in streams of babble in play, with a pleasant acoustic quality and appropriate prosody.

Charlie was interested in communicating and noise-making with a handbell and also a toy drum which he tapped whilst walking. He was described as enjoying looking at picture books and music such as the Wiggles. He engaged in a number of non-verbal communication strategies such as pointing, taking adults by the hand and waving. There was clear evidence of his understanding the nexus between communication and social interaction.

Subscale C, **Eye and Hand Coordination,** indicated that Charlie's fine motor skills were on the cusp of becoming purposeful problem-solving skills. For example, he enjoyed straight-scribbling with a marker pen and was also able to imitate a vertical stroke on one occasion.

Although Charlie could place one block on top of one of the box lids, he was not yet putting blocks on top of each other as a precursor to tower building. Charlie enjoyed taking wooden rings off a pole, but not one at a time. This meant that it was not easy to put them back the same manner way, limiting his efforts to two rings onto the pole. He was not yet able to connect Duplo blocks together, another example of his early manipulation skills preceding his problem-solving skills.

In subscale D, **Personal-Social-Emotional**, Charlie's skills and interactions included sustained eye contact, reactive and reciprocal smiles, physical affection and a desire to explore his image in a mirror. He was beginning to indicate body parts upon himself and clearly enjoyed interactive games such as "peekaboo" and rolling a ball backwards and forwards.

Charlie was described as beginning to understand his toileting needs at a physical level, for example, showing a change of demeanour when it was "time". He was able to initiate his own play activities and to clap his hands in pleasure. He was beginning to drink from an open cup with help and to finger-feed.

Subscale E, **Gross Motor**, involved Charlie moving about the office without difficulty. He knelt on the floor independently without excessive "W-sitting", rose to standing without too much difficulty and squatted to play with and pick up objects. He was able to climb and descend stairs by clinging to a railing with both hands. He enjoyed picking up a ball and attempting to throw it although the ball went backwards rather than forwards. Charlie sat himself at a small chair and desk with no apparent difficulties with stability. When he moved about my room, there were no occasions on which he tripped or fell. He was also skilled at clinging to furniture and side-stepping when necessary.

Test used 2: Adaptive Behaviour Assessment System 3 (ABAS 3)

0–5 years (parent form)

Charlie's parents kindly completed an adaptive behaviour assessment questionnaire as a means of "cross-checking" his developmental skills. His scored results are tabulated below and discussed in terms of their relationship with results obtained from the Griffiths III assessment.

Composite Scores	Score Range	Percentile	Classification
GAC	72–78	5	Low
CONCEPTUAL	67–75	3	Low
SOCIAL	74–84	8	Low
PRACTICAL	71–79	5	Low

Specific skill area	Scaled score	Classification
Communication skills	1	Extremely low
Community use	5	Low
Functional pre-academics	6	Below average
Home living	6	Below average
Health and safety	5	Low
Leisure	7	Below average
Self-care	5	Low
Self-direction	7	Below average
Social	6	Below average
Motor	5	Low

Outcomes

The scores tabulated above indicate Charlie is functioning below average for age, with an overall rating of "low" functional skills. Individual skills indicate that Charlie has extremely delayed speech and language skills. In other areas such as early learning, home living, play time and choice-making and social interaction, he was scored as functioning in the "below average" range.

When combined together, Charlie's results on Griffiths III and on the Adaptive Behaviour Assessment System 3 confirm that he meets DSM-5-TR criteria for a diagnosis of mild global developmental delay. This assessment is a form of "benchmarking" Charlie's current skills, and whether they are well-formed and established, or "emerging". It will be interesting and important to note the speed and ease with which Charlie learns and consolidates new skills, particularly through his therapeutic assistance and preschool or childcare. He clearly presents as a child with considerable potential to improve.

Recommendations

At assessment, it was discussed that Griffiths III is an assessment tool which can be repeated every 6 months, and this is important as a means of monitoring a young child's progress through therapy and assistance. The more therapeutic assistance children receive by way of speech pathology and occupational therapy, preschool or childcare also has a beneficial impact upon a child's ability to sit and complete tasks in such tests as Griffiths III, and a first assessment such as this one with Charlie should be conceptualised as a "benchmark" assessment. It is generally recommended that at least a six-month interval should take place between assessments.

Case Study 4:   Possible Autism Spectrum Disorder

Child's Name: John
Chronological Age: 29 months

Background information

John was two and half years old, and in his second short-term foster/out-of-home placement. He was referred by his current foster parents and consultant paediatrician for assessment of possible autism spectrum disorder as defined by DSM-5-TR. John's developmental paediatrician was concerned about developmental delay, particularly John's severely delayed receptive and expressive language skills. The paediatrician was planning to undertake formal developmental assessment with John in the near future.

John's hearing has been assessed as within normal limits. He may have hip dysplasia, apparently a familial condition. John was described as being very awkward and clumsy and having many falls. Concerns about possible autism spectrum disorder stemmed from:

- A speech pathology assessment indicating severely delayed and disordered expressive and receptive language skills, poor eye contact and joint attention skills, motor and verbal imitation skills, and poor non-verbal communication strategies such as pointing and gesturing.
- Frequent temper tantrums and "shutdown mode" episodes when denied what he wanted.

- Self-injurious behaviours such as head banging and biting, as well as covering ears in new and unfamiliar situations.

John was described as a fussy eater, with a preference for bland foods. Complex sleep patterns were described including waking and screaming loudly. Some but not all of these behaviours were noted at John's early learning centre. Genetic testing had been commenced with results pending. No background knowledge about John's birth parents and family background was provided.

Diagnostic assessment

Test used 1: Autism Diagnostic Observation Schedule 2, Toddler Module
Outcomes

Level of Concern	Comment
Moderate-to-severe concern	Not applicable
Mild-to-moderate concern	Not applicable at this stage
Little-to-no concern	Considerable progress noted in recent months.

Behavioural observations

John was observed and engaged with for approximately 60 minutes. His behavioural presentation was not consistent with autism spectrum disorder. His foster mother described the rapid progress which had occurred in his current fostering arrangement, and this progress was confirmed through assessment:

- John vocalised frequently during assessment, with babble and early word usage and imitation reminiscent of a younger child. His voice had a pleasant acoustic quality and prosody, and no stereotypic or unusual sounds were heard. He was now using and imitating single words, responding promptly to the call of his name, initiating "joint attention" through eye contact, pointing, vocalising and gesturing, expressions and engaging in simple interactive games such as "peekaboo".
- Some functional and imitative play was observed.
- John was now affectionate with his foster parents, interested to a degree in other children and able to anticipate and respond to the care and affection he was receiving.
- John spontaneously engaged in non-verbal communication to establish joint attention. This included pointing coordinated with eye contact, facial expression and vocalisation. He enjoyed giving "high-fives" and waved "goodbye" when prompted. Facial expressions were varied and appropriate.
- There was no evidence of stereotypic movement patterns such as arm flapping, toe walking, body rocking or unusual head swaying.
- There were no facial grimaces or tics or unusual sounds. There was no indication of unusual or non-functional rituals or routines. John did not respond in any unusual manner to sensory stimuli in the assessment room.

In summary, John did not meet the threshold for a diagnosis of autism spectrum disorder as defined by DSM-5-TR. He presented as having made significant progress socially and emotionally in his current foster family. It is frequently a consideration with "out-of-home"

268   *Diagnosing Young Children with Neurodevelopmental Disorders*

parenting that problematic early language and social skills, play skills and behavioural/social skills and emotional lability may be noted early in their new domestic circumstances.

Test used 2: Adaptive Behaviour Assessment System 3, 0–5 years

Specific skill area	Scaled score	Classification
Communication skills	1	Extremely low
Community use	3	Extremely low
Functional pre-academics	5	Low
Home living	1	Extremely low
Health and safety	3	Extremely low
Leisure	2	Extremely low
Self-care	1	Extremely low
Self-direction	3	Extremely low
Social	1	Extremely low
Motor	6	Below average

Outcomes

John's current foster parents had completed a questionnaire-based assessment of his current adaptive behaviour/daily living skills prior to this assessment. This formed the basis of a detailed discussion about John's current level of need and the types of assistance which may benefit him. This questionnaire when scored confirmed that John was functioning significantly below average in all areas of daily living, with scores in the "extremely low" range.

These results were consistent with an overall developmental age of approximately 17 months, highlighting the likelihood of a significant global developmental delay.

Summary and recommendations

John presented as a young child who had made significant progress through the security and consistency of care he was receiving in his current foster care arrangement. His early signs of autism spectrum disorder had resolved, and it can be argued that these early symptoms may have reflected a number of circumstantial factors such as early neglect and subsequent attachment difficulties. He is now in an excellent and supportive caring situation, which is hopefully to be maintained. John is regularly monitored for his health and welfare by his paediatrician who will be conducting formal developmental assessment in the near future.

A firm recommendation is that an application for funding be sought for John's therapeutic assistance on the basis of a diagnosis of global developmental delay as defined by DSM-5-TR, as this is very likely to be the outcome of further upcoming assessment.

Case Study 5:   Specific Language Disorder

Child's Name: Kellie
Chronological Age: 4 years 10 months

Kellie is a four-year-old girl approaching her fifth birthday and has a significant history of speech, language and communication delay and disorder. She is under the care of a speech pathology service, but it has not been possible to conduct formal psychometric assessment as her difficulties specifically relate to delayed and disordered semantic and pragmatic language skills. There is a significant family history of speech and language delay of no specific aetiology. Kellie was referred by her paediatrician for developmental assessment prior to commencing school. Her preschool is concerned that Kellie may present with an autism spectrum disorder; however, her paediatrician has expressed doubts about this and instead suspects that she may present with "developmental dyspraxia". Prior to assessment Kellie's speech pathologist provided through telephone discussion and written report the following information:

- Despite using more words and word combinations than previously, with content broadening and grammatical complexity improving, Kellie continued to present with significantly delayed and disordered language, particularly with semantic and pragmatic skills.
- At approximately three years of age, she was described as having virtually "no successful communication". Kellie was described as attempting to "control" or "lead" speech pathology sessions, thereby interfering with attempts at formal assessment. Her speech pathologist remains unconvinced that Kellie presents with either autism spectrum disorder or oral dyspraxia.
- Kellie's preschool has noted their concerns about her behaviour and progress, including difficulties with fine and gross motor coordination and planning skills, emotional regulation skills, attention and concentration skills, early academic skills and her ability to engage expressively or receptively through language.

Diagnostic assessment outcomes

Upon meeting Kellie, it was immediately apparent that she was not "ready" for formal table-top psychometric assessment of either cognitive abilities or general developmental skills. She presented as "playfully defiant" throughout the assessment session, in a manner reminiscent of a developmentally younger child.

Kellie was initially shy and anxious, with an unusual habit of covering her eyes when approached or spoken to. A decision was taken not to place her under any undue pressure to "perform". Instead, detailed observations were made during play and conversation with and around Kellie as she explored the assessment room, played with her own toys, interacted when she felt the need to and became increasingly friendly. By the end of the 2.5-hour session, Kellie was sharing fun and excitement. The following points were noted from this observation period, augmented by information provided by Kellie's mother:

- Kellie presented with significantly delayed and disordered speech and language skills although her words were quite articulate. She understood the nexus between social interaction and speech and was clearly attempting to engage through her language although this was particularly disordered in both expressive and receptive skills, grammatical accuracy, vocabulary selection, word order, maintenance of topic and accurate listening.
- Kellie made appropriate use of non-verbal communication skills such as pointing and eye contact and coordinated these with speech. She also used other gestures to express her needs and to respond as best she could to spoken communication.

- Kellie presented with a pleasant voice, with good use of expression and prosody. Unusual or self-stimulatory noises were not heard, nor were there obvious signs of echolalia or unusual accents.
- Kellie engaged in spontaneous and ongoing symbolic social role-play with dolls, toy animals, telephones, eating utensils and other items from her collection as well as from the office. Her play was not consistent with the stereotypic play associated with autism spectrum disorder.
- Kellie did not present with stereotypic movement patterns associated with autism spectrum disorder, such as arm flapping, toe walking, facial grimaces or tics.
- Kellie's anxiety and the covering of her eyes were unusual, but it was described by her mother that there was a significant family history of anxiety.

In summary, Kellie's presentation was not consistent with that of autism spectrum disorder as defined by DSM-5-TR. Her presentation would however indicate that Kellie meets criteria for a language disorder (315.39). ICD-11 provides a more detailed and descriptive breakdown of various types of language delay and disorder found in young children. In the case of Kellie, ICD-11 criteria is met for the following:

1. Developmental language disorder with impairment of receptive and expressive language (6A01.2).
2. Developmental language disorder with impairment of mainly pragmatic language (6A01.23).

ICD-11 defines this disorder in the following manner:

Developmental language disorder is characterised by persistent deficits in the acquisition, understanding, production or use of language (spoken or signed), that arise during the developmental period, typically during early childhood, and cause significant limitations in the individual's ability to communicate.

The individual's ability to understand, produce or use language is markedly below what would be expected given the individual's age. The language deficits are not explained by another neurodevelopmental disorder or a sensory impairment or neurological condition, including the effects of brain injury or infection.

Kellie did not present as a child who would at this stage cooperate in a standardised psychometric assessment of developmental skills such as Griffiths III or Bayley-4. However, this observation session with Kellie indicates the following:

- Kellie presents with fine motor coordination and planning skills which are mildly delayed. Most of this delay relates to her use of pencil and paper. Observation of her skills in this area indicates that when she does engage with pencil and paper, it is at approximately a three-year-old level. She holds pencils in an immature and awkward fashion and is not yet consistently drawing circles or more complex shapes such as crosses or squares.
- Kellie presents with a social, emotional and behavioural presentation which is immature for her age. Her emotional regulation skills, oppositional and refusal behaviours and social engagement skills are also consistent with a developmental age of approximately three years.

- Kellie's speech pathologist has confirmed significant delay and disorder in her speech, language, semantic and pragmatic skills.
- It is noted that Kellie is more interested in playing at preschool with younger children and not those of her own age. Again, it is estimated that her ability to communicate and function socially through language is significantly delayed, again at an approximate three-year level of development.

DSM-5-TR criteria refer to the diagnosis of "global developmental delay" when a child is delayed in a number of areas of developmental skill and functioning but cannot complete formal psychometric assessment. Kellie therefore meets DSM-5-TR criteria for a diagnosis of mild global developmental delay. On the basis of these diagnoses, it was discussed that Kellie was eligible for support funding through relevant government agencies. Kellie currently receives speech pathology services, but her delayed fine motor coordination and planning skills suggest that she would benefit also from occupational therapy services.

Case Study 6:   Co-morbid Autism Spectrum Disorder and Attention Deficit Hyperactivity Disorder

Child's Name: Vik
Chronological Age: 4 years 6 months

Background

Vik was diagnosed by his consultant paediatrician at age 3 and a half years with autism spectrum disorder as defined by DSM-5-TR, with level III "Very Substantial" support needs. He has also been described as having attention deficit hyperactivity disorder despite his young age, but medication was not prescribed because of his youth. Government support funding is provided for Vik's family for speech pathology, occupational therapy and other early intervention services. A developmental assessment was requested because Vik's family were requesting enrolment in a special school requiring a formal assessment of either intellectual functioning or developmental delay, including an assessment of adaptive behaviour skills. Vik also needed confirmation of his diagnosis of autism spectrum disorder for an upcoming review of his current support funding.

Diagnostic assessment outcomes

Test Used 1: Autism Diagnostic Observation Schedule 2 (Module 1)
DSM-5-TR Diagnosis: Autism spectrum disorder
Level of Support Required: Level 3 "Very Substantial"

Vik presented at assessment in an extremely excited and agitated mood symptomatic of both autism spectrum disorder and attention deficit hyperactivity disorder. He frenetically explored the psychologist's office, climbing onto and over furniture, floor and cupboards, equipment and toys. He calmed at times, but not for long. It took the combined efforts of the psychologist and Vik's parents to steady and manage his behaviour sufficiently to keep him safe and attempt formal developmental assessment tasks.

Vik sat briefly at a table or in his parents' laps for these tasks, but his hyperactivity and excitement did not decline. An "executive decision" was taken for Vik's mother to complete an Adaptive Behaviour Assessment System 3 questionnaire whilst his father and the psychologist attempted as many assessment tasks as possible with Vik. The following points were noted:

- Vik vocalised continuously throughout the assessment, this consisting mainly of echoed words and phrases, sometimes repeated immediately and at other times completely out of context, but clearly related to past contexts. His spoken words were generally the names of toys, objects, pictures or colours and occasional "action word" such as "climb". In this way, he spontaneously named with great accuracy. Some "counting" words were also noted. Vik's voice was pleasant, with only occasional stereotypic sounds and acoustic qualities.
- Vik was sometimes able to make eye contact and point to what he wanted. At other times, Vik took adults by the hand, placing them on what he wanted. He clapped on one occasion when happy, gave "high-fives" when requested and also waved "goodbye" but in a backward direction.
- Vik did not respond consistently to the call of his name but responded quickly to music or when his mother sang.
- Vik enjoyed simple interactive physical games such as "mock attack", tickles and finger prods. He anticipated these games with laughs and smiles.
- Vik sometimes gave objects to his parents for help, but not for showing or sharing.
- On report, Vik was beginning to show some interest in other children.
- When Vik was excited and happy, he jumped up and down and flapped his arms. He did not show unusual facial expressions, grimaces or "tics".
- Vik's play was severely restricted and odd. It included lining up and sorting by colour. He did demonstrate some emerging imitation skills.
- Vik was described by his parents as being capable of self-injurious behaviours such as scratching his skin.

Overall the Autism Diagnostic Observation Schedule 2 (Module 1) confirmed that Vik continued to meet DSM-5-TR criteria for a diagnosis of autism spectrum disorder, with support needs rated by the same criteria as level 3 "Very Substantial". This assessment also confirmed that Vik met DSM-5-TR criteria for a diagnosis of attention deficit hyperactivity disorder.

Test used 2: Bayley-4

With the invaluable help of his parents, an attempt was made to assess Vik using the Bayley-4. His current level of hyperactivity and distractibility severely impeded his ability to focus on tasks, remain seated and attempt tasks in a meaningful manner, and therefore, the assessment was incomplete. His scores are therefore best considered as an underestimation and "basal" at this stage. It is a strong recommendation from this assessment that Vik be reassessed at a time when his behaviour and attention are more conducive to a more complete assessment.

In this respect, enrolment in a specialist school environment is vital for Vik as a means of "stabilising" his attention and task completion skills. Sufficient tasks and guided observations were made however to confirm that Vik met criteria for a diagnosis of global developmental delay as defined by DSM-5-TR and that the impact of his delay was moderate.

Bayley scales of infant and toddler development, fourth edition (bayley-4)

Area	Standard score	Percentile	Interpretation	
Bayley-4 cognitive composite	3	0.1	Extremely low	
Bayley-4 language composite	3	0.1	Extremely low	
Domain	Scaled score	Percentile	Age equivalent	Interpretation
Bayley-4 cognitive scale	4	0.2	25 months	Moderately delayed
Bayley-4 receptive language scale	4	0.2	26	Moderately delayed
Adaptive behaviour scale and social-emotional				
Area	Standard score	Percentile	Interpretation	
Bayley-4 communication composite	46	0.2	Extremely low	
Bayley-4 daily living skills composite	59	0.5	Extremely low	
Bayley-4 socialisation	52	0.1	Extremely low	
Bayley-4 adaptive behaviour	59	0.3	Extremely low	
Bayley-4 social emotional scale				
Domain	Scaled score	Percentile	Age equivalent	Interpretation
Bayley-4 receptive	1	Below 0.1	16 months	Extremely low
Bayley-4 expressive	2	0.1	20 months	Extremely low
Bayley-4 personal	2	Below 0.1	22 months	Extremely low
Bayley-4 interpersonal relationships	1	Below 0.1	16 months	Extremely low
Bayley-4 play and leisure	1	Below 0.1	18 months	Extremely low

Despite of the logistical difficulties associated with assessing Vik, the following skills were noted:

- Vik performed best on physical and visual tasks such as completing simple puzzles involving circles, squares and triangles.
- Vik showed only fleeting interest in materials such as blocks.
- Vik's severely delayed language meant that he could not demonstrate understanding of concepts such as "big" or "little".
- He was not able to make symbolic drawings but could match colours, shapes and patterns.
- Although Vik vocalised throughout assessment, his communication was not functional, reciprocal or conversational. At best, he could name a small number of toys, objects, colours and pictures.
- Vik was able to scribble on paper and imitate an early phase circle.
- He was able to remove and replace wooden rings from a ring pole and stack some blocks into a tower.
- Vik showed little interest in Duplo materials or play dough.

- Vik was not toilet-trained but was beginning to show some awareness of his needs.
- He was beginning to pull down and pull up elasticised pants and take off shoes.
- Vik ate with his fingers and had a narrow range of food preferences.
- He was able to recognise himself in a photograph, but not in a mirror.
- Vik was affectionate with his parents and friendly with the psychologist, but cuddles and physical contact were only brief. He did enjoy physical contact games such as tickling and prodding.
- Vik was capable of kneeling correctly on the floor and rising without using his hands.
- He spontaneously jumped in association with his arm flapping and was skilful at climbing onto and over furniture.
- Vik did not attempt to abscond from the office. Vik was more skilful at climbing stairs than descending. He was also able to kick a ball and sit on a ride-on toy.

Vik's adaptive behaviour skills were confirmed as being in the "Extremely Low" range of abilities but with an uneven profile of skills. His early interest in naming objects and pictures, understanding numbers and using vocabulary to describe objects by colour was reflected in his emerging and potential pre-academic skills. Vik's early gross motor coordination skills were also noted. Core symptoms of autism spectrum disorder such as language disorder and difficulties with social interaction were reflected in his scores, as were his restricted play skills, health and safety conceptualisation and decision-making skills. Vik's profile was entirely consistent with his diagnosis of autism spectrum disorder with level 3 "Very Substantial" support needs, and with his moderate global developmental delay. Thus, the following diagnoses were confirmed:

- Autism spectrum disorder as defined by DSM-5-TR with level 3 "Very Substantial" support needs.
- Moderate global developmental delay as defined by DSM-5-TR.
- Attention deficit hyperactivity disorder as defined by DSM-5-TR.

Summation

Vik presented with a complex array of developmental concerns and clearly met DSM-5-TR criteria for three co-morbid conditions: Autism spectrum disorder with level 3 "Very Substantial" support needs, moderate global developmental delay and attention deficit hyperactivity disorder. On this basis, it is felt that Vik would greatly benefit from enrolment in a special school of his parents' choosing so that the routine and structured curriculum of such schools could be applied to his current inability to attend to and complete tasks and to begin to learn more effectively. It is often said of special education curricula that the first goal is to establish attentional skills and task completion skills, and in Vik's case, there is a clear and pressing priority for this to be achieved.

Case Study 7: A Case of "Unintended Neglect"

Name of Child: Aidan
Chronological Age: 3 years 9 months

Background

Aidan was referred at 3 years 9 months by his consultant paediatrician. He was described with delayed speech, language and social skills. It was stated that he had been subject to "unintended neglect". Reference was made to Aidan having been cared for over long periods by his non-English speaking grandmother and described also as having a significant mental health disorder. He was attending an early childhood centre and receiving support there.

Aidan was of good health, with normal vision and hearing. The consultant paediatrician was concerned about possible autism spectrum disorder or global developmental delay. Background information included:

- Speech pathology assessment indicating good preverbal and gestural skills, single words and two-word phrases.
- Difficulty making eye contact, unusual social response and some echolalic language.
- Recommended parental involvement in a Hanen Program to help them stimulate his language and communication skills.
- The early childhood centre employing social role modelling; visual augmentative support systems to reinforce rules, routines and preparation for change; and direct teaching of new skills.
- Significant progress through these remediations, including the beginning of symbolic language and communication skills such as pointing, emerging thematic play, reduced echolalia and increased social interaction.

Diagnostic assessment outcomes

Tests Used 1: Autism Diagnostic Observation Schedule 2, Module 1
DSM-5-TR Diagnosis: Not on autism spectrum

Aidan was initially observed in the psychologist's office over a 40-minute period and then for an additional 40 minutes in his early childhood centre. This second observation period allowed contextual information to be gained, both through watching Aidan's ability to play and interact within a normal childcare environment and through discussion with his teachers and carers. The following points were noted:

- Aiden was happy and enthusiastic although strong-willed and self-directed.
- Delayed but improved speech and language was noted although there were some instances of echolalia.
- Developing vocabulary skills, including pronouns, descriptive and definitional words, were noted, and these were increasingly occurring in context.
- Aidan used increased eye contact, physical gesture, varied facial expression and social "acts".
- Elements of pretend play with emerging thematic content were observed, including social role-play.
- There was one isolated instance of stereotypic play, but ongoing non-functional play was also observed.
- Aidan engaged in imitation of new play themes and "play language".
- Some sensory processing difficulties such as licking objects was noted.
- No stereotypic movements were observed.

Psychometric assessment

Test used 2: Griffiths III

Aiden was often impulsive and of short attention during this assessment. He appeared to lack experience with some of the assessment materials even though they were a typical sample of toys and objects which would be found in family homes. Over the duration of the assessment, Aidan quite quickly adapted to these new materials and was clearly enjoying these "learning experiences".

Overall Developmental Age: 28–34 months

- Assessment confirmed a diagnosis of mild global developmental delay as defined by DSM 5-TR. However, it was felt that Aiden's short attention span and impulsivity affected his "true" potential.

Subscale A: Foundations of Learning: 29–35 months

- Difficulties with verbal tasks and his short attention span and impulsive behaviours compromised Aidan's performance on these tasks.
- He was developing good skills with insert puzzles, for example, methodical "scanning" skills.
- Aidan enjoyed playing with boxes of coloured blocks, unpacking and repacking them, stacking blocks, boxes or lids, attempting to imitative play and colour-matching.
- Aidan used language terminology of size, for example, "big", "bigger" and "little".
- Aidan counted orally and with fingers and demonstrated good matching skills. No symbolic drawings were noted.

Subscale B: Language and Communication: 31–37 months

- Aidan showed impressive naming and defining skills and use of associative language and sounds.
- There was spontaneous use of pronouns and gender terminology.
- Aidan enjoyed of picture book, both for his own pleasure and for the shared social opportunity it provided.

Subscale C: Eye and Hand Coordination: 27–33 months

- Aidan had not developed clear hand dominance as yet but was effectively using his hands for stacking, inserting, pressing, scribbling and imitating vertical and horizontal lines.
- Aidan attempted to cut and fold paper but appeared inexperienced with these activities.
- Throughout formal assessment and childcare observation, Aidan demonstrated good core stability skills when sitting at a table for prolonged periods.
- It was noted that an occupational therapy assessment and programme had been recommended by early education centre personnel.

Subscale D: Personal-Social-Emotional: 30–36 months

- Overall, Aidan presented as delightful but stubborn and interactive but self-directed. It was easy to engage with him but more on "his terms".
- He has good self-calming skills.
- Emerging independence skills for toileting, undressing, eating and self-care were noted and reported.

Subscale E: Gross Motor: 26–32 months

- Aidan was very active, nimble and well-coordinated. He engaged in running, jumping, stair climbing and early ball skills such as kicking and throwing.
- Some "W-sitting" was noted, and it was observed that Aidan needed to use his hands on the floor when rising from kneeling.
- Aidan was now riding a tricycle, throwing balls with some strength and beginning to catch balls although he tended to turn his head as the ball approached.

Summary

In summary, Aiden did not present as meeting DSM-5-TR criteria for autism spectrum disorder. Previously noted symptoms were resolving through increased focus upon his language and communication skills, social interaction opportunities and play themes. Some "residual" behaviours remained, and it was prognosticated that his encouraging progress and improvement reinforced the paediatrician's initial description of "unintended neglect". Prognoses for such children are positive when underlying issues of under-stimulation are addressed.

Aiden was assessed and presented with a mild global developmental delay as defined by DSM-5-TR. Aiden presented with considerable potential to improve. An occupational therapy assessment and programme was recommended to support his fine motor coordination and planning skills, play skills and attention and concentration skills.

Case Study 8: Denial of Entry Visa. Submission to Government Medical Officer

Child's Name: Mogali
Chronological Age: 5 years 5 months

Submission

To whom may concern, Commonwealth Department of Health:

This submission pertains to a decision of a commonwealth medical officer to disallow an application for a temporary visa for the child "Mogali" under "Public Interest Criteria" on the grounds that she may present with a disabling condition which will incur costs upon the government in excess of the allowable limits for such circumstances.

This submission has been requested by both a consultant paediatrician and the adoptive parents of Mogali, on the basis of her suggested intellectual disability, the differences between special education and disability provisions in her home country and proposed temporary residence, and the necessary reappraisal of the expense of services Mogali's parents would be seeking on behalf of Mogali should the adoptive fathers temporarily reside and work in this country.

Author's credentials

The author of this submission is an educational and developmental psychologist with many years of experience and has an extensive background in the assessment, diagnosis and support of children with a range of neurodevelopmental disorders, intellectual disabilities, specific genetic disorders, global developmental delays and physical disabilities. This background includes senior psychologist and team leader roles in both government and non-government disability service agencies and training supervisory roles in these employments.

Mogali's assessment and diagnostic history

Assessment 1

Mogali was adopted by her parents at approximately 4 months of age. Prior to her adoption, she was assessed by a paediatrician as being healthy and developing normally, but at approximately two and a half years of age, it was apparent that she was lagging behind in her milestone development. According to available reports, she was initially assessed using Griffiths III and found to have significant delays in speech and language, gross and fine motor skill milestones.

Early intervention therapies such as speech and occupational therapy and physiotherapy were recommended and commenced at parental expense.

It is important to note at this point that developmental tests such as Griffiths III are comprehensive "screening instruments" to highlight immediate and short-term intervention needs such as the therapies mentioned and are not necessarily predictive of future educational and intellectual outcomes. They are not measures of intellectual development or intelligence.

Assessment 2

At a later date, when 4 years of age, Mogali was assessed by a child psychiatrist. Report findings suggested that Mogali showed signs of foetal alcohol spectrum syndrome, inattention consistent with a diagnosis of attention deficit hyperactivity disorder, mild anxiety, a mild intellectual disability and disinhibited social engagement disorder.

This last diagnosis is often made in relation to children who have been adopted or fostered. Recommendations for management included stimulant medication and continued speech pathology and occupational therapy programs and the addition of play therapy programs and access to a "less academic" educational environment.

Assessment 3

Mogali's next assessment was conducted when she was 5 years of age. An "independent psychometrist" using the Wechsler Preschool & Primary Scale of Intelligence, fourth edition (WPPSI-IV), reported that obtained results indicated functioning in the low "borderline" range of intellectual ability, with a relatively uneven profile of skills. However, her academic skills were significantly delayed with reference to specific assessments of reading vocabulary and comprehension, spelling and mathematical skills.

Assessment 4

In late 2023, Mogali was interviewed and reviewed online by a consultant paediatrician in the adoptive family's proposed residency. The paediatrician acknowledged the limitations of "remote" diagnostic and review formats but stated that in his view, Mogali did not present with signs of foetal alcohol spectrum disorder, and nor did she present with obvious dysmorphic signs. He did not feel that Mogali displayed signs of disinhibited social engagement disorder, and noted that although she was initially anxious, Mogali was able to take part interactively, pleasantly and cooperatively in this online review.

The paediatrician noted Mogali's previous results on assessments of intellectual functioning and her positive response to stimulant medication of her inattentive behaviours. It was the paediatrician's view that Mogali would be highly unlikely to be offered enrolment in a special school programme in the family's proposed country of temporary residence.

Assessment 5

Mogali's adoptive parents kindly completed an Adaptive Behaviour Assessment questionnaire, as such assessments are a mandatory component of any consideration of diagnoses of intellectual disability and of consideration of specific special education and school options for children in many countries, government and non-government school systems and for consideration or application for specific government financial support schemes for children with disabilities.

Adaptive Behaviour Assessment System 3, 5–21 years (parent form)

Composite	Score range	Percentile	Classification
GAC	90–96	32	Average
Conceptual	83–93	21	Below average
Social	97–107	55	Average
Practical	90–98	34	Average

Specific skill area	Scaled score	Classification
Communication skills	10	Average
Community use	10	Average
Functional academics	4	Low
Home living	9	Average
Health and safety	9	Average
Leisure	9	Average
Self-care	9	Average
Self-direction	10	Average
Social	12	Average

Scoring of this adaptive behaviour assessment questionnaire indicated that Mogali is perceived as functioning at an appropriate degree of competency in all areas of functioning with the exception of academic performance. She was developing appropriate self-care and self-management skills, was accessing community facilities and activities appropriate to her age and was learning appropriate social, domestic and communication skills, and health and hygiene practices. Her difficulties with academic and school-based activities were significantly delayed, and consistent with previous psychometric assessments undertaken in her home country.

Educational history

Mogali is currently enrolled in a private special school although clarification by per parents suggest that this is a coaching college run by a teacher with some special education experience. Comments by Mogali's current teacher indicate that she is making progress, that she is less anxious than previously and that she is increasingly applying learning strategies to improve her reading and spelling. Short-term memories difficulties were cited as a limiting factor to her continued progression. Information from Mogali's adoptive parents and other sources indicate that this private school is apparently the best available option to support her learning needs in the absence of other support class and programme options which may be more appropriate.

Discussion

To fully understand this situation, it is important to consider a number of factors, particularly the manner in which psychometric assessment results are interpreted and classified, and the different types of educational and therapeutic support services available in different countries.

Firstly, there is the conceptualisation and classification of intellectual disabilities. These are detailed in the Diagnostic and Statistical Manual, currently in its fifth edition (DSM-5-TR). This defines intellectual disability as follows:

> "Intellectual disability (Intellectual Developmental Disorder) is a disorder with onset during the developmental period that includes both intellectual and adaptive functioning deficits in conceptual, social, and practical domains. The following three criteria must be met:
>
> a Deficits in intellectual functioning confirmed by both clinical assessment and individualised, standardised intelligence testing.
> b Deficits in adaptive functioning that result in failure to meet developmental and socio-cultural standards for personal independence and social responsibility.
> c Onset of intellectual and adaptive deficits during the developmental period."

On the basis of this diagnostic criteria, Mogali cannot be diagnosed with an intellectual disability. Her adaptive behaviour skills are in the average range, with the exception of her academic skills. Her scores on tests of intelligence are indeed significantly below average, but that outcome alone is not sufficient for a diagnosis of intellectual disability. Mogali clearly presents with a specific learning disability, but not an intellectual disability in its defined terms. The ramifications of this finding relate to specific support service eligibility in Mogali's family case. On this basis, they would not be able to access support funding through the financial support schemes available even if granted the relevant short-term visas.

The second implication of this finding relates to the types of contrasting educational support services available in different countries. In her home country, Mogali attends a privately run special school as the only alternative choice there would be special schools for children with moderate-to-severe disabilities. Mogali is not eligible for any such schools in the adoptive family's preferred short-term residence, whether government or non-government.

What is available for Mogali in the proposed country of residence are specific support classes and learning support programs in regular, "mainstream" government schools once a child has reached a specific minimum age. The proposed country of residence is also served by many private schools, mainly denominational such Roman Catholic, Christian, Baptist, Arabic and Lutheran. These schools do receive specific government funding for their learning support programs, but very few of such schools offer special support classes.

Finally, the adoptive family is planning to live in the short term in this country on the basis of the adoptive parents' being seconded to positions in the commercial financial sector of that country. These jobs are in the senior consultant category and are richly rewarded through salaries, bonuses and entitlements. Mogali's ongoing therapeutic needs such as speech pathology, occupational therapy and academic support can therefore be funded privately through the family's own resources and personal health insurance. There will be no additional financial impost placed upon the adoptive parents' proposed country.

Conclusion and summation

On the basis of all the relevant and supplied information about Mogali, her academic support needs and her alignment with the types of services, she would be able to access in her family's proposed country; it is my view that Mogali would not impose a financial burden upon the government to the degree suggested in the determination made by the senior medical officer. It is my view that Mogali does not present with "special education needs" commensurate with the quoted financial costing. On that basis alone, it is my view that the child Mogali should be granted a visa to reside in this country during the duration of her parents' secondment and temporary employment in this country. They have already demonstrated their willingness to pay for any educational and therapeutic support services Mogali may require from their own resources. I trust this report is received and considered in good faith, and I would of course be happy to speak further to its contents if necessary.

Case Study 9: Expert Witness Testimony in Divorce Settlement, a Girl with a Rare Chromosomal Disorder

Child's Name: Helen
Chronological Age: 4 years 1 month

Author's credentials

The author of this submission is an educational and developmental psychologist with many years of experience and has an extensive background in the assessment, diagnosis and support of children with a range of neurodevelopmental disorders, intellectual disabilities, specific genetic disorders, global developmental delays and physical disabilities. The author has specific experience in the support and management of young children with rare chromosomal abnormalities such as that at the centre of this legal action. This background includes senior psychologist and team leader roles in both government and non-government disability service agencies and training supervisory roles in these employments.

Background

Helen is four-year-old girl with a rare genetic syndrome, technically a micro-deletion at chromosome 22q11.2 but more commonly known as velocardiofacial syndrome (VCFS). This syndrome, which occurs in 1 in 4,000 live births, is known to be associated with various developmental abnormalities, including:

- Developmental delays and intellectual disability.
- Behavioural and emotional difficulties.
- Cardiac issues, some involving surgical intervention.
- Pharyngeal and palate dysfunction, some involving surgical intervention.
- Attentional deficit.
- Possible autism spectrum disorder.
- Seizure disorders.
- Psychiatric illnesses.

Additionally, there can be any number of health and medical complications, ranging from blood platelet disorders, severe leg cramps, spinal cord abnormalities and vision and hearing deficits. VCFS is not an inherited condition and is not the result of any specific familial histories. Helen is the focus of divorce proceedings where disputation is centred upon possible support costs. She is currently funded through various government disability subsidy schemes and attends a special school for children with various disabilities: Intellectual, sensory and physical.

Her support funding currently does not fully cover all medical and therapeutic treatments, requiring her parents to pay out of pocket for these. As a part of these proceedings, it was requested that a current assessment of developmental disabilities be undertaken and estimates made as to the long-term prognosis and expense of her therapeutic treatments so that family court determinations can be made in the final divorce settlement. Helen attended assessment in my rooms for an updated developmental assessment with two purposes in mind:

1. To complete an assessment applicable for school enrolment when she is age-appropriate stage of readiness.
2. To establish her current levels of disability.

Previous medical proceedings

- Helen was treated surgically at age 15 months for a cardiac anomaly known as "Tetralogy of Fallot", which can occur relatively frequently in children with VCFS. This surgery was successful, and her cardiac status is now stable.
- Helen has not yet required surgery such as skin grafts for her mild "pharyngeal incontinence", whereby intricate repairs need to be rendered to her pharyngeal flap. This is extremely complex surgery and is sometimes recommended to be undertaken in the United States of America.
- Helen has a significant spinal cord distortion which is managed as best as possible through physiotherapy treatment, but it has been discussed that surgical intervention such as the insertion of supporting and straightening rods may need to be undertaken.
- Helen does not present with seizure disorders at this stage. She is being monitored for the possibility of later psychosocial dysfunction such as the onset of depression,

anxiety and "prodromal" signs of psychosis. These conditions are particularly common amongst individuals with VCFS.

Previous assessments

- Previous assessments of Helen undertaken at a specialist children's hospital indicated that at age 23 months, she presented with a moderate global developmental delay, with skills at approximately a 13-month level.
- Recent speech pathology reports indicated the aim to increase the length of spoken phrases and range of expressive vocabulary. Also noted was the aim to improve Helen's speech intelligibility and to reduce her hypernasality. There are also minor feeding and swallowing difficulties to be remediated.
- Physiotherapy reports highlighted the need to improve Helen's stationary and dynamic balance, walking skills, postural strength and endurance and joint mobility.
- Occupational therapy reports focused upon Helen's ability to sit for prolonged periods and to manipulate objects such as scissors and pencils.

Most recent developmental assessment

Helen was assessed in my rooms using a standard developmental assessment tool, Griffiths 3. Overall, she was found to be functioning at approximately a two-and-a-half-year age equivalent, consistent with a moderate global developmental delay. This numerical result is deceptive in that it masks the "qualitative" aspects of her functioning whereby Helen was obviously in considerable distress whilst attempting tasks. She was very easily physically fatigued due to the strain of sitting and maintaining adequate postural control when not able to use her hands for support. This occurred for example when trying to coordinate her hands when using scissors. Helen's physical and emotional support needs were clearly very elevated, and it was a testament to her determination that she was able to complete as many tasks as she could.

Implications for future education, support and financing

This assessment confirmed that Helen was functioning in the moderate range of global developmental delay as defined by DSM-5-TR, with a strong determination to complete tasks even when these were clearly difficult and uncomfortable for her. The prognosis for those with VCFS is extremely problematic, with the distinct possibility of necessary surgical interventions, ongoing therapeutic needs such as speech pathology, occupational therapy and physiotherapy. Helen will require these supports well into the foreseeable future, and there is every likelihood that her support needs will increase and not diminish.

In relation to the question of distribution of maintenance costs between Helen's parents upon the finalisation of these proceedings, I am unable to provide an exact amount, suffice it to say that they will be in the higher range and ongoing.

Case Study 10:   Parental Relinquishment of a Child with a Rare Genetic Disorder

Child's Name: Maggie
Chronological Age: 6 years

Author's credentials

The writer of this report is an educational and developmental psychologist of 40 years' experience, with an extensive background in the domain of children with neurodevelopmental delays and disorders, specific rare genetic disorders and comorbid psychiatric disorders, including research into such conditions.

Smith–Magenis syndrome

As this report concerns a young child with Smith–Magenis Syndrome, a rare genetic disorder, the following background information is provided about the syndrome to assist in understanding the child's parents decision to relinquish their parental responsibilities for her to the government.

Overview

- Smith–Magenis syndrome is an extremely rare genetic disorder caused by a "microdeletion" of genetic material on chromosome 17 (17p11.2). It occurs in approximately 1 in 25,000–50,000 live births. It is not inherited, nor is it the result of any particular parental behaviours or environmental agents.
- Smith–Magenis syndrome presents with prominent "dysmorphic" facial and physical features. Early health can be compromised by failure to thrive, and there can be cardiac defects, renal, brain, eye and spinal abnormalities and hearing loss.
- A defining feature of Smith–Magenis syndrome is severe sleep disturbances caused by "phase shift" in circadian rhythms, whereby the individual's melatonin is produced during the day rather than at night. Moderately delayed intellectual skills and delayed language skills are common in Smith–Magenis syndrome.
- There is often a hoarse voice, a high threshold to pain, increased incidence rate of autistic-type features (reduced empathy, repetitive questioning, insistence on sameness and restricted activities) and high levels of anxiety. A repetitive physical movement pattern known as a "self-hug" is extremely common.

Behaviour and psychopathology

A defining feature of Smith–Magenis syndrome is the presence of severely maladaptive, violent, aggressive and destructive behaviours, including:

- Severe sleep disturbance is present in 65–100% of individuals with Smith–Magenis syndrome.
- There is an 80% occurrence of problematic impulsive behaviours and attention deficit hyperactivity.
- Traits of autism spectrum disorder are present in at least 75% of individuals with the syndrome.
- Physical aggression, destructive behaviours and self-harm occur in at least 70% of individuals with the syndrome.
- Soiling and smearing of faeces is frequently reported, as are maladaptive behaviours such as "inserting" foreign objects into bodily orifices.
- These extreme behavioural challenges frequently lead to family breakdown, and an extremely high incidence of "relinquishment" of parental responsibilities to government authorities is found.

- Children with Smith–Magenis syndrome are most likely to be educated in special schools for children with moderate-to-severe intellectual disabilities or schools for children with autism spectrum disorder.

Specific background information, Maggie

Maggie was assessed in 2022 by a professor of genetics and head of a genetics clinic and found to have the microdeletion for Smith–Magenis syndrome. Maggie spent some time in her local school before her behaviours and support needs rendered this enrolment untenable. She now attends an autism spectrum disorder–specific school on the basis of the following comorbid conditions:

- An intellectual disability with a wide scatter of skills.
- Adaptive behaviour/daily living skills in the "extremely low" range.
- Autism spectrum disorder as defined by DSM-5-TR with level 3 "Very Substantial" support needs.
- Attention deficit hyperactivity disorder.

Maggie is funded through the relevant government support schemes for a number of services including speech pathology, occupational therapy, play therapy and respite care access. She is under the medical care of a consultant paediatrician at the family's local general hospital. A recent review adjusted her medication regime which consists of:

- Vyvance and Intuniv for her attention deficit hyperactivity disorder.
- Sertraline for high levels of anxiety.
- Risperidone for her extremely aggressive, violent and destructive behaviours.
- Melatonin for her severely disrupted sleep cycles.

As a direct result of her Smith–Magenis syndrome, Maggie's challenging behaviours have accelerated extremely quickly in recent months, with many critical incidents being reported at both her home, her school, her respite care facility and her various service providers. These behaviours have included:

- Severe aggression directed towards family members, children and staff school, respite and community access workers and carers. These have included hitting, kicking, hair/scalp pulling and spitting.
- There have been attempts at absconding.
- Serious property damage includes punching holes in Gyprock walls, breaking of windows and windscreens in cars and other transports.
- Self-harm include insertion of foreign objects.
- Soiling and smearing of faeces is reported.
- Verbal abuse of staff and support personnel is also reported.

Maggie was recently excluded from her school programme due to her challenging behaviours, pending the outcome of a medication review, and it is anticipated she will return to school in the near future. The relationship between Maggie's family and her respite care service provider has also broken down as a result of her challenging behaviours, leaving her parents in a most fraught situation where they can no longer access any relief from the daily stress and trauma of caring for her and managing her behaviours. As a result, Maggie's family have come to the most difficult decision that any parents can possibly arrive at, to relinquish parental responsibility of Maggie to the state. They do not take this decision lightly but as a matter of "forced choice" for a number of reasons:

1 Smith–Magenis syndrome is perhaps the most behaviourally challenging disabling condition known. It is exceedingly rare but consistent in its course and impact.
2 No parents have specific training in the management of Smith–Magenis syndrome prior to a child's birth; in fact, this syndrome cannot currently be assessed or diagnosed in utero. It is a totally unexpected "one in 50,000" event with no specific cause and no specific cultural, socioeconomic or ethnic association. It occurs "de novo", unexpectedly and with no pre-warning.
3 Maggie's parents have done their utmost best to raise Maggie, to manage her severely challenging behaviours and to negotiate the complexities of the health, education and welfare systems into which they have become involved. This was not what they planned, hoped or expected when they brought Maggie into the world.
4 Maggie's parents and her sibling have endured many crises and traumas as a direct result of her genetic disorder and consequent behavioural challenges. There have been physical attacks, emotional outbursts, severe damage to their property and disruption to their married lives, study and employment. There have been deleterious impacts upon their health and emotional well-being.

It is well documented that with Smith–Magenis syndrome, the relinquishment of parenting responsibilities to the state is a common outcome and a "forced choice", and so it is of Maggie's parents. This is not a case of parents "abandoning" their children through any lack of love or commitment, rather it is a realisation that they have done their very best to parent and support their child when expert skills and knowledge are required but not necessarily available. On this basis, the following issues need to be considered:

- Maggie's parents should be treated with all due respect when relinquishment is being considered, discussed and organised.
- That consideration be given to addressing the emotional and physical trauma which Maggie's family have endured in their attempts to support and manage her severely challenging behaviours. Should Maggie's parents feel the need for external support and debriefing such as counselling and psychological assistance, this should be funded through the relevant government services and funding sources.
- Similarly, Maggie's parents have endured ongoing episodes of destructive aggression upon their house and property, and consideration should be given to the funding the necessary repairs to or replacement of property resulting from these aggressive/destructive outbursts.

Upon relinquishment Maggie will need to be relocated to a suitable facility such as a group home. To make this move successful the following needs to occur or be considered:

1 All staff at Maggie's new residence should be briefed about the nature of Smith–Magenis Syndrome and its attendant behavioural challenges before Maggie moves there.
2 Specific staff members should be selected on the basis of their skills and experience in supporting students with severely challenging behaviours.

3 Before Maggie has any engagement with her new abode, the following procedures should be discussed and followed:

   a A comprehensive audit and review of all security procedures, for example security of all doors, gates and windows, implements and utensils which may be present such as kitchen equipment, and any other procedures relating to absconding into the broader community.
   b Detailed training for all staff, particularly in relation to maintaining "constant vigilance" in relation to Maggie.
   c Incorporation of any specific information from those already familiar with Maggie and her behavioural challenges and trajectory.
   d For example, personnel from either Maggie's school or respite facility may have learned through experience and observation to "predict" Maggie's behavioural escalation on the basis of such factors as changes in voice, levels of agitation, skin tone, verbalisations, or specific activities. An understanding and awareness of these subtle changes and contexts may enable staff to predict a behavioural episode or outburst, thereby enabling pre-emptory actions to either prevent or minimise outbursts. than to respond to them after the event.

4 Maggie should not commence in any new residential or respite placement full-time. Rather, she should undergo a planned and gradual transition, including "orientation visits" with an experienced and familiar carer or support staff. These visits should be of short duration and place no pressure on Maggie to "perform". These visits should gradually increase in duration, with a gradual increase in duration and complexity.
5 It is strongly recommended that there be an increased allocation of staffing to support and monitor Maggie. Ideally, Maggie should be supervised on a 1:1 or 1:2 basis for as long as possible, with a "waking shift" in the context of Maggie's "reversed" sleep cycle.
6 Maggie's behaviour and progress should be closely monitored and shared with all support personnel on a regular basis.
7 Changes in personnel such as "supply" staff should only occur as a last resort, and as much preparation as possible for "new" personnel should be given prior to their contact with Maggie, in much the same way as a "handover" of medical notes occurs in hospital settings.
8 It is recommended that staff allocated to teach and support Maggie should wear personal duress alarms at all times when in close proximity to her.
9 It is vital that ongoing contact be maintained with other professionals involved with Maggie, for example, her consultant paediatrician who needs to have awareness of the effectiveness or otherwise of Maggie's current medication regime.
10 Genetic disorders such as Smith–Magenis syndrome often present with autistic behaviours as part of their profile, but not all of their behaviours are consistent with autism spectrum disorder. In the case of Smith–Magenis syndrome, there are some behaviours which are effectively "hard-wired" genetically and not likely to change. Priority should not be given to these specific behaviours unless they are challenging in nature.
11 Individuals with Smith–Magenis syndrome do respond to the types of teaching and communication strategies often applied to children with autism spectrum disorder, for example:

   a The use of visual-augmentative materials such as pictures and symbols.
   b Schedule boxes, timetables, lists and calendars.

c Highly repetitive and predictable routines.
  d The use of clear, concrete and simple communication, including choice of words and instructions, "count-downs", ordered and hierarchical instructions.

Summations

It has been this psychologist's experience that in the context of children with Smith–Magenis syndrome, relinquishment of parental responsibility to the State is a most frequent occurrence. It is always a saddening and regretful experience, and I would be happy to speak more directly with those involved if that were seen as necessary or advantageous.

Case Study 11:   Observational "Triage" at a Childcare Centre, Possible Autism Spectrum Disorder

Child's Name: Samantha
Chronological Age: 4 years

Background information:

Samantha is a 4-year-old child who was referred by her parents in collaboration with her childcare centre staff over concerns about her social, communication and play development. This childcare centre has had previous experience with children with autism spectrum disorder and requested urgent observations of Samantha before the family would consent to further assessment. At the time of this observation session Samantha had not been assessed by a paediatrician although this was planned for the near future.

Prior to observing Samantha her parents kindly completed the Parent Form 2–5 years Autism Spectrum Rating Scales form, and information from this is tabulated and charted below:

Scale	T score 90% C.I.	Percentile	Classification	Interpretive guideline
Total Score				
Total Score	62 (59–64)	88	Slightly elevated	Has many behavioural characteristics similar to children diagnosed with an autism spectrum disorder
ASRS Scales				
Social/ communication	62 (58–65)	88	Slightly elevated	Has difficulty using verbal and non-verbal communication appropriately to initiate, engage in, and maintain social contact
Unusual behaviours	59 (55–62)	82	Average score	No problems indicated

(Continued)

Case studies and reports 289

Scale	T score 90% C.I.	Percentile	Classification	Interpretive guideline
DSM-5 SCALE				
DSM-5 Scale	64 (60–67)	92	Slightly elevated	Has symptoms directly related to the DSM-5 diagnostic criteria for an autism spectrum disorder
TREATMENT SCALES				
Peer socialisation	77 (69–79)	99	Very elevated	Has limited willingness and capacity to successfully engage in activities that develop and maintain relationships with other children
Adult socialisation	67 (56–70)	96	Elevated score	Has limited willingness and capacity to successfully engage in activities that develop and maintain relationships with adults
Social/emotional reciprocity	57 (52–61)	76	Average score	No problems indicated
Atypical language	59 (50–64)	82	Average Score	No problems indicated
Stereotypy	59 (51–64)	82	Average score	No problems indicated
Behavioural rigidity	58 (52–62)	79	Average score	No problems indicated
Sensory sensitivity	56 (48–61)	73	Average score	No problems indicated
Attention/self-regulation	46 (41–52)	34	Average score	No problems indicated

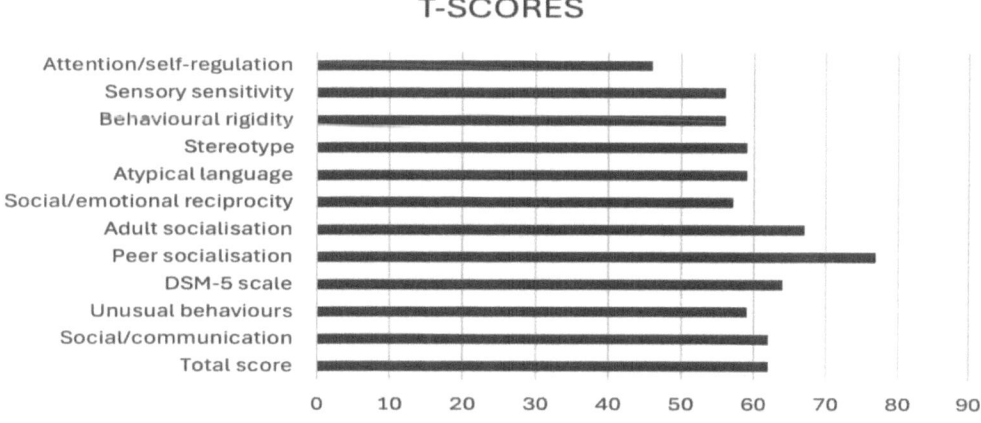

Interpretation

Scoring of the Autism Spectrum Rating Scale did not of itself indicate that Samantha may meet criteria for a diagnosis of autism spectrum disorder as defined by DSM-5-TR. Concerns were noted in relation to her current ability to communicate and interact with her age peers and with her adult carers. There were however no indications of atypical or stereotypic language or word use, stereotypic play or object use, attention or self-regulation skills, or sensory processing abilities.

Observations

Samantha was observed over a 45-minute period at her childcare centre. She tended to present as shy and "careful" in relation to her interactions with other children, preferring to play on her own and only communicate when necessary. On observation her play skills included normal use of toys such as dolls, puzzles and kitchen utensils, and she enjoyed reading age-appropriate books. Samantha did not engage in any unusual or repetitive play and no physical stereotypies were noted. She did not present with unusual or concerning responses to her sensory environment. Samanthan did not present with anxieties and followed routines appropriately. There were no excessive displays of emotionality.

Discussion

This observational triage, supplemented by completion of a detailed questionnaire encompassing the features and criteria of autism spectrum disorder, did not at this stage indicate sufficient concern about autism spectrum disorder to warrant a comprehensive diagnostic assessment. However it must be noted that girls do tend to present later with concerns about autism spectrum disorder. A recommendation from this observational session and questionnaire-based triage is that a follow-up review of Samantha be undertaken as she approaches the end of this year so that any changes in her presentation can be noted.

Case Study 12: Profound Intellectual Disability Post-hydrocephalus

Name of Child: Saleeb
Chronological Age: 5 years 6 months

Background

This observational assessment of Saleeb was undertaken at a hospice for severely to profoundly disabled children, when they are unable to attend school and to be assessed on standard psychometric assessments. It was undertaken at the behest of the local school authority who were concerned as to whether or not Saleeb would be able to attend the school for specific purposes in their district as school enrolment is compulsory.

Medical history

At his birth Saleeb was diagnosed with Spina Bifida, a neural tube defect where a baby's spine and spinal cord fail to develop properly during pregnancy. Upon birth, treatment involves surgery close to the defect, but complications can arise, including hydrocephalus when excess cerebrospinal fluid builds up in the ventricles (cavities) deep within the brain, thus creating harmful pressure on the brain's tissues. One of the two treatment options when this occurs involves a tube known as a "shunt" which is surgically inserted into the brain and connected to a flexible tube placed under the skin to drain the excess fluid into either the chest cavity or the abdomen so it can be absorbed by the body.

Saleeb underwent this surgery immediately after his birth, however complications arose shortly after this, when the shunt became blocked and severe hydrocephalus resulted. A secondary infection then set in, causing irreparable brain damage. His condition deteriorated rapidly and it was not expected that he would survive, however he did, and has since been cared for in a hospice for children with severe to profound intellectual disabilities and developmental delays. Saleeb is described as totally bed-ridden, and non-sentient. He receives nursing care, is stomach-fed, and requires manual lifting and rolling to alleviate pressure sores.

Assessment observations

Saleeb was observed from his bedside, using the Developmental Assessment for Severely Disabled (DASH-3) protocol as a guide. It was determined that Saleeb was profoundly disabled across all areas assessed by the DASH-3. He did not respond to voice or tactile stimuli such as touch, other than some signs of muscular relaxation when gently stroked. He also appeared to register some sensation when air was gently blown on him. Saleeb did not make any meaningful communication sounds, and only minimal vocal noises were heard. There was no evidence of his having awareness of his surroundings. Saleeb lay peacefully and quietly with no signs of distress.

Discussions with attending hospice personnel confirmed that Saleeb was entirely dependent upon their daily care for all basic needs-tube feeding, toileting, bathing and medicating. He was described as being too fragile medically to be transported from the hospice.

Conclusion

Saleeb, although of an age where he should be attending school, is considered far to disabled and medically fragile to attend his nearest school for specific purposes. He does not respond consistently to any meaningful stimuli and is not safe to travel. Exemption should be granted from any compulsory school attendance, including schools catering for the developmental support needs of children with severe disabilities.

DASH-3 score summary

Subtest	Developmental age
Social-emotional scale	Too low to assess
Language scale:	Too low to assess
Sensory motor scale:	Too low to assess
• Gross motor	
• Sensory	
• Hand skills	
Activities of daily living scale:	Too low to assess
• Feeding	
• Dressing	
• Toileting	
• Home routines	
• Travel and safety	

(Continued)

Subtest	Developmental age
Academics scale:	Too low to assess
• Preacademic skills	
• Academic skills	
• Numerical reasoning	
• Reading	
Overall developmental age:	Too low to assess

Case Study 13:   Pre- and Post-assessment for Program Evaluation

Child's Name: Juanita
Chronological Age: 40 months

Background

Juanita is a 3 years and 4 months old child who was diagnosed by her paediatrician as meeting DSM-5-TR criteria for autism spectrum disorder with Level 2 "very substantial" support needs. This diagnosis was submitted to relevant State funding authorities and she was allocated "set plan" financial support to undertake a 12-month programme of applied behaviour therapy (ABA) support through a registered programme provider. She was assessed at the beginning of the programme and then reassessed on exit from the programme to evaluate its success. Details of this assessment are provided below:

Standardised developmental assessment

Developmental assessments were conducted to determine Juanita's skills and progress across the past 10 months of the ABA intervention program. The Mullen scales of early learning is a developmental assessment where the child participates in a range of developmental activities. It assesses a child's skills in four areas:

- Visual reception.
- Fine motor.
- Receptive language.
- Expressive language.

Scores on the MSEL are categorised as falling with the ranges of Low, Below Average, Average, Above Average, or High. Scores can also be expressed as "age equivalents" (AEs). It is important to note that a child's scores on this assessment do not necessarily provide a perfect indication of their skills. Scores can be influenced by the motivation, health, attention span, mood, and behaviour of the child on the day of the assessment. It was noted that Juanita's attention did fluctuate throughout the assessment. The tables below summarise Juanita's performance on the Mullen scales of early learning at and after the first year of intervention, with Table 28.1 indicating the change in Juanita's age equivalent scores.

Table 28.1 Mullen scales programme intake and exit results

Mullen scales of learning pre- and post-programme results in months

Scales	Intake assessment	Exit assessment
Chronological age	30	40
Visual receptive	20	30
Fine motor	22	31
Receptive language	2	22
Expressive language	15	17

Juanita has made clear progress in the past 10 months in a number of developmental areas. She has made 11 months of gains in visual-spatial skills, 9 months of progress in her fine motor skills and 20 months of progress in receptive language. Expressive language is challenging for Juanita and she has made 1 month of progress in this area. Her communication has grown substantially through alternative means. For example, she now successfully uses proloquo2go, a computer application, to express her wants and needs. Her strengths and areas of difficulty across the different learning domains are discussed in greater detail below.

Visual Reception Subscale: The Visual Reception subscale measured Juanita's ability to process visual-spatial information to learn about the world around her. Juanita could pay close attention to items and match items by shape and size and notice very subtle differences, such as black and white line drawings of slightly different flowers. She struggled to remember items shown to her. Letter matching was also challenging.

Fine Motor Subscale: The Fine Motor subscale assessed Juanita's movement and coordination of small body parts, particularly in the hands and fingers. Juanita showed great interest in drawing and copied a number of different shapes very well, she struggled when the drawings became more complex such as a circle in a circle. Juanita enjoyed manipulating small toy coins to fit into a money box. She found it difficult to imitate block structures and imitate more precise movements with her hands such as touching her fingers together.

Receptive Language Subscale: Receptive Language subscale tests a child's understanding of spoken language, including attention to speech and knowledge of words. Juanita's receptive language has seen huge growth in the past 9 months. She demonstrated an ability to identify items and body parts. She struggled with more advanced concepts such as functions of items and prepositions such as in, on, under and behind.

Expressive Language Subscale: The Expressive Language subscale measures Juanita's ability to use spoken language to communicate and express ideas. Juanita has made limited progress expressively with her gains measured via the assessment of 1 month. She was observed throughout the assessment to communicate very effectively on her iPad via an application called proloquo2go.

These results provide clear evidence that early and intensive intervention has been effective in teaching Juanita new skills across the past nine months. She will require the continuation of her current intensive and structured environment to maintain her skills and to continue to develop her skills across all domains. The language domains should have a strong focus; her receptive language has seen the largest growth however it remains one of her most challenging areas of development.

Vineland adaptive behaviour scales-survey interview form (VABS)

The Vineland Adaptive Behaviour Scale is a parent interview designed to measure a child's adaptive behaviour in everyday life. It examines four domains: Communication, Daily Living Skills, Socialisation, and Motor Skills. Scores are described as percentile ranks and can be described as falling in the ranges Low, Moderately Low or Adequate. A percentile rank is a number between 1 and 99, with 50 being the average score for a child that age. For example, a score of 14 would mean that the child has performed better than 14% of other children the same age.

Juanita's father answered the questions for the Vineland interview at intake and after 9 months of intervention. Juanita's scores on the Vineland are below in Table 28.2:

Juanita currently displays adaptive skills that fall between the Low to Moderately Low range among children her age. The results show that her Daily Living Skills and Motor Skills domains fall within the Moderately Low range, with scores that are in the 4th and 5th percentile respectively. This is significant progress since her intake assessment, where her level of skills in these domains fell below the 1st percentile. These domains are now considered areas of personal strength compared to other adaptive domains. Juanita's skills in the Communication and Socialisation domains fall in the Low range, with scores that both fall below the 1st percentile compared to same-aged peers.

These are areas that are particularly challenging for Juanita when compared to other adaptive domains. However, she has made important progress in these areas.

Communication: Receptively, Juanita is able to recognise verbal labels for some preferred items (e.g., blueberries, paint paper), and is also able to identify some things through pointing or retrieving them (e.g., objects, body parts, action words), and is beginning to understand some 'wh' questions. Juanita is also now beginning to follow some simple, 1-step instructions however, this does depend on her level of motivation/attention at the time. Juanita has difficulty understanding "yes" and "no", and also shows significant challenges in regulating her attention in daily activities.

Expressively, Juanita does not use vocal speech to communicate, and primarily uses her body (i.e., gestures and body movements) to express her wants and needs in everyday life. She is now producing vocalisations more frequently in her daily life compared to intake, and can produce several different one syllable sounds, and on occasion, has said "Mama" or "Dada". There were some items where Juanita is indicated to have shown a decrease in how frequently she shows these skills since intake including repeating words she hears, labelling objects, and saying one-word requests. The examiner can follow up to determine if this is an accurate reflection of Juanita's skills across time, or if this is reflective of an error in scoring/administration.

Table 28.2 Pre- and post-test results, Vineland Adaptive Behaviour Scale

Vineland adaptive behaviour scale:
Results at programme entry and exit (8-month duration)

Assessment	Communication	Daily living	Socialisation	Motor skills
At entry	Below 1st Percentile Low	Below 1st Percentile Low	Below 1st Percentile Low	Below 1st Percentile Low
On exit after 8 months	Below 1st Percentile Low	4th Percentile Low	Below 1st Percentile Low	5th Percentile Low

Daily Living Skills: Juanita is showing increased independence in some areas of daily living. She is now able to feed herself with a spoon without spilling and is learning to use a fork. She is becoming more independent with toilet training during the day, and is learning to pull up her pants, put on her shoes, and wash her hands independently. Currently, she still requires support with wiping after toileting, and washing and personal hygiene routines (e.g., face washing, wiping/blowing her nose, drying her hands after washing them) along with close supervision to ensure she remains on-task across the toileting routine. Juanita requires some support to keep herself safe at home and in the community. She is learning to remain within a close distance to caregivers when in public spaces, and be careful around hot or sharp objects at home.

Socialisation: Juanita displays a limited range of emotions in daily life, and Javeeth notes that she does not frequently smile or laugh. Juanita is beginning to show affection towards family members and sometimes initiates interactions with her parents, and will reach out to her father's hand to initiate play. Juanita also tends to check in to see whether her parents are nearby.

Juanita's play interests include sand, paint, and slides. She is beginning to be more responsive when her parents are playful with her, and also shows interest in her surroundings and is able to play near other children. However, Juanita does not yet participate in back and forth play in a way that might be expected with children or adults.

Juanita is now better able to cope with transitions and separating from her parents in daily life compared to intake. Changes in routine can still be challenging, however, she is sometimes able to cope when these arise, and tends to recover more quickly when encountering a minor disappointment. Transitioning away from preferred activities or needing to wait for items can also still be quite challenging for Juanita. Juanita is also now able to request for help, and accept help when she needs it.

Motor Skills: Juanita is now able to run without falling, jump off the ground with two feet, and navigate slippery or uneven surfaces. She is also no able to walk up and down stairs with alternating feet, and kick a ball. She is still learning to throw and catch, jump forwards, and climb up and down high objects safely. In terms of fine motor skills, Juanita can now hold and manipulate small objects, open doors, and is learning to hold a crayon/pencil for drawing.

Vineland-3 growth scale value:

The growth scale value (GSV) on the Vineland-3 measures change and tracks individual progress across time, without comparing a child to their same-aged peers. It allows us to consider the amount of progress a child makes, in comparison to their scores in the past. The Vineland-3 GSV scores allow us to look at statistically significant changes in a child's progress across the last two time points. Juanita displays statistically significant improvements in a number of areas of adaptive functioning after 12 months of intervention. Growth has been significant in the following areas:

- Receptive.
- Personal (self-care skills).
- Play and Leisure.
- Coping Skills.
- Gross Motor.
- Fine Motor.

Taken together, Juanita's developmental assessment results demonstrate that she has benefited from early and intensive intervention and that this structure of learning is helping her work towards achieving her nominated goals. She will require the continuation of this intensive and structured intervention programme in the coming 12 months.

Bibliography

Alfonso, V., Engler, C., and Turner, R. (2022), Essentials of the Bayley 4 Assessment, Wiley.

Aylward, G. (2020), Bayley-4: Clinical Use and Interpretation, Academic Press.

Preston, P. (2005), Testing Children-A Practitioner's Guide to the Assessment of Mental Development in Infants and Young Children, Hogrefe and Huber.

Stroud, L., and Green, E. (2022), Griffiths III: A Case Study Book for Practitioners, Hogrefe Ltd.

Part VI
Follow-up

29 Follow-up and support

After referral, assessment, feedback, diagnosis and reporting have been finished, what is the role of psychologists when young children and families are concerned? Is it ongoing counselling and support for families or therapeutic intervention with a young child, establishing and planning behavioural support plans or providing advocacy and advice when needed? Are cases simply filed away as "finished", or is there ongoing involvement?

The nature of "follow-up" can be a decision made by a psychologist's employers; for example, psychologists in specific employment contexts may work to a set of conditions which dictate to greater or lesser degrees the post-assessment roles they may engage in and the services they may offer. Or psychologists may have a greater degree of autonomy as to how they support children and families post-assessment:

- Some psychological assessment and diagnostic clinics may, for example, offer reassessment and review services for existing clients up to certain ages and stages in the life of a young child, for example, until the commencement of formal schooling.
- Individual psychologists may wish to extend their roles into services such as behavioural support planning, particularly when there may be systemic needs for such programs to be written professionally.
- Some may offer therapies and programs themselves if they are skilled and qualified in specific techniques.
- Others may pursue specific roles such as organising and conducting family support programs such as parent support groups or siblings programs.
- Advocacy and consultative services on behalf of referred families may be part of the "follow-up" post-assessment, ensuring that service providers such as childcare centres, therapists and school settings know the needs of a particular child and the relative importance and priority of service delivery or enrolment.
- Follow-up may be immediate or soon after assessment, and diagnosis has occurred or may be after a period of time in which families have had the chance to process the information given, to make specific enquiries and arrangements regarding service provision or to simply attend to other matters.

Families themselves will often decide which services they need from their psychologist. Parents of young children with neurodevelopmental disorders will experience differing emotions and reactions to diagnostic information. Some will accept readily that the assessment and diagnostic process is an end in itself, facilitating access to programs and support funding so that intervention and assistance can begin. Perhaps these families will not need to maintain contact with their psychologist.

Other families may wish to seek advice and guidance on an ongoing basis about their child, his/her behaviours and progress, selection of support programs and therapies and significant decisions such as which school their child should attend when the time comes. There are parents who will be greatly saddened and distressed by diagnostic outcomes and the practicalities of raising a young child with a disorder and will seek ongoing support to guide them through difficult emotional times. Whether psychologists offer their support on a regular appointment-orientated basis or spontaneously respond to need is a clinical as well as an "operational" decision to be made.

There will be psychologists who offer highly specific post-assessment follow-up: Time to reflect on the assessment and diagnostic process, clarifying points of concern or confusion and specific question-and-answer opportunities. And there are psychologists who see their role as "finished" once the process of assessment, diagnosis, discussion and report writing is complete.

Psychologists who are employed in "disability-specific" contexts, for example, schools or services for children with autism spectrum disorder, cerebral palsy or physical or sensory disabilities, may be involved in ongoing education, information and training programs for families and staff, facilitating "capacity building" for their families, and even for the broader community. Some psychologists will incorporate home visits in their role, either individually or as part of therapy "teams". The roles for psychologists in early childhood disability are indeed varied.

As well as supporting individual parents, psychologists in these settings may of their own volition establish "parent groups" and even "siblings' groups" to foster communication and sharing of ideas, experiences, resources and expertise. Sometimes these groups simply serve a social support function, allowing parents to spend time together for activities which have nothing to do with their busy roles as parents of young children with neurodevelopmental disorders.

For the siblings of children with neurodevelopmental disorders, mixed emotions can range from pride in a brother or sister's achievements, fear of aggressive behaviours, frustration at their inability to play and share or embarrassment at their brother or sister's behaviour in public places. The opportunity to voice these experiences in a safe and supported environment, away from their home lives, can be liberating. Emotions and reactions they may have felt inhibited from sharing at home with their parents can be given a voice, and the discovery that other children share the same concerns can give rise to new friendships through shared experience.

In our increasingly diverse and multicultural world, parents and grandparents can hold very different attitudes and understandings towards childhood disability. Grandparents and other important family members may hold more traditional beliefs than their children who may feel more educated and enlightened, and this can be a source of intergenerational conflict, particularly when grandparents are being called upon to share the role of childcare. Psychologists may be called upon to mediate between parties when calmness and clarity is required, to explain the nature of a neurodevelopmental disorder and the best means by which all family members can play a supportive role.

Reassessments are frequently required for young children once diagnosed. With the passing of time and the impact of appropriate therapies and services, their profiles and needs will change, and this progression often needs to be monitored. A common occurrence is the need to reassess a child when completing one course of "treatment" and commencing another or transitioning from preschool settings to more formal educational facilities. Psychometric assessments have clearly stated "test-retest" intervals to avoid incidental "learning effect" to occur and potentially invalidate assessment outcomes. Questionnaire-based assessments sometimes have "parallel forms"—two versions of the same items but with different wordings or subtly differing items. Alternatively, psychologists may need access to the nearest equivalent assessment tool to conduct repeat assessments. Knowledge of these matters is another component of a psychologist's core skills.

Parents of children with developmental concerns share with parents of "neurotypical" children the need to pass through various "transitions" in the lives of their children, for example, reaching school enrolment age, whether this be mainstream schooling or special education facilities. Decisions will need to be made, and new processes learned and mastered to ease over that new hurdle. All "systems" require evidential reports and application forms, a clerical and bureaucratic task psychologists are often called upon to complete.

Children with neurodevelopmental disorders transition through different phases of development which can presage significant behavioural change. For example, the approach of puberty is an important and sometimes dramatic developmental shift in a child's life, and parents frequently feel confused and concerned about how best to deal with these new challenges. In fact, there is evidence that children with neurodevelopmental disorders can reach puberty and its attendant behavioural challenges earlier than expected. Parents often recontact trusted professionals such as psychologists at these points of transition. Parents may seek advice on highly specific behavioural challenges such as a child with a chronic sleep disorder or a behavioural pattern only occurring at home and not in the child's day program.

Parents and families change as well, learning through their efforts and experiences to cope better with the demands of parenting a child with a neurodevelopmental disorder. They will have "new stories" to tell but also have new questions to ask, new challenges to face and new insights into their "journeys" thus far. Some will have reached a stage where they can reflect upon their initial experiences of negotiating the assessment and diagnosis phase of their child's life and realise that they have only paid attention to the needs of their child, neglecting their own until they have the opportunity to revisit their own emotional state. There can be unresolved grief, anger, bitterness and even trauma to address or pride and satisfaction in the roles they have played and the successes they can share.

Some psychologists choose to practise and work "longitudinally", that is, they regard their referred families as "clients for life" and maintain an "open-door" policy for their families so that, at these transition points, they can return if they wish to where their "journeys" often began. Psychologists who practise in this manner benefit considerably from the unique opportunity to watch a young child and his/her family grow "with" their disorder, thus enriching their professional knowledge base and understanding of child development even further.

It is often stated that successful psychological collaborations with clients stem from the quality of the relationship which is established early between practitioner and client. When empathy, trust and understanding are created in this manner and when a family's needs are understood and responded to in timely and appropriate ways, the benefits are rich and reciprocal.

Bibliography

Bartolo, P. A. (2002), "Communicating a Diagnosis of Developmental Disability to Parents: Multi-professional Negotiation Framework", Child: Care, Health and Development, 28(1), pp 65–71.

Bowen, C., and Snow, P. (2017), "Making Sense of Interventions for Children with Developmental Disorders", J&R Press.

Gilmore, L. (2018), "Supporting Families of Children with Rare and Unique Chromosome Disorders", Research and Practice in Intellectual and Developmental Disabilities, 5(1), pp 8–16.

Siddiqui, S. U., Van Dyke, C. D., Donohoue, P., and McBrien, D. M. (1999), "Premature Sexual Development in Individuals with Neurodevelopmental Disabilities", Developmental Medicine & Child Neurology, 41(6), pp 392–395.

Tharinger, D. J., Finn, S. E., Hersh, B., and Wilkinson, A. (2008), "Assessment Feedback with Parents of Pre-adolescent Children: A Collegiate Approach", Professional Psychology Research and Practice 39(6), pp 600–609.

The Royal Children's Hospital Melbourne, "Puberty in Young People with Disabilities".

Tsai, S. J., Lue, W. Y., Yu, C. H., Chen, T. J., and Chen, M. H. (2024), "Autism and Risk of Precocious Puberty: A Cohort Study of 22,208 Children", Research in Autism Spectrum Disorders, 114, 102390.

Tudor, M. E., and Lerner, M. D. (2014), "Intervention and Support for Siblings of Youth with Developmental Disabilities: A Systematic Review", Clinical Child and Family Psychology Review, 18, pp 1–23.

Part VII
Pondering the future

30 Pondering the future of neurodevelopmental disorders

Our current generation has become far more accustomed to change than previous generations. The worlds of science, information technology, health diagnosis and treatment, communications, and transport have been revolutionised by inventions, achievements, industry, politics and breakthroughs. Attitudes, values, cultural mores, religions and faiths have changed dramatically. Some would say such progress is for the betterment of societies; others highlight the conflicts and complications which have arisen as a result of change. How will the new technologies and sciences, inventions, laws and legislations, policies and procedures, attitudes and beliefs impact upon our understanding of neurodevelopmental disorders, their causation and presentation, support and treatment? There are no definitive answers to these questions and issues, but there is opportunity to wonder, to prognosticate, to analyse trends already occurring and to attempt to make predictions.

The genetics of neurodevelopmental disorders

The science of genetics is advancing at an extraordinary pace. Since the ground-shaking revealing of the "double helix" of DNA by James Watson, Francis Crick and Rosalind Elsie Franklin in 1953, the understanding of our humanity changed forever. Research continued apace. The genetic underpinning of Down syndrome in 1959 opened the world's eyes to the study of genetic errors. The number and type of such errors, which have always existed but were until recently invisible to the world of science, have increased enormously. "New" genetic disorders are announced on a regular basis. It was not so long ago that genetic microdeletions and microduplications came to light, followed by genetic mutations. Genetic science now refers to "sub-microdeletions and duplications", and even to "pre-mutations". Many questions arise from these advances and, although hypothetical in nature, do impact upon the understanding of neurodevelopmental disorders:

- How many more genetic factors in the causation and course of neurodevelopmental disorders will be discovered or clarified?
- Will the cause of existing neurodevelopmental disorders with as yet no known genetic substrate be linked to genetic factors as yet unobservable?
- If so, will these conditions follow the path of Rett syndrome and cease to be classified as "neurodevelopmental disorders" in tomes such as DSM-5-TR? Or will there need to be new means of classifying these disorders and syndromes?
- What impact if any will such an occurrence have upon management and treatment options, support funding and service access?

- Will there be the possibility of genetic errors being "re-engineered" to prevent the development of these disorders, for example through in utero processes?
- Will there be negative consequences to heightened awareness and understanding of genetic disorders? For example, would this perhaps lead to mandatory population genetic screening as a means of prevention, or will this instead cause ethical and legal problems such as the confidentiality of such genetic data and its accessibility to other agencies such as insurance companies?
- Or will such discoveries lead to a return to such social policies as eugenics, where certain genetic traits and errors are eradicated?

Government and agency policies on neurodevelopmental disorders

The recognition and acceptance of disabilities in recent decades has been long fought for and hard-won. The impact upon the lives of families with disabilities amongst their number has been overwhelmingly positive through inclusionary policies and procedures for education, employment, financial support, community access, leisure time and recreation.

There are still anomalies, restrictions, prejudices, prohibitions, barriers, misunderstandings and confusions around the rights of individuals with disabilities, and one question to pose is whether the subtle difference between "equality" and "equity" has been fully understood in disability legislation and law.

In the workforce, for example, it is becoming increasingly frequent for corporations to have "diversity policies". Some sectors of employment even have affirmative action policies such as quotas for employing people with neurodevelopmental disorders and other disabilities. In film and television, for example, it is increasingly frequent to note an actor with a disability playing an important role. In some offices, factories and retail outlets, people with disabilities such as neurodevelopmental disorders will have specific arrangements made to facilitate their well-being in the workforce—extra rest breaks when necessary, adapted facilities such as bathrooms and desks and adapted technologies such as voice-activated computers. And sectors of the workforce now acknowledge and appreciate the unique skills and contributions of "neurodiverse" people.

These policies and procedures have changed the lives of many people with disabilities for the better, but one does not have to look far to find anomalies and gaps in these processes, and even examples of unabashed discrimination. Consider the following examples:

- Guide dogs for the visually impaired and care dogs for people with neurodevelopmental disorders not being allowed in certain modes of transport, for example, hire taxis.
- Wheelchairs not being permitted on certain aircraft and no viable alternatives being offered.
- People with neurodevelopmental disorders such as autism spectrum disorder having to undertake work roles that are unsuited to their individual and often unique skill sets, and which can exacerbate their often heightened levels of anxiety and social estrangement.
- Buildings and transport hubs still existing without easy access for people with physical disabilities and limited mobility.

These examples suggest that is not a clear misunderstanding of the difference between equality and equity. Who will be responsible for the consequences of these discrepancies? How far can legislations, acts of parliament, laws and policies actually delve into the community and workplace, and who will resource the many adaptations and changes to bring about real "equity"?

Financial assistance for families and individuals with neurodevelopmental disorders

Nations which have developed and enacted financial support schemes for individuals with disabilities have sometimes been surprised by the rapid uptakes of these schemes and supports. Some are now questioning the viability and sustainability of these programmes, resorting to various cost-cutting measures such as increasingly stringent eligibility requirements, restrictions on the types and amount of services provided, and even attempts at redefining the nature of certain disabilities to render individuals ineligible entirely or only eligible for restricted financial benefits. This process by definition undermines the central tenets of disability legislation-choice, freedom, and equity.

There are many ways to compare individual nations' financial commitment to funding disability support and intervention programmes and to at least partially reimburse families for the expenses they incur. Some countries simply report their total expenditure on disability and other social benefit programmes, but of course, these "uncorrected" numbers are a distortion which simply favour more populated and more developed countries. "Proportional" statistics such as per capita funding, percentage of gross national product or gross net income are a more accurate comparative statistic—do the biggest and richest countries necessarily commit more funding, or do smaller or lesser able nations "punch above their weight?"

The most recent The Organisation for Economic Co-ordination and Development (OECD) statistics on percentage of national gross domestic product expended on disability (2019) may make surprising reading in relation to which countries are more or less willing to contribute to support programmes for families (Table 30.1).

No doubt some of these figures may only be low at face value and reflective of specific factors such as the methodology of data collection and classification. One question stemming from these fiscal realities will be of the choices governments make between long-term commitment to those with disabilities and the many other priorities of statehood: Housing, defence, the environment, climate change, health and education. There

Table 30.1 Percentage of Gross Domestic Product expenditure on disability benefits

Highest and least spenders on disability as percentage of GDP

Highest 10 (%)		Lowest 10 (%)	
OECD average	2.0	OECD average	2.0
Denmark	4.5	Mexico	0.0
Norway	4.5	Costa Rica	0.4
Sweden	3.4	Turkey	0.5
Belgium	3.2	Canada	0.7
Finland	3.2	Korea	0.7
Iceland	3.1	Chile	0.8
Australia	2.9	United States	1.0
Israel	2.9	Japan	1.1
Netherlands	2.8	United Kingdom	1.3
Estonia	2.3	Greece	1.3

Source: OECD.

are already challenges to schemes such as the Australian National Disability Insurance Scheme (NDIS) which is generous and far-reaching in its support brief, but which is also experiencing expediential cost overruns, perhaps because of its comprehensive format and commitment. How would the political "optics" appear and be explained away by governments if people with disabling conditions were suddenly deprived of the funding and support services provided to them after so many decades of inaction?

Governments in "developed" western countries are also vital to the financial support of developing nations for their economic well-being and development, including education and welfare programmes and services. The western world assumes a moral responsibility to less "well-off" countries, both politically and socially, but if they themselves are under the pressure of fiscal constraints, will this eventually impact upon their ability and willingness to support less developed countries? If so, will there be a "flow-on" effect on social funding and welfare in the low-to-middle-income nations?

In her controversial book *The Genetic Lottery: Why DNA Matters for Social Equality*, Clinical Psychologist and Professor Kathyryn Paige Harden from the University of Texas describes the cumulative effect of poverty, malnutrition, disease, unemployment and service deprivation as an example of "long-chain causal genetics", whereby this endless cycle of disadvantage repeats itself over and over. She argues for "equity" over "equality" with a simple example of a poster found on an elementary school classroom wall: "Fair isn't everybody getting the same thing. Fair is everybody getting what they need in order to be successful".

In other words and in the context of "lesser developed countries", more aid money needs to be contributed by the "developed" nations to address this cycle of disadvantage (Table 30.2).

Again, there may be compelling reasons why some of the wealthiest nations in the world provide less than others for aid programmes, but the "lesser developed countries" may feel a compulsion to question why this is so. The challenges for the "disabled" community have always been substantial and constant. The world has come a very long way since people with disabilities were misunderstood, ridiculed, stigmatised and forgotten and is a richer and better world because of the increased levels of respect, tolerance, understanding and inclusion that are now enshrined not just in constitutions and acts of

Table 30.2 Percentage of gross national income (GNI) expenditure on overseas aid

Highest and least spenders on overseas aid as a percentage of GNI			
Highest 10 (%)		*Lowest 10 (%)*	
Luxembourg	1.05	Slovakia	0.12
Norway	1.02	Poland	0.12
Sweden	0.99	Czech Republic	0.13
Denmark	0.71	Greece	0.14
Germany	0.6	Poland	0.15
Netherlands	0.59	Korea	0.15
United Kingdom	0.5	Portugal	0.16
France	0.44	United States	0.16
Switzerland	0.44	Spain	0.21
Finland	0.42	Italy	0.24

Source: OECD.

parliament but also in fabric and psyche of its nations and peoples. It would be a tragedy to relinquish the enormous gains made.

Bibliography

Harden, K. P. (2021), The Genetic Lottery: Why DNA Matters for Social Equality, Princeton University Press.
OECD Family Database, Social Policy Division, "Child Disability", https://www.oecd.org/en.html.
OECD (2024), "Public Expenditure on Disability and Sickness Cash Benefits in % GDP", https://www.oecd.org/en.html.
United Nations Department of Economic and Social Affairs Disability and Development Report, (2018), United Nations New York.
United Nations Trade and Development (2024), "UN List of Least Developed Countries".

Appendix A1

Table A.1 Global disability laws, acts and legislations

Country	Legislation	Inception
Afghanistan	Law on Disability Rights and Privileges	?
Albania	Law No. 8626 on the Status of Paraplegic and Tetraplegic	2000
Algeria	Act on the protection and promotion of persons with disabilities	2002
Andorra	Law guaranteeing the rights of persons with disabilities	?
Angola	Law 21/12, Law on persons with disabilities	2012
Antigua and Barbuda	Disabilities and Equal Opportunities Bill	2017
Argentina	Law 22431 Comprehensive protection system for the disabled	1981
Armenia	Law of the Republic of Armenia "On social protection of persons with disabilities in the Republic of Armenia"	1993
Australia	National Disability Insurance Scheme	2013
Austria	Federal Disability Equality Act (BGBl.I No. 82/2005	2005
Azerbaijan	Law on prevention of disabilities and impaired health of children and rehabilitation and social protection of the disabled and children with impaired health	?
Bahamas	Persons with disabilities (equal opportunities) Act	2014
Bahrain	Law No. 74 of 2006 regulating the care and employment of persons with disabilities	2006
Bangladesh	Disability Welfare Act	2001
Belarus	Law of the Republic of Belarus, No. 1244-XII, "on the social protection of Disabled Persons of the Republic of Belarus"	1991
Belgium	Reform Act on disability and introducing a new protected status in accordance with human dignity	1987
Bolivia	General Law for Persons with Disabilities	2012
Bosnia and Herzegovina	Law on pensions and disability insurance	?
Brazil	Law No. 13, 146 on inclusion of people with disabilities	2015
Brunei Darussalam	Old Age and Disability Pension Law 1955/Revised Version	1984
Bulgaria	Law on the Integration of Persons with Disabilities	2005
Burkina Faso	Law No. 12-2010/AN on the protection and promotion of the rights of persons with disabilities	2010
Cambodia	Law on the Protection and Promotion of the Rights of Persons with Disabilities	?
Cameroon	2010/002 on the protection and promotion of persons with disabilities	2010

(Continued)

Table A.1 (Continued)

Country	Legislation	Inception
Canada	The Accessible Canada Act	2019
Chad	Law No. 007/PR/2007 Bearing Protection for Disabled Persons	2007
Chile	Law 20,422 establishing rules on equal opportunities and social inclusion of persons with disabilities	2010
China (Mainland)	Law Of The People's Republic Of China On The Protection Of Persons With Disabilities	2008
China (Hong Kong)	Disability Discrimination Ordinance (Cap.487) (DDO)	?
China (Macau)	Law 9/83/M on the suppression of architectural barriers	?
Colombia	Enacting Law 1618, through which the provisions are established to ensure the full exercise of the rights of persons with disabilities (2013)	2013
Cook Islands	Disability Act of 2008	2008
Costa Rica	Act 7600 on Equal Opportunities for Persons with Disabilities (1996)	1996
	Law No. 9379 on the Promotion of Personal Autonomy of Persons with Disabilities (2016)	2016
Croatia	Law on the Croatian Registry of Persons with Disability (2001)	2001
Democratic People's Republic of Korea	Law on the Protection of Persons with Disabilities	?
Denmark	Incorporated In The Danish Equality Act	2010
Dominican Republic	Law No. 5-13 of 5 January 2013 on Organic Equal Rights of Persons with Disabilities	2013
Ecuador	Organic Law on Disabilities	2012
El Salvador	Law of Equality of Opportunities for Persons with Disabilities	?
Ethiopia	Proclamation of the Rights to Employment for Persons with Disabilities No. 568/2008	2007
Fiji	Fiji National Council for disabled Persons Act 1994	1994
Finland	Disability Services Act 380/1987	1987
	Act on Intellectual Disabilities 519/1977	1977
France	Law 2005-102 on equal rights, opportunities, participation and citizenship to individuals with disabilities	2005
Gabon	Act No. 19/95 of 13 February 1996 on Social Protection for Persons with Disabilities	1996
Georgia	Law of Georgia of 16 October 1997 №959 on Social Protection of Persons with Disabilities	1997
Germany	The General Equal Treatment Act	2006
Ghana	Persons with Disability Act, 2006 (Act 715)	2006
Guatemala	Decree No. 135-96 on the law on the care for persons with disabilities	?
Haiti	Law on the Integration of Persons with Disabilities (2012)	2012
Honduras	Law on equity and integral development for people with disabilities (2005)	2005
Hungary	Disability Act XXVI of 1998 on the rights and equal opportunities of persons with disabilities	1998
India	Rights Of Persons With Disabilities Act	2016
Indonesia	Persons with Disabilities Act 2016	2016
Iran	Comprehensive Law on the Protection of Persons with Disabilities of 2004	2004

(*Continued*)

Table A.1 (Continued)

Country	Legislation	Inception
Iraq	Act No. 38 of 2013 on Care of Persons with Disabilities and Special Needs	2013
Israel	Equal Rights for Persons with Disabilities Law 5758-1998 (the "Equal Rights Law")	1998
Italy	Law 104/92	1992
Jamaica	Disabilities Act 2014	2014
Japan	Basic Act for Persons with Disabilities (August 2011)	2011
Jordan	Law No. 20 for the year 2017 on the Rights of Persons with Disabilities	2017
Kazakhstan	Law No. 39 of 13 April 2005 on Social Protection of disabled Persons	2005
Kenya	Persons With Disabilities Act No. 14 of 2003	2003
Latvia	Disability Law	?
Lithuania	Law of the Republic of Lithuania on Social Integration of Persons with Disabilities	2015
Luxemburg	Law No. 169 of 28 July 2011 on the rights of persons with disabilities	2011
Malaysia	Persons with Disabilities Act 2008	2008
Maldives	Protection of the Rights of Persons with Disabilities and Provision of Financial Assistance (Law No. 8/2010)	2010
Malta	Equal Opportunities (Persons with Disability) Act	?
Marshall Islands	Rights of Persons with disabilities Act, 2015	2015
Mauritius	Constitution Article 16	?
Mexico	General Law for the Inclusion of Persons with Disabilities (2011)	2011
Monaco	Law No. 1.410 of 02 December 2014 for the protection and autonomy and promotion of the rights of persons with disabilities	2014
Mongolia	Law on the Human Rights of Persons with Disabilities 2016	2016
Montenegro	Law on prohibition of discrimination	?
Myanmar	Pyidaungsu Hluttaw Law No. 30/2015 – Law on the Rights of Persons with Disabilities	2015
Nepal	Act No. 2039 of 1982 on the Protection and Welfare of the Disabled Persons	1982
Netherlands	Act on Equal Treatment on the Grounds of Disability or Chronic Illness	?
New Zealand	New Zealand Public Health and Disability Act 2000	2000
Nicaragua	Law No. 763 on the Rights of Persons with Disabilities (2011)	2011
Niger	Ordinance No. 2010-028 of 20 May 2010	2010
Nigeria	Discrimination Against Persons with Disabilities (Prohibition) Act 2018	2018
Norway	Anti-Discrimination and Accessibility Act (No. 42 of 2008).	2008
Oman	Welfare and Rehabilitation of Persons with Disabilities Act 2008	2008
Palau	The Disabled Person's Anti-Discrimination Act	?
Panama	Law 15 of 31 May 2016 amending Law 42 of 1999 on Equalisation of Opportunities for Persons with Disabilities	2016
Paraguay	Law 122/90 establishing rights and privileges for persons with disabilities	?

(Continued)

Table A.1 (Continued)

Country	Legislation	Inception
Peru	General Law for the Inclusion of Persons with Disabilities (2012)	2012
Philippines	Republic Act No. 7277 – Magna Carta for Persons with Disabilities	?
Poland	Act on Vocational and Social Rehabilitation and Employment of Disabled People	?
Portugal	Framework Act 38/2004 of 18 August – General Basis of the Legal System for Prevention, Habilitation, Rehabilitation and Participation of Persons with Disabilities	2004
Qatar	Persons with Special Needs Act No. 2 of 2004	2004
Republic of Korea	Act on the Prohibition of Discrimination of Disabled Persons	?
	Act on Welfare of Persons with Disabilities	
Republic of Moldova	Law No. 60 of 30.03.2012 on the social inclusion of persons with disabilities	2012
Republic of North Macedonia	The Rulebook on Assessing Specific Needs of Persons with Physical or Mental Disabilities	?
Romania	Law no. 448/2006 Regarding the Protection and Promotion of the Rights of Disabled Persons	2006
Russian Federation	Law No. 181-FZ of 24 November 1995 on Social Protection of the Disabled (as amended on 02 July 2013)	2013
Rwanda	Law No. 01/2007 of 20 January 2007 Relating to the Protection of Persons with Disabilities in General	2007
Saudi Arabia	Disability Law 2000	2000
Senegal	Social orientation law no.2010-15 of July 6, 2010	2010
Serbia	Law on Prevention of Discrimination against Persons with Disabilities (LPDPD) – Official Gazette of RS No. 33/06	?
Sierra Leone	Persons with Disability Act, 2011	2011
Slovenia	The Equalisation of Opportunities for Persons with Disabilities Act (ZIMI)	?
South Africa	Disability Inclusion Act 2018 SA	2018
Spain	Act No. 13/1982 of 7 April 1982 on social integration of the handicapped	1982
	Act No. 51/2003 of 2 December 2003 on equality of opportunity, non-discrimination and universal accessibility for persons with disabilities	2003
Sri Lanka	1996 Protection of the Rights of Persons with Disabilities Act No. 28	1996
Sudan	Persons with Disabilities Act of 2009	2009
Sweden	The Act Concerning Support And Service For Persons With Certain Functional Impairments (LSS)	2014
Switzerland	Federal Act on the Elimination of Discrimination against People with Disabilities	?
Tanzania	Persons with Disabilities Act (2010)	2010
Thailand	The Persons with Disabilities Empowerment Act B.E. 2550 (2007)	2007
Togo	Act No. 2004-005 of 23 April 2004 on the social protection of disabled persons	2004
Trinidad and Tobago	Equal Opportunity Act of 2000	2000

(*Continued*)

Table A.1 (Continued)

Country	Legislation	Inception
Tunisia	Law No. 83 of 15 August 2005 on the advancement and protection of persons with disabilities	2005
Turkey	Turkish Disability Act (TDA) No. 5378 of 2005	2005
Uganda	Persons with Disabilities Act (2006)	2006
Ukraine	Law "On Basics of Social Protection for the Disabled in Ukraine"	?
United Arab Emirates	Law No. (3) of 2022 Concerning the Rights of Persons with Disabilities in the Emirate of Dubai	2022
United Kingdom	The Care Act For Disabilities	2010
United States Of America	American With Disabilities Act	2008
Uruguay	Law No.29973 – General Law on Persons with Disabilities	?
Venezuela	18,651 Comprehensive Protection Act of Persons with Disabilities (2010)	2010
Vietnam	Law on Persons with Disabilities (No. 51/2010/QH12)	2010

Source: United Nations Department of Economic and Social Affairs-Disability

Appendix A2
United Nations Convention on the Rights of Persons with Disabilities (UNCRPD)

a The principles of the UNCRPD aim to ensure those countries who become a signatory to and ratify the Convention are kept accountable. The principles of the current convention are:

1 Respect for inherent dignity, individual autonomy including the freedom to make one's own choices, and independence of persons.
2 Non-discrimination.
3 Full and effective participation and inclusion in society.
4 Respect for difference and acceptance of persons with disabilities as part of human diversity and humanity.
5 Equality of opportunity.
6 Accessibility.
7 Equality between men and women.
8 Respect for the evolving capacities of children with disabilities and respect for the right of children with disabilities to preserve their identities.

Key issues

The UNCRPD addresses several key issues that people with disability face. This includes:

1 **Discrimination:** Persons with disabilities have the right to be treated equally and without discrimination in all areas of life. This includes education, employment, and access to goods and services.
2 **Accessibility:** Persons with disabilities have the right to access things like buildings, public transport, and information and communication technologies.
3 **Emergencies:** All necessary measures are met to ensure the protection and safety of people with disability during situations of armed conflict, humanitarian emergencies, and natural disasters.
4 **Participation and inclusion:** Persons with disabilities have the right to participate fully in all aspects of society and to be included in decision-making processes that affect their lives.
5 **Respect for inherent dignity:** People with disabilities have the right to be treated with respect and dignity, have an inherent right to life, and must have their privacy protected.
6 **Support for independent living:** People with disabilities have the right to access the resources and support they need to live independently and participate fully in society.

Appendix A3
United Nations Convention on the Rights of Persons with Disabilities 2006

Article 18 – Liberty of movement and nationality

1. States parties shall recognise the rights of persons with disabilities to liberty of movement, to freedom to choose their residence and to a nationality, on an equal basis with others, including by ensuring that persons with disabilities:

    a Have the right to acquire and change a nationality and are not deprived of their nationality arbitrarily or on the basis of disability.
    b Are not deprived, on the basis of disability, of their ability to obtain, possess and utilise documentation of their nationality or other documentation of identification, or to utilise relevant processes such as immigration proceedings that may be needed to facilitate exercise of the right to liberty of movement.
    c Are free to leave any country, including their own.
    d Are not deprived, arbitrarily or on the basis of disability, of the right to enter their own country.

2. Children with disabilities shall be registered immediately after birth and shall have the right from birth to a name, the right to acquire a nationality and, as far as possible, the right to know and be cared for by their parents.

Appendix A4
Overview of selected national early childhood development programs, children with disabilities

Table A.4 Selected national disability service programs

Nation	Australia	USA	UK	Brazil	India	South Africa	Nigeria
Program or policy	Early Childhood Targeted Action Plan in the Australia's Disability Strategy 2021–2031 National Disability Insurance Scheme	Early Head Start & Head Start IDEA Part C Early Intervention Programme and Part B Preschool Education Program Preschool Development Grant Birth to Five	Early Years Foundation Stage (EYFS) Children with Special Educational Needs and Disabilities (SEND)	Special Education Guidelines for Early Childhood Education	Rashriya Bal Swasthya Karyakram (RBSK)	The National Integrated Early Childhood Development Policy	The National Policy for Integrated Early Childhood Development (IECD) in Nigeria
Target group	Children 0-9 years	All children with disabilities, emphasis on low income	All children with disabilities	All children aged 0–6 years	All children aged 0–years	All children 0–school entry age	All children aged 0–5 years
Services	Detection, assessment and diagnosis, counselling, financial support	Detection, assessment and diagnosis, individual service plans, support	Education and care of young children, developmental assessments	Early detection and management	Early detection and intervention	Birth screening and follow-up for intervention	Early detection and management
Service providers	Commonwealth, state, territory and local governments, and the non-government sector	Public agencies, private nonprofit and for-profit organisations, tribal governments and school systems	Health Visitors and registered Early Years Providers, e.g., nurseries, childminders	Public and private sector Early Childhood caregivers in Health Centres, Clinics Pre-School/Day Care facilities	District Early Intervention Centres and Mobile intervention units for diagnosis and therapies	Health Professionals, Educationists, and Early Childhood practitioners accredited by the Dept of Social Development	Public and private-sector Early Childhood caregivers in Health Centres, Clinics and Pre- School/Day Care facilities

Appendix A5
American Psychological Association guidelines on assessing individuals with disabilities

- **Guideline 1:** Psychologists strive to learn about various disability paradigms and models and their implications for service provision.
- **Guideline 2:** Psychologists strive to examine their beliefs and emotional reactions toward various disabilities and determine how these might influence their work.
- **Guideline 3:** Psychologists strive to increase their knowledge and skills about working with individuals with disabilities through training, supervision, education, and expert consultation.
- **Guideline 4:** Psychologists strive to learn about federal and state laws that support and protect people with disabilities.
- **Guideline 5:** Psychologists strive to provide a barrier-free physical and communication environment in which clients with disabilities may access psychological services.
- **Guideline 6:** Psychologists strive to use appropriate language and respectful behavior toward individuals with disabilities.
- **Guideline 7:** Psychologist strive to understand both the common experiences shared by persons with disabilities and the factors that influence an individual's personal disability experience.
- **Guideline 8:** Psychologists strive to recognise social and cultural diversity in the lives of persons with disabilities.
- **Guideline 9:** Psychologists strive to learn how attitudes and misconceptions, the social environment, and the nature of a person's disability influence development across the lifespan.
- **Guideline 10:** Psychologists strive to recognise that families of individuals with disabilities have strengths and challenges.
- **Guideline 11:** Psychologists strive to recognise that people with disabilities are at an increased risk for abuse and address abuse-related situations appropriately.
- **Guideline 12:** Psychologists strive to learn about the opportunities and challenges presented by assistive technology.

Testing and assessment

- **Guideline 13:** In assessing persons with disabilities, psychologists strive to consider disability as a dimension of diversity together with other individual and contextual dimensions.
- **Guideline 14:** Depending on the context and goals of assessment and testing, psychologists strive to apply the assessment approach that is most psychometrically sound, fair, comprehensive, and appropriate for clients with disabilities.

- **Guideline 15:** Psychologists strive to determine whether accommodations are appropriate for clients to yield a valid test score.
- **Guideline 16:** Consistent with the goals of the assessment and disability-related barriers to assessment, psychologists in clinical settings strive to appropriately balance quantitative, qualitative, and ecological perspectives, and articulate both the strengths and limitations of assessment.
- **Guideline 17:** Psychologists in clinical settings strive to maximise fairness and relevance in interpreting assessment of data of clients who have disabilities by applying approaches which reduce potential bias and balance and integrate data from multiple sources.

Interventions

- **Guideline 18:** Psychologists strive to recognize that there is a wide range of individual response to disability, and collaborate with their clients who have disabilities, and when appropriate, with their clients' families to plan, develop, and implement psychological interventions.
- **Guideline 19:** Psychologists strive to be aware of the therapeutic structure and environment's impact on their work with clients with disabilities.
- **Guideline 20:** Psychologists strive to recognise that interventions with persons with disabilities may focus on enhancing strengths wellbeing as well as reducing stress and ameliorating skill deficits.
- **Guideline 21:** When working with systems that support, treat, or educate people with disabilities, psychologists strive to keep clients' perspectives paramount and advocate for client self-determination, integration, choice, and least restrictive alternatives.
- **Guideline 22:** Psychologists strive to recognise and address health promotion issues for individuals with disabilities.

Reference

American Psychological Association (2020), "Guidelines for Assessment of and Intervention with Persons with Disabilities", https://www.apa.org/pi/disability/resources/assessment-disabilities.

Appendix A6
International Test Commission

ITC Guidelines for Translating and Adapting Tests (second edition), version 2.4, 2016

Test Adaptation Guidelines

PC-1 (1) Obtain the necessary permission from the holder of the intellectual property rights relating to the test before carrying out any adaptation.

PC-2 (2) Evaluate that the amount of overlap in the definition and content of the construct measured by the test and the item content in the populations of interest is sufficient for the intended use (or uses) of the scores.

PC-3 (3) Minimise the influence of any cultural and linguistic differences that are irrelevant to the intended uses of the test in the populations of interest.

TD-1 (4) Ensure that the translation and adaptation processes consider linguistic, psychological, and cultural differences in the intended populations through the choice of experts with relevant expertise.

TD-2 (5) Use appropriate translation designs and procedures to maximise the suitability of the test adaptation in the intended populations.

TD-3 (6) Provide evidence that the test instructions and item content have similar meaning for all intended populations.

TD-4 (7) Provide evidence that the item formats, rating scales, scoring categories, test conventions, modes of administration, and other procedures are suitable for all intended populations.

TD-5 (8) Collect pilot data on the adapted test to enable item analysis, reliability assessment, and small-scale validity studies so that any necessary revisions to the adapted test can be made.

C-1 (9) Select sample with characteristics that are relevant for the intended use of the test and of sufficient size and relevance for the empirical analyses.

C-2 (10) Provide relevant statistical evidence about the construct equivalence, method equivalence, and item equivalence for all intended populations.

C-3 (11) Provide evidence supporting the norms, reliability, and validity of the adapted version of the test in the intended populations.

C-4 (12) Use an appropriate equating design and data analysis procedures when linking score scales from different language versions of a test.

A-1 (13) Prepare administration materials and instructions to minimise any culture- and language-related problems that are caused by administration procedures and response modes that can affect the validity of the inferences drawn from the scores.

A-2 (14) Specify testing conditions that should be followed closely in all populations of interest.

SSI-1 (15) Interpret any group score differences with reference to all relevant available information.

SSI-2 (16) Only compare scores across populations when the level of invariance has been established on the scale on which scores are reported.

Doc-1 (17) Provide technical documentation of any changes, including an account of the evidence obtained to support equivalence, when a test is adapted for use in another population.

Doc-2 (18) Provide documentation for test users that will support good practice in the use of an adapted test with people in the context of the new population.

Appendix A7

Working with interpreters: A practical guide for psychologists" Australian Psychological Society professional practice (selected sections)

3. Why use an interpreter?

Without effective communication between client and psychologist, there will be limitations in the psychologist's capacity to:

- Develop a therapeutic relationship.
- Understand the point of view of the client.
- Understand the cultural context of the client.
- Conduct an assessment.
- Formulate a diagnosis.
- Reach an agreement on an appropriate psychological intervention plan.
- Provide psychological intervention.
- Monitor and evaluate the effectiveness and any adverse effects of psychological intervention.

4.1 Assessing the need for an interpreter

- simply ask the client if they want or need an interpreter.
- ask the client to answer some simple questions or summarise something you have said in their own words.

When arranging and booking an interpreter:

- clarify the appropriate language and dialect.
- consider the client's ethnicity and religion.
- enquire whether the client needs a male or a female interpreter.

5.1 Ethical considerations

Psychologists who use interpreters should:

- (a) take reasonable steps to ensure that the interpreters are competent to work as interpreters in the relevant context.
- (b) take reasonable steps to ensure that the interpreter is not in a multiple relationship with the client that may impair the interpreter's judgement.
- (c) take reasonable steps to ensure that the interpreter will keep confidential the existence and content of the psychological service.

- (d) take reasonable steps to ensure that the interpreter is aware of any other relevant provisions of this Code.
- (e) obtain informed consent from the client to use the selected interpreter.

8. Administration of psychometric tests

- Allow the interpreter time to familiarise themselves with the psychometric instrument and clarify terminology, rather than requesting spontaneous translation during consultation.
- Explain standardised assessment procedures to the interpreter and allocate time to practice standardised administration of the instrument.
- In the debriefing session with the interpreter, discuss whether there were any difficulties with the translation of items, make a note of them and consider the implications on the validity of the results for that item.
- Consider the results in light of the individual's social status, education level and developmental history when interpreting scores.

Cultural considerations when administering psychometric assessments:

- Refugees from some countries may have had minimal or no formal education, but may demonstrate higher level skills in tasks of daily functioning.
- Consider administering a battery of processes that assess functioning in addition to formal cognitive assessment, as knowledge and skills required by some instruments are heavily reliant on education and experience of the host culture.

Appendix A8
British Psychological Society

Working with interpreters: Guidelines for psychologists

Psychologists should:

- Consider undertaking a language needs analysis for the service population and consider how to best meet identified needs.
- Consider undertaking a training course in working with interpreters or, if working with an interpreter unexpectedly, read the guidelines and allocate time to consider the issues or discuss them with a more experienced colleague prior to your first session with an interpreter.
- Consider attending a d/Deaf1 awareness training in advance of working with a registered sign language interpreter (RSLI).
- Check the interpreter is qualified and appropriate for the consultation/meeting.
- Allocate 10–15 minutes in advance of the session to brief the interpreter about the purpose of the meeting and to enable them to explain any cultural issues that may have bearing on the session.
- Be mindful of issues of confidentiality and trust, when working with someone from a small language community (including the d/Deaf community). The service user may be anxious about being identifiable and may mistrust the interpreter's professionalism and the psychologists may need to address this directly.
- Consider matching service user and interpreter for age, gender and ethnicity and should discuss this in advance with service users so that their preferences can be taken into account rather than assumed.
- State clearly that they alone hold clinical or organisational responsibility for the meeting.
- Create a good atmosphere where each member of the group feels able to ask for clarification if anything is unclear.
- Commit to a collaborative, working relationship based on trust and mutual respect across all parties.
- Be aware of the wellbeing of the interpreter and mindful of the risk of vicarious traumatisation. Consider what support they will be offered, and if they are subcontracted from an outside agency, be aware that there is often little support provided by their employer.
- Allocate 10–15 minutes at the end of the session to debrief the interpreter about the session and offer support and supervision as appropriate.
- Ensure that all written translations used have been back translated to ensure they are fit for purpose.

- Exercise extreme caution when considering the use of translated assessment measures.
- When employing simultaneous interpreting, consider the additional concentration necessary and include regular breaks where possible.
- Be aware that meetings conducted with an interpreter may take longer and take account of this when booking appointments.
- Use their often unique positions in different organisations to advise on best practice when working with interpreters.
- Offer an interpreter in situations where one family member has good English but others do not.

Appendix A9
DSM-5-TR, and ICD-11 diagnostic criteria, developmental delay (Code 6a00)

"This diagnosis is reserved for individuals under the age of 5 years when the clinical severity level cannot be reliably assessed during early childhood. This category is diagnosed when an individual fails to meet expected developmental milestones in several areas of intellectual functioning and applies to individuals who are unable to undergo systematic assessments of intellectual functioning, including children who are too young to participate in standardized testing. This category requires reassessment after a period of time."

Appendix A10
DSM-5-TR and ICD-11 intellectual developmental disorder (intellectual disability), (ICD-11 code 6A00)

Intellectual developmental disorder (intellectual disability) is a disorder with onset during the developmental period that includes both intellectual and adaptive functioning deficits in conceptual, social, and practical domains. The following three criteria must be met:

a Deficits in intellectual functions, such as reasoning, problem solving, planning, abstract thinking, judgement, academic learning, and learning from experience, confirmed by both clinical assessment and individualised, standardised intelligence testing.
b Deficits in adaptive functioning that result in failure to meet developmental and sociocultural standards for personal independence and social responsibility. Without ongoing support, the adaptive deficits limit functioning in one or more activities of daily life, such as communication, social participation, and independent living, across multiple environments, such as home, school, work, and community.
c Onset of intellectual and adaptive deficits during the developmental period.

Table A.10 DSM-5-TR levels of intellectual disability

Severity level	Conceptual domain	Social domain	Practical domain
Mild	Preschool: May be no obvious conceptual differences School: Learning difficulties, with support needed in one or more areas Adult: Impairments in abstract thinking, executive functioning, short-term memory, and functional use of academic skills	• Immature social interactions • Concrete and immature communication • Emotional regulation difficulties • Limited understanding of risk, including gullibility	• Support needed with complex daily living tasks in comparison to peers • Support needed in judgement of appropriate recreational time • Employment in jobs not requiring conceptual skills • Support needed in making health care and legal decisions • Support needed when raising a family

(*Continued*)

Table A.10 (Continued)

Severity level	Conceptual domain	Social domain	Practical domain
Moderate	Preschool: Slow development of language and preacademic skills School: Academic progress markedly impaired and slow to develop Adults: Elementary level academic skills, support needed in daily life and occupation. Ongoing assistance in daily living skills, including surrogates assuming responsibility	• Spoken language much less complex than for age-peers • Inaccurate understanding of social cues • Limited social judgement and decision-making • Significant social and communication support needed	• Considerable extra time and support needed to learn independence skills • Employment in non-conceptual areas with considerable support needed • Additional support needed for leisure-time activities • Presence of maladaptive behaviours
Severe	Limited attainment of conceptual skills Little understanding of writing, numeracy Extensive caretaker support necessary throughout life	• Single word or simple phrase speech only • Limited gestures • Nonsymbolic communication • Communication on 'here and now'	• Support and supervision required for all activities of daily living • Maladaptive behaviour, including self-injury, often present
Profound	Lack of symbolic processes Physical impairment in functional use of objects	• Very limited understanding of symbolic communication. Expression of need through non-verbal, non-symbolic communication	• Dependent on others for all daily living activities • Frequent inability to participate in leisure and vocational activities • Maladaptive behaviours often present

Appendix A11
Diagnostic criteria for autism spectrum disorder, DSM-5-TR (F84.0) and ICD-11 (6AO2.Z)

For a person to be diagnosed with autism spectrum disorder, they must meet criteria A, B, C and D.

a Persistent deficits in social communication and social interaction across multiple contexts, as manifest by all of the following, currently or by history:

   1 Deficits in social-emotional reciprocity, ranging, for example, from abnormal social approach and failure of normal back and forth conversation; to reduced sharing of interests, emotions, or affect; to failure to initiate or respond to social interactions.
   2 Deficits in nonverbal communicative behaviours used for social interaction, ranging, for example, from poorly integrated verbal and non-verbal communication; to abnormalities in eye contact and body language, or deficits in understanding and use of gestures; to a total lack of facial expressions and nonverbal communication.
   3 Deficits in developing, maintaining, and understanding relationships, ranging, for example, from difficulties adjusting behaviour to suit various social contexts; to difficulties in sharing imaginative play or in making friends to absence of interest in peers.

   Specify current severity:

Severity is based on social communication impairments and restricted, repetitive patterns of behaviour.

b Restricted, repetitive patterns of behaviour, interests, or activities as manifest by at least two of the following, currently or by history:

   1 Stereotyped or repetitive motor movements, use of objects, or speech (e.g., simple motor stereotypes, lining up toys or flipping objects, echolalia, idiosyncratic phrases).
   2 Insistence on sameness, inflexible adherence to routines, or ritualised patterns of verbal or nonverbal behaviour (e.g., extreme distress at small changes, difficulties with transitions, rigid thinking patterns, greeting rituals, need to take same route or eat same food every day). Highly restricted, fixated interests that are abnormal in intensity or focus (e.g., strong attachment to or preoccupation with unusual objects, excessively circumscribed or perseverative interests).
   3 Hyper-, or hyporeactivity to sensory input or unusual interest in sensory aspects of the environment (e.g., apparent indifference to pain/temperature, adverse response to specific sounds or textures, excessive smelling or touching of objects, visual fascination with lights or with movement).

Specify current severity:

Severity is based on social communication impairments and restrictive, repetitive patterns of behaviour.

c Symptoms must be present in the early developmental period (but may not become fully manifest until social demands exceed limited capacities, or may be masked by learned strategies in later life).
d Symptoms cause clinically significant impairment in social, occupational, or other important areas of current functioning.
e These disturbances are not better explained by intellectual disability (intellectual developmental disorder) or global developmental delay. Intellectual disability and autism spectrum disorder frequently co-occur; to make comorbid diagnoses of autism spectrum disorder and intellectual disability, social communication should be below that expected for general developmental level.

Table A.11 DSM-5-TR levels of support, autism spectrum disorder

Levels of severity for autism spectrum disorder

Severity level	Social communication	Restricted, repetitive behaviours
LEVEL 3, "REQUIRING VERY SUBSTANTIAL SUPPORT"	Severe deficits in verbal and nonverbal social communication skills causes severe impairments in functioning, very limited initiation of social interactions, and minimal response to social overtures from others. For example, a person with few words or intelligible speech who rarely initiates interaction, and, when he or she does, makes unusual approaches to meet needs only and responds to only very direct social approaches	Inflexibility of behaviour, extreme difficulty coping with change, or other restricted/repetitive behaviours markedly interfere with functioning in all spheres. Great distress/difficulty changing focus or action
LEVEL 2, "REQUIRING SUBSTANTIAL SUPPORT"	Marked deficits in verbal and nonverbal social communication skills; social impairments apparent even with supports in place; limited initiation of social interactions; and reduced or abnormal responses to social overtures from others. For example, a person who speaks simple sentences, whose interaction is limited to narrow special interests, and who has markedly odd nonverbal communication	Inflexibility of behaviour, difficulty coping with change, or other restricted/repetitive behaviours appear frequently enough to be obvious to the casual observer and interfere with functioning in a variety of contexts. Distress and/or difficulty changing focus or action
LEVEL 1, "REQUIRING SUPPORT"	Without supports in place, deficits in social communication cause noticeable impairments. Difficulty initiating social interactions, and clear examples of atypical or unsuccessful responses to social overtures of others. May appear to have decreased interest in social interactions. For example, a person who is able to speak in full sentences and engages in communication but whose to-and-fro conversation with others fails, and whose attempts to make friends are odd and typically unsuccessful	Inflexibility of behaviour causes significant interference with functioning in one or more contexts. Difficulty switching between activities. Problems of organisation and planning hamper independence

Appendix A12
DSM-5-TR and ICD-11 criteria for speech, language and communication disorders

Language disorder (DSM-5-TR code F80.2, ICD-11 code 6AO1.2)

a Persistent difficulties in the acquisition and use of language across modalities (i.e., spoken, written, sign language, or other) due to deficits in comprehension or production that include the following:

   1 Reduced vocabulary (word knowledge and use).
   2 Limited sentence structure (ability to put words and word endings together to form sentences based on the rules of grammar and morphology).
   3 Impairments in discourse (ability to use vocabulary and connect sentences to explain or describe a topic or a series of events or have a conversation).

b Language abilities are substantially and quantifiably below those expected for age, resulting in functional limitations in effective communication, social participation, academic achievement, or occupational performance, individually or in any combination.
c Onset of symptoms is in the early developmental period.
d The difficulties are not attributable to hearing or other sensory impairment, motor dysfunction, or another medical or neurological condition and are not better explained by intellectual disability (intellectual developmental disorder) or global developmental delay.

ICD-11 definitions

1 Developmental language disorder with impairment of receptive and expressive language (6A01.2).
2 Developmental language disorder with impairment of mainly pragmatic language (6A01.23).

"Developmental language disorder is characterised by persistent deficits in the acquisition, understanding, production or use of language (spoken or signed), that arise during the developmental period, typically during early childhood, and cause significant limitations in the individual's ability to communicate. The individual's ability to understand, produce or use language is markedly below what would be expected given the individual's age. The language deficits are not explained by another neurodevelopmental disorder or a sensory impairment or neurological condition, including the effects of brain injury or infection."

Social (pragmatic) communication disorder (DSM-5-Rr Code F80.82)

a Persistent difficulties in the social use of verbal and nonverbal communication as manifested by all of the following:

1. Deficits in using communication for social purposes, such as greeting and sharing information, in a manner that is appropriate for the social context.
2. Impairment of the ability to change communication to match context or the needs of the listener, such as speaking differently in a classroom than on a playground, talking differently to a child than to an adult, and avoiding use of overly formal language.
3. Difficulties following rules of conversation and storytelling, such as taking turns in conversation, rephrasing when misunderstood, and knowing how to use verbal and nonverbal signals to regulate interaction.
4. Difficulties understanding what is not explicitly stated (e.g., making inferences) and nonliteral or ambiguous meanings of language (e.g., idioms, humour, metaphors, multiple meanings that depend on the context for interpretation).

b The deficits result in functional limitations in effective communication, social participation, social relationships, academic achievement, or occupational performance, individually or in combination.

c The onset of the symptoms is in the early developmental period (but deficits may not become fully manifest until social communication demands exceed limited capabilities).

d The symptoms are not attributable to another medical or neurological condition or to low abilities in the domain of word structure and grammar, and are not better explained by autism spectrum disorder, intellectual disability (intellectual development disorder), global developmental delay, or another mental disorder.

Appendix A13
DSM-5-TR and ICD-11 criteria for disorders of motor function

Developmental coordination disorder (DSM Code F82), (ICD-11 Code 6a04)

a The acquisition and execution of coordinated motor skills is substantially below that expected given the individual's chronological age and opportunity for skill learning and use. Difficulties are manifested as clumsiness (e.g., dropping or bumping into objects) as well as slowness and inaccuracy of performance of motor skills (e.g., catching an object, using scissors or cutlery, handwriting, riding a bike, or participating in sports).
b The motor skills deficit in Criterion A significantly and persistently interferes with the activities of daily living appropriate to chronological age (e.g., self-care and self-maintenance) and impacts academic/school productivity, prevocational and vocational activities, leisure, and play.
c Onset of symptoms is in the early developmental period.
d The motor skills deficits are not better explained by intellectual disability (intellectual developmental disorder) or visual impairment and are not attributable to a neurological condition affecting movement (e.g., cerebral palsy, muscular dystrophy, degenerative disorder).

Stereotypic movement disorder (DSM-5-TR Code F98.4), (ICD-11 Code 8aoz)

a Repetitive, seemingly driven, and apparently purposeless motor behavior (e.g., hand shaking or flapping, body rocking, head banging, self-biting, hitting own body).
b The repetitive motor behavior interferes with social, academic, or other activities and may result in self-injury.
c Onset is in the early developmental period.
d The repetitive motor behavior is not attributable to the physiological effects of a substance or neurological condition and is not better explained by another neurodevelopmental disorder or mental disorder (e.g., trichotillomania [hair-pulling disorder], obsessive-compulsive disorder).

Specify if:

With self-injurious behavior (or behavior that would result in an injury if preventative measures were not used).

Without self-injurious behaviour

Specify if:

Associated with a known medical or genetic condition, neurological disorder, or environmental factor.

Specify current severity:

Mild: Symptoms are easily suppressed by sensory stimulus or distraction.
Moderate: Symptoms require explicit protective measures and behavior modification.
Severe: Continuous monitoring and protective measures are required to prevent serious injury.

Appendix A14

Table A.14 Fine motor skills developmental sequence

	1 Yr Old	2 Yr Old	3 Yr Old	4 Yr Old	5 Yr Old
Grasping behaviour	*Pincer grip by 18 months *Can pick up small objects by opposition of thumb, forefinger and middle finger	*Similar, but more control of movement	*Can grasp more with finger movement, and less initial palm contact with the object	*Grasps small objects with thumb and middle finger, with index finger extended *Picks up very small objects with thumb and index finger	*Pincer grasp is refined by adult-type flexion of the index finger and middle finger, and fingers contact the object on the diagonal and not vertical angle
Releasing behaviour	*Before 1 yr: Release only achieved by pushing object against another surface *By 1 yr can release objects on a table top *By 18 months can place cubes in a cup, but still must contact cup	*Releases cubes or small objects still with marked finger extension, but can place them more accurately	*Can build cube towers and use hands more accurately than 2 yrs *Tend to press objects into place and release is still poorly coordinated	*Can release small objects into a container with speed and accuracy *Can release objects like cubes without pressure and without exaggerated opening of the hand	*Marked improvement in dexterity *Frequently holds cubes with the fingertips and releases objects by extension of finger tips

(Continued)

Table A.14 (Continued)

	1 Yr Old	2 Yr Old	3 Yr Old	4 Yr Old	5 Yr Old
Pre-writing and drawing behaviour	*Spoons and long, thin objects held with fingertips *When using these objects as tools, regression to palmar grasp *Uses palmar grasp for holding crayons *Full arm action when trying to draw	*Palmar grasp used less for crayons, grasp varies from thumb to the left and all fingers on the right of the crayon *OR palmar grasp, but index finger extended down crayon	*Most hold crayon in pincer-type grasp between thumb and index finger, but middle finger extends down shaft further than index finger	*Pencil or crayon held in adult fashion but tendency to grasp with the three radial fingers with middle finger still more extended down shaft. Firm grip *Finger and wrist movement present	*Change in pencil grasp to normal adult one *Achieved by grasping shaft with thumb and index finger, while middle finger now supports pencil near tip
Performance criteria	*Can build tower of two small cubes *Still holds many objects with palmar grasp *Can crudely drop and throw objects only with marked finger extension	*Can unwrap lollies *Can screw and unscrew lids of jars *Can imitate vertical dot line, scribble and thread beads *Can neatly place two cubes in a row. Can build six-block tower, but has very slow placing and release action	*Copies circles *Cuts with scissors *Draws simple human figure *Unfastens clothes *Can build a bridge out of three cubes Builds a tower of 9 or 10 cubes *Strings beads	*Draws simple house *Human figure has more detail than 3 yrs *Likes constructive building *Copies a cross *Frequently uses both hands, separately *Traces diamond path with minimal error	*Can wind thread onto a bobbin *Copies squares, triangles and letters *Can rapidly touch each finger in turn to thumb *Can lace shoes

Appendix A15

Gross motor developmental stages

Table A.15 Sequence of gross motor skills

Walking

12–24 months approx	• Stiff movement, frequent falls, considerable "sideways sway" • High bent knee-forward stepping action, flat foot contact with ground • Wide base of support. "Out-toeing" of feet • High rigid bent arm position. Trunk inclined forwards from the hips • Arms high above waist, bent at elbow ("high-guard" position)
24 months	• Erect body, absence of sway with each step • Knee "lock" on ground contact, moderate width base of support • Heel-to-toe foot contact with ground, moderate out-toeing • Consistent walking speed, stride length and action. Arms by side with little swing
4–5 years	• Body erect with little sideways or up/down movement • Base of support narrower than trunk, heel-toe contact with ground. Smooth transfer of weight facilitated by pelvic rotation. Double knee lock during two steps • Consistency in action of leg movement and stride width • Arms by side, some contralateral swing

Running

18–24 months	• No airborne phase. Stiff, bouncy action • Limited knee bend, feet close to ground with out-toeing
2–3 years	• Presence of airborne phase. Longer stride and more fluid action • Greater knee bend on moving forwards. Flat foot contact with ground • Marked pelvic rotation, but foot position straighter • Arms at waist height, but movement restricted. Some ability to start, stop, turn
3 and a half-5 years	• Extended airborne phase • Smooth forward progression, less vertical movement than horizontal • Knee bend to 90 degrees. Feet lifted high off ground. Back leg swing • Pelvic rotation in some children • Arm swing forwards and back with bent elbow. Arms counterbalance leg actions

Jumping

18–30 months	• Body upright in jump. One foot take-off and landing. Brief airborne phase • Beginning of "winging" arm action-both arms move back during airborne phase • Little or no head movement. Vertical take-off and landing by 27 months

(Continued)

Table A.15 (Continued)

Jumping	
30–39 months	• Squat before take-off. Trunk angled forwards
	• Legs straight on take-off then bend backwards during flight and bent on landing
	• 2 foot take-off and landing. Marked "winging" of arms
4–5 and a half years	• Body inclined 45 degrees on take-off from squat. Head adjustment to position changes
	• Well-coordinated leg action on take-off. Legs straight then backwards during flight
	• Arms swing from behind body to horizontal or sidewards
Throwing	
2–3 years	• Facing square to target. Slight body sway simultaneous with arm action
	• Little or no leg movement. Feet slightly apart, parallel to target
	• Throw dependent for force on back and forward arm movements
3 and a half-5 years	• Child square on to target. Little/no leg movement, feet together and parallel
	• Characteristic trunk rotation, to right on backswing and left on forward swing (RH)
	• Throw starts with forward arm swing. Forearm extended forwards before release

Appendix A16
Language development in young children

Table A.16 Language development sequence

6–12 months					
Listening	*Vocabulary*	*Sentences*	*Verbal grammar*	*Concepts*	*Questions*
Attends to sounds and voices Recognises facial expressions, tones of voice	Babbling (ma-ma, da-da) Takes turns vocalising Recognises names of some objects	No specific milestones	No specific milestones	No specific milestones	No specific milestones
1–2 years					
Responds to familiar requests (e.g. come here) and own name Understands gestures (e.g. wave for 'bye')	Babbling (ma-ma, da-da) Takes turns vocalising Recognises names of some objects	No specific milestones	No specific milestones	No specific milestones	Can understand one key word in a sentence (e.g. Where's your nose?)
2–3 years					
Follows 2-part instructions (e.g. Go to your room and get your shoes) Points to main body parts, items of clothing, toys and food when asked	Names actions (e.g. go, run) By 2 years, vocabulary is 250–300 words By 3 years uses 1000 words	Minimum of 2–3 words in a sentence (e.g. "Daddy go work" Still talks to self in long monologues	Talks about present events. Uses regular plurals, e.g. 2 dogs Articles 'a'/'the'. Progressive- "The boy is jumping." Pronouns, "you, I, me, mine" Regular Past Tense- "I climbed". Possessive's, e.g. "Daddy's car"	Position: On; off; in; out; up; down; under; top; open; shut Size: Big; small/little; long Quantity: 1; 2 Other: Stop; go/start; loud; quiet; heavy; soft; fast; hot; cold	Understands and asks What and Where questions

(*Continued*)

Table A.16 (Continued)

Listening	Vocabulary	Sentences	Verbal grammar	Concepts	Questions
3–4 years					
Follows three-part instructions (e.g. point to the cat, the dog and the monkey) Understands longer, more complex sentences	By 4 years uses nearly 1500 words	Minimum of 3–4 words Tells you what they are doing Tells you the function or use of an object	Begins to talk about past events **Auxiliaries:** The girl **is** skipping. **Pronouns: He** is running. **Connector:** I want a car **and** a train. **3rd Person Singular:** He want**s** the ball. **Contracted Negative:** Isn't, doesn't. **Contracted Copula:** He's happy. **Past Participle:** It's broken.	Position: Top, behind; first; near. Size: Short (length) emerging; short (height) Quantity: 3; every; none Other: Hard; slow; light (weight); many colours	Understands Who questions Asks What, Why, When and How questions
4–5 years					
Follows the meaning of others' conversations	Continuing to expand Can generally understand colour and shape words (e.g. red, square) Can sort objects by simple categories (e.g. animals, food)	Minimum of 4–5 word sentences	Talks past and future events **Pronouns** "his, hers, theirs" **Comparative and Superlative**, e.g. big, bigger, biggest **Use of "is" vs "are" Past Tense,** e.g. "I was running" **Connector,** e.g. "because" **Adverb** "ly"- quickly **Irregular Plurals,** e.g. mice, men	Position: Middle; around; away from; between; through; next to/ beside; last Size: Short (length); short (height); tall; fat. Quantity: 4; most; few. Other: Same; different (size); different (function)	Understands How questions Asks meanings of words

Appendix A17
United Nations less developed countries (LDCs) as of 2024

Table A.17 United Nations "Less Developed Countries" 2024

Afghanistan	Guinea	Rwanda
Angola	Guinea-Bissau	Sao Tome et Principe
Bangladesh	Haiti	Senegal
Benin	Kiribati	Sierra Leone
Burkina Faso	Lao People's Democratic Republic	Solomon Islands
Burundi	Lesotho	Somalia
Cambodia	Liberia	South Soudan
Central African Republic	Madagascar	Sudan
Chad	Malawi	Timor-Leste
Comoros	Mali	Togo
Democratic Republic of the Congo	Mauritania	Tuvalu
Djibouti	Mozambique	Uganda
Eritrea	Myanmar	United Republic of Tanzania
Ethiopia	Nepal	Yemen
Gambia	Niger	Zambia

Selection criteria

1. Income correction
2. Human assets (health) index
   a. Mortality under 5 years
   b. Maternal mortality rate
   c. Prevalence of stunting
3. Education index
   a. Lower secondary school completion rate
   b. Adult literacy rate
   c. Gender parity index
4. Economic vulnerability index
   a. share of agriculture, forestry and fishing in GDP
   b. remoteness and landlockedness
   c. merchandise export concentration
   d. instability of exports of goods and services.
5. Environmental vulnerability index
   a. share of population in low elevated coastal zones
   b. share of the population living in drylands
   c. instability of agricultural production
   d. victims of disasters

Appendix A18
The New Zealand Psychological Association Guidelines for the use of artificial intelligence (AI)

1. Psychologists to consider the unique cultural context of Aotearoa New Zealand when using AI in their practice.
2. Psychologists are encouraged to view their obligations in understanding an AI tool as similar to those when using psychometric measures.
3. Psychologists to consider their obligations under Te Tiriti and the principles of Māori Data Sovereignty when using AI tools.
4. Psychologists to consider the potential biases in results from an AI tool and avoid perpetuating any form of discrimination based on biased data sets.
5. Psychological services and opinions that a registered psychologist offers should not be exclusively delegated to AI.
6. Psychologists should only use AI tools that they have assessed as being ethically robust and transparent about the parameters of data sharing.
7. Psychologists should consider the principles of the Privacy Act 2020 and a privacy impact assessment when using AI tools in their work.
8. Psychologists should be transparent about the use of AI and inform those with whom they work that they are using AI if the AI tool performs a significant part of the service, and/or if the person(s) would reasonably expect to know when consenting to a service.
9. The onus is on the psychologist to ensure the person(s) with whom they are working understands the role of any AI, to the extent the person requires to make an informed choice at the outset of a psychological service or research.
10. Person(s) working with a psychologist should not be disadvantaged if they do not wish to have AI tools used in their care or their data entered into an AI system.

Appendix A19
Adapted and translated assessments

Table A.19 Adapted and "new assessment tools for specific cultures"

Assessment	Mode	Country of Origin
Ages and Stages for China ASQ-C	Adapted from ASQ	China
Ages and Stages Questionnaire-Talking about Raising Aboriginal Kids Second Edition (ASQ-TRAK2)	Adapted from ASQ	Australia
Autism Diagnostic Observation Schedule-2, Afrikaans adaptation	Adaptation	South Africa
Autism Diagnostic Observation Schedule-2, Brazilian Portuguese adaptation	Adaptation	Brazil
Autism Diagnostic Observation Schedule-2, Taiwanese adaptation	Adaptation	Taiwan
Autism Diagnostic Observation Schedule-2, Module 3, modifications for visual impairment	Adaptation	United Kingdom
Autism Stigma and Knowledge Questionnaire 2nd Edition (ASK-Q-2)	Specific Test	United States of America
BRIEF2 for Russia	Adapted from BRIEF2	Russia
Child Development Assessment Questionnaire (QAD-PIPASS), Brazil	Specific Test	Brazil
Child Development Review (CDR) Questionnaire	Adapted from original American version, 1990	Caribbean
Children Neuropsychological And Behavior Scale (CNBS-R2016), China	Specific Test	China
Developmental Assessment Scale for Indian Infants (DASII)	Adapted from Bayley Scales	India
Developmental Disorder-Children Disability Assessment Schedule (DD-CDAS)	Adapted from World Health Organisation Disability Assessment Schedule for Children (WHODAS-child)	Pakistan
Global Scales For Early Development (GSED) For Children	Specific Test	World Health Organisation
Griffiths Development Scales-Chinese (GDS-C)	Adapted from Griffith Mental Development Scales 1996	China
Indian Scale For Assessment of ASD (ISAA)	Specific Test	India

(Continued)

Table A.19 (Continued)

Assessment	Mode	Country of Origin
International Clinical Epidemiology Network Diagnostic Tool for autism spectrum disorder (Indt-asd)	Specific Test	India
Kaufman Assessment Battery For Children II (KABC-II)	Adapted For Use in Rural Zimbabwe	Malawi
Kilifi Developmental Checklist (KDC) and Kilifi Developmental Inventory	Specific Test	Kenya
Malawi Developmental Assessment Tool (MDAT)	Adaptation	Zimbabwe
Modified Checklist for Autism in Toddlers (M-CHAT-R/FM)	Adaptation	Northern Sotho
Social Responsiveness Scale German Adaptation	Adaptation	Germany
Social Responsiveness Scale Taiwanese Adaptation	Adaptation	Taiwan
Trivandrum Development Screening Chart	Specific Test	India

Appendix A20

Table A.20 Screening tests for general population usage

Motor Skills Screening	Communication/Social/Speech Language Screening
Alberta Infant Motor Skills (AIMS)	Battelle Developmental Inventory Screening Test (BDI II)
Bruininks-Oseretsky Test of Motor Proficiency (BOT-2)	Battelle Developmental Inventory Screening Test (BDI II)
General Movement Assessment (GMs)	Clinical Adaptive Test/Clinical Linguistic Auditory Milestone Scale (CAT/CLAMS)
Movement Assessment Battery for Children (MABC II)	Denver Developmental Screening Test – II (DDST II)
Movement Assessment of Infants (MAI)	Early Language Milestone Scale (ELMS)
Parent Evaluation of Developmental Status (PEDS)	Fluharty Preschool Speech and Language Screening Test
Neurological Sensory Motor Development Assessment (NSMDA)	Language Development Survey (LDS)
Peabody Developmental Motor Scales (PDMS II)	Levett-Muir Language Screening Test
Test of Infant Motor Performance (TIMP)	Parent Language Checklist (PLC)
Test of Gross Motor Development (TGMD)	Paediatric Language Acquisition Screening Tool for Early Referral (PLASTER)
Infant Development Inventory (IDI)	Screening Kit of Language Development (SKOLD)
	Sentence Repetition Screening Test (SRST)

Glossary of terms

Adaptive behaviour The collection of conceptual, social and practical skills learned by people to enable them to function in their everyday lives.
American public laws A public bill or joint resolution that has passed both chambers of American Government (Congress and Senate) and been enacted into law. Public laws have general applicability nationwide. The part of law that governs relationships between legal persons and a government, between different institutions within a state, between different branches of governments, and relationships between persons that are of direct concern to the society. Public law comprises constitutional law, administrative law, tax law and criminal law, as well as all procedural law.
Amniocentesis A procedure in which amniotic fluid is removed from the uterus for testing or treatment. Amniotic fluid is the fluid that surrounds and protects a baby during pregnancy. This fluid contains foetal cells and various proteins.
Apgar scores Apgar scores are clinical indicators of a baby's condition shortly after birth. The score is based on five characteristics of the baby: Skin colour, pulse, breathing, muscle tone and reflex irritability. Each characteristic is given between 0 and 2 points, with a total score between 0 and 10 points.
Bell curve The Bell Curve represents statistically a "normal distribution", that is a normal distribution of sample scores with an arithmetic average and an equal distribution above and below average.
Brain connectivity Brain connectivity refers to anatomical links of statistical dependencies or of causal interactions between distinct units within a nervous system. The units correspond to individual neurons, neuronal populations or anatomically segregated brain regions. Reference is made to "hypoconnectivity syndromes" and "hyperconnectivity syndromes" in neurological literature.
Cell packing The number of cells grouped in the various regions of the brain.
CGH tests Comparative genomic hybridisation (CGH), also referred to as chromosomal microarray analysis (CMA), and array CGH (aCGH), is a method of genetic testing that may identify small deletions and duplications of the sub telomers, each pericentromeric region and other chromosome regions.
Chromosome A chromosome is a long DNA molecule with a part or all of the genetic material of an organism.
Comorbidity The simultaneous presence of two or more diseases or medical conditions in a patient.
CT scan A computerised tomography scan (CT or CAT scan) uses computers and rotating X-ray machines to create cross-sectional images of the body. These images provide more detailed information than normal X-ray images. They can show the soft tissues, blood vessels and bones in various parts of the body.
De novo New or previously undetected, for example the occurrence of a genetic disorder in a family not previously affected by the disorder.
Degenerative Refers to the process by which tissue deteriorates and loses its functional ability due to traumatic injury, ageing and wear and tear, or where behaviours and skills previously mastered and demonstrated gradually cease to be observed.
Deletion syndromes Chromosomal deletion syndromes result from deletion of parts of chromosomes. Chromosomal deletion syndromes typically involve larger deletions that are visible

using karyotyping techniques. Smaller deletions result in microdeletion syndromes and sub-micro deletions, which are detected using fluorescence in situ hybridisation (FISH).

Demylenation disorders Demyelinating disorders are any conditions that damage myelin. When this happens, scar tissue forms in its place. Brain signals do not move across scar tissue as quickly, so the nerves do not work as well as they should.

Developmental age equivalents Developmental age equivalents are an individual's ability, skill, knowledge or measurement expressed as the age at which most individuals reach the same level (age norm). The Age Norm is the average score of a particular test completed by children of a given chronological age.

Developmental quotients A development quotient (DQ), most frequently used with infants or preschool children, is a numerical indicator of a child's growth to maturity across a range of psychosocial competencies. On standardised tests of development, age equivalent scores for each domain may be converted to ratios or quotients, for example to derive a social or language DQ.

Diagnosis The art or act of identifying a disease or condition from its signs and symptoms.

Diagnostic and Statistical Manual (DSM) The Diagnostic and Statistical Manual is the handbook used by healthcare professionals in much of the world as the authoritative guide to the diagnosis of mental disorders. The current edition is the Diagnostic and Statistical Manual 5 Text Revision (DSM-5-TR).

DMG Dimethylglycine (DMG) is a derivative of the amino acid glycine, and it has been studied as a dietary supplement in children with autism spectrum disorder.

DNA Deoxyribonucleic acid is a molecule composed of two polynucleotide chains that coil around each other to form a "double helix" carrying genetic instructions for the development, functioning, growth and reproduction of all known organisms and many viruses.

Dopamine Dopamine is a hormone and a neurotransmitter that plays several important roles in the brain and body. It is an organic chemical of the catecholamine and phenethylamine families. Dopamine constitutes about 80% of the catecholamine content in the brain.

Duplication syndrome A chromosomal duplication is a type of mutation that involves the production of one or more copies of a gene or region of a chromosome. Microduplications, or submicroscopic duplications, are chromosomal duplications that are too small to be detected by light microscopy using conventional cytogenetics methods.

Dysmorphic A dysmorphic feature is an abnormal difference in body structure. It can be an isolated finding in an otherwise normal individual, or it can be related to a congenital disorder, genetic syndrome or birth defect.

Dyspraxia Dyspraxia is a neurological disorder that impacts an individual's ability to plan and process motor tasks. Individuals with dyspraxia often have language problems, and sometimes a degree of difficulty with thought and perception.

Echolalia Echolalia is the unsolicited repetition of vocalisations made by another person. In its profound form, it is automatic and effortless. Echolalia is often an associated symptom of autism spectrum disorder.

EEG An electroencephalogram (EEG) is a test that detects electrical activity in the brain using small, metal discs (electrodes) attached to the scalp. It is used in the assessment of epilepsy and other convulsive disorders.

Equality Equality means that the law and government treat everyone the same, irrespective of their status or identity.

Equity Equity means that, in some circumstances, people need to be treated differently in order to provide meaningful equality of opportunity.

Ethnic diversity The existence of people from a variety of cultural and diverse backgrounds within a single area. Ethnicity refers to a group's shared cultural norms beliefs and practices, while diversity refers to what makes people different based on age, gender and culture.

Epilepsy A disorder in which nerve cell activity in the brain is disturbed, causing seizures. Epilepsy may occur as a result of a genetic disorder or an acquired brain injury, such as a trauma or stroke. During a seizure, a person experiences abnormal behaviour, symptoms and sensations, sometimes including loss of consciousness. There are few symptoms between seizures. Epilepsy is usually treated by medication and in some cases by surgery, devices or dietary changes.

Eugenics Eugenics is the practice of attempting to improve the human species by selectively mating people with specific desirable hereditary traits. It aims to "breed out" disease, disabilities and so-called undesirable characteristics from the human population.

Factor scores A factor score is a numerical value that indicates a person's relative spacing or standing on a latent factor. Factor analysis is a statistical method used to describe variability among observed, correlated variables in terms of a potentially lower number of unobserved variables called factors.

Fish test Fluorescence in situ hybridisation (FISH) is a test that "maps" the genetic material in a person's cells. This test can be used to visualise specific genes or portions of genes.

Genes A gene is the basic physical and functional unit of heredity. Genes are made up of DNA. Some genes act as instructions to make molecules called proteins. However, many genes do not code for proteins. In humans, genes vary considerably in size.

Genetic expression Genetic expression is the process by which information from a gene is used in the synthesis of a functional gene product. These products are often proteins, but in non-protein-coding genes such as transfer RNA or small nuclear RNA genes, the product is a functional RNA.

Genetic mutation Genetic mutations are changes in the genetic sequence, and they are a main cause of diversity among organisms. These changes occur at many different levels, and they can have widely differing consequences.

General adaptive composite score In psychometric assessment of adaptive behaviour skills, a General Adaptive Composite or GAC is the score which compares a person's global adaptive skills to the adaptive skills of others in the same age group from the standardisation sample.

Generalised intelligence General intelligence, also known as the g factor, is a psychometric construct from the assessment of cognitive abilities and human intelligence. General intelligence summarises positive correlations among different cognitive tasks, reflecting the fact that an individual's performance on one type of cognitive task tends to be comparable to that person's performance on other kinds of cognitive tasks. The terms IQ, general intelligence, general cognitive ability, general mental ability and simply intelligence are often used interchangeably to refer to this common core shared by cognitive tests.

ICD 11 The International Classification of Diseases 11th Edition (ICD 11) is the global health information standard for mortality and morbidity statistics. ICD is used in clinical care and research to define diseases and study disease patterns, as well as manage healthcare, monitor outcomes and allocate resources.

Intrauterine Refers to the intrauterine environment inside the mother's womb or uterus.

Megabase pairs A megabase pair (Mbp) is a unit of length of nucleic acids, equal to one million base pairs or to 1000 kilobase pairs.

Melatonin Melatonin is a hormone primarily released by the pineal gland that regulates the sleep–wake cycle. As a dietary supplement, it is often used for the short-term treatment of insomnia.

MRI Magnetic resonance imaging is a medical imaging technique used in radiology to form pictures of the anatomy and the physiological processes of the human body. MRI scanners use strong magnetic fields, magnetic field gradients and radio waves to generate images of the organs in the body.

MMR The MMR vaccine is a vaccine against measles, mumps and rubella. The first dose is generally given to children around 9 months to 15 months of age, with a second dose at 15 months to 6 years of age, with at least 4 weeks between the doses.

Mosaicism Mosaicism is when a person has two or more genetically different sets of cells in his or her body.

Multifactorial Refers to traits and conditions that are caused by more than one gene occurring together. Diseases and conditions that are caused by more than one factor interacting are multifactorial.

Neonatal Relating to newborn children.

Neonatal intensive care units (NICU) A neonatal intensive care unit at a hospital (NICU) has specialist medical staff and equipment to care for premature and sick newborn babies. The NICU has highly trained staff and advanced life support equipment designed to meet the unique needs of newborn babies.

Neurodevelopmental disorders Neurodevelopmental disorders are a group of conditions with onset in the developmental period. The disorders typically manifest early in development, often before the child enters grade school, and are characterised by developmental deficits that produce impairments of personal, social, academic or occupational functioning. The neurodevelopmental disorders frequently co-occur. For some disorders, the clinical presentation includes symptoms of excess as well as deficits and delays in achieving expected milestones.

Percentile In statistics, a percentile is a score below which a given percentage of scores in its frequency distribution fall or a score at or below which a given percentage fall.

Perinatal Perinatal refers to the period from the conception of a child through to the first year after birth.

Phenotype A phenotype is an individual's observable traits, such as height, eye colour and blood type. In developmental disability contexts, a phenotype also refers to consistently occurring behavioural traits or symptoms. The genetic contribution to the phenotype is called the genotype. Some traits are largely determined by the genotype, while other traits are largely determined by environmental factors.

Predictive validity Predictive validity is the degree to which a correct prediction or forecast of a system's state can be made either qualitatively or quantitatively. Reference is made in psychometric assessment to predictive validity in terms of correlation between an assessment and later outcomes.

Psychometrics Psychometrics is a field of study concerned with the theory and technique of psychological measurement. Psychometrics refers to psychological measurement. Generally, it refers to the field of objective measurement of skills and knowledge, abilities, attitudes, personality traits and educational achievement.

Rasch modelling The Rasch model, named after Georg Rasch, is a psychometric model for analysing categorical data, such as answers to questions on a reading assessment or responses to test items in psychometric assessments. In the Rasch model, the probability of a specified response (e.g. right/wrong answer or "pass/fail" criteria) is modelled as a function of person and item parameters. In psychometric assessment, the Rasch Model is used to place test items in an appropriate hierarchical order of difficulty.

Secretin A hormone that regulates water homeostasis throughout the body and influences the environment of the duodenum by regulating secretions in the stomach, pancreas and liver. Reference is made to the use of secretin from pigs as a possible treatment for autism spectrum disorder.

Semantic-pragmatic disorders Semantics refer to the relationship between words or sentences and their meanings. Pragmatics refer to the ability to make effective use of language in context. Social (pragmatic) communication disorders can be diagnosed in individuals who have difficulty using verbal and/or nonverbal communication that is appropriate for the social context.

Serotonin Serotonin is the key hormone that stabilises mood, feelings of well-being and happiness. This hormone impacts the entire body. It enables brain cells and other nervous system cells to communicate with each other, and also assists with sleeping, eating and digestion.

Silent seizures (also referred to as absence seizures) Absence seizures or silent seizures involve brief, sudden lapses of consciousness. They are more common in children than in adults. A sufferer of such seizures may appear to be staring blankly into space for a short period of time, before quickly returning to normal alertness. Absence seizures can be controlled with anti-convulsant medications. Some children who have them also develop other seizures. Silent seizing is felt to occur frequently in autism spectrum disorder.

Spectrum disorders A spectrum disorder is a developmental disorder that includes a range of linked conditions or symptoms, varying in severity of impact, frequency or duration. The different elements of a spectrum either have a similar appearance or are thought to be caused by the same underlying mechanism.

Standard deviation A standard deviation is a measure of the amount of variation of a set of values. A low standard deviation indicates that the values tend to cluster around the mean of the set, while a high standard deviation indicates that values being spread out over a wider range.

Standard error of measurement The standard error of measurement estimates how repeated measures of an individual on the same test tend to be distributed around his/her "true" score.

Standard scores Standard scores represent the number of standard deviations by which the value of a raw score is above or below the mean. Raw scores above the mean have positive standard scores, while those below the mean have negative standard scores.

Stereotypies A stereotypy is a repetitive or ritualistic movement, posture or sound or utterance. They may be simple movements such as body rocking, or complex, physical rituals.

Stimulant medication Stimulant medications stimulate the central nervous system by increasing the activity of certain chemicals in the brain. They are most frequently used in the treatment of attention deficit hyperactivity disorder (ADHD) and narcolepsy (a sleep disorder). They may also be used in the treatment of depression or acquired brain injury.

Symptomatology The set of symptoms characteristic of a medical condition or disorder exhibited by a patient.

Syndrome A syndrome is a set of medical signs and symptoms which are correlated with each other and often associated with a particular disease or a disorder.

T scores A T-score is a standardised score that is calculated from the total distribution of scores within a population sample. T-scores enable the comparison of individual scores against norms from an equivalent age and gender group.

Test reliability, validity and stability The statistical qualities of psychometric tests that ensure that they measure what they are intended to measure (validity), with results that are stable over time, (reliability), can detect changes in conditions (responsiveness) and can predict future outcomes and subsequent test performance.

Theory of mind Theory of mind is a term referring to an individual's degree of capacity for empathy and understanding of others.

Tic disorders Tics are sudden twitches, movements or sounds that occur repeatedly and unintentionally.

Translocation syndrome A translocation syndrome occurs when an extra copy of a chromosome is attached to another chromosome.

Trisomy A trisomy is a chromosomal condition characterised by an additional chromosome.

Volumetric studies Brain size can be measured by weight and sometimes by volume through MRI scans. A volumetric MRI scan measures volumes of the key brain structures: Hippocampus, ventricles and other brain structures, and compares the volumes to standard norms based on age, gender and cranial volume.

Index

Note: Page numbers in *italics* and **bold** refer to figure and table, respectively.

15q11-q13 syndrome (Prader-Willi syndrome) 41, 43, 58–59
17p11.2 syndrome (Smith-Magenis Syndrome) 41, 43, 45, 46, 57, **57**
22q11.2 syndrome (velocardiofacial syndrome) 43, 53–56
45X/45XO syndrome (Turner syndrome) 53
47XXy/46XX syndrome 52, 348
47XXY syndrome (Klinefelter syndrome) 43, 52
48XXXY syndrome 52
48XXYY syndrome 42, 52
49XXXXY syndrome 52

ABAS-3 (Adaptive Behavior Assessment System, 3rd Edition) 143–144, **144**
absence seizures 349
acceptance 89–90
activities of daily living 141, 147, 232
adaptive behavior 140, 346
Adaptive Behavior Assessment System, 3rd Edition (ABAS-3) 143–144, **144**
adaptive behaviour questionnaires 141–145
Adaptive Behaviour Scale (Bayley-4) 131
ADHD (attention deficit/hyperactivity disorder) 32–34, 58, 349
"A Different Kind of Perfect" 2, 85
ADI-R (Autism Diagnostic Interview-Revised) 167–168, 233
ADOS 2 (Autism Diagnostic Observation Schedule, 2nd Edition) 169–170, 198, 233
alcohol 44, 64–66
American Psychological Association (APA) 212; Code of Ethics 81; guidelines on assessing individuals with disabilities 318–319
amniocentesis 19, 346
Angelman syndrome 41
anger 87–88
"anthropometric laboratory" 11
anticonvulsants 224
antipsychotics 224
anxiety medications 224
APGAR scores 19, 346
array CGH (aCGH) 46, 346
Asperger, Hans 28–30
Asperger's disorder 28–30
ASRS (Autism Spectrum Rating Scales) 165–166, 234
assessment 75–83; APA guidelines 318–319; clinical practice 185–186; considerations in 82; definition of 75; issues in 80–81; methods 82; parental experience of 77–83; pre-assessment preparation 187–192; principles for engagements in 81; procedures in 230, 235; purposes of 75; questionnaires and checklists 138–147; role of psychologists in 76; settings 82, 187; skills needed in 76; systemic reasons for 75, 96–106
assessment process 193–199; background information 193; and diagnosis 228; "from referral to diagnosis to action" flowchart 228; initial contact 194; issues during 196–197; questions in 193–195; suggestions in 194–195, 197–199
assessment room 189–190, *190*
Association for Research in Infant and Child Development (ARICD) 212
Association of Infant and Child Development 212
atlantoaxial instability 51
attention deficit/hyperactivity disorder (ADHD) 32–34, 58, 349
Attwood, Tony 28
Australian Psychological Society 80, 211
autism 11
Autism Diagnostic Interview-Revised (ADI-R) 167–168, 233

352 *Index*

Autism Diagnostic Observation Schedule, 2nd Edition (ADOS 2) 169–170, 198, 233
autism spectrum disorder 25–32, **26**, 60–61; assessment 161–171; case summary 266–268; diagnostic formulation of 233–238; direct interaction assessments 168–171; DSM 5 criteria for 329–330, **330**; ICD-10/11 criteria for 329–330; levels of severity for 329–330, **330**; levels of support **330**; screening checklists for 162–168
Autism Spectrum Rating Scales (ASRS) 165–166, 234
"Automatic entry" conditions 97–98
"Avenues of Learning" 13, 114, *126*, *128*; foundations of learning subscale 127; subscales 125

"Baby Scales" 125, 127
background information 193, 230, 234; in reports 247, 248; sample reports 263, 266–267, 271
balance skills 119
bargaining 88
Baron-Cohen, Simon 44
Bayley-4 117, 118, 122; format changes 132; history 130–131; predictive validity 202; subscales 131; training 197–198
Bayley, Nancy 13, 130–131, 202
Bayley Scales of Infant Development 130–131
behaviour, in reports 248
Bell curve 111–113, *113*, 346
Binet, Alfred 12
Boardmaker 208
Brachmann-de Lange syndrome 43
brachycephaly 245
brain: abnormalities 55–56, 60; connectivity 346; and fetal alcohol spectrum syndrome 64
British Psychological Society Code of Conduct 81
"burden of proof" 104

California First-Year Mental Scale 13, 130–131
California Infant Scale of Motor Development 130–131
California Pre-school Mental Scale 130–131
camptodactyly 245
capacity-building 98, 300
case summaries 252–296; autism spectrum disorder 266–268; global developmental delay 263–266; microdeletion syndrome 283–288; unintended neglect 274–277
Cattell, James 12
"cell packing" 30, 346
Centrelink Carers Allowance 97, **98**

"charter schools" 105
Child Behavior Checklist 146–147
Child Health and Mental Retardation Act 14
Childhood Autism Rating Scale, 2nd Edition 163–164
childhood disintegrative disorder 29
child onset pervasive developmental disorder 25
chromosomal disorders 40–48
chromosomal microarray analysis (CMA) 346
chromosome 9p deletion syndrome 245
chromosomes 41–42, 346; extra 42, 49–58; missing 49–58
clinical practice 185–186
CMA (chromosomal microarray analysis) 346
cognition coping 90
cognitive adaptation 90
cognitive revelation 15
Cognitive Scale (Bayley-4) 131
communication 244; components of *244*; written 244
communication devices 207–208
communication skills 121
comorbidity 229, 346
comparative genomic hybridization (CGH) 46, 346
Complex Tasks Index (Miller Assessment) 136
computer-generated scoring 245–247
computerized tomography scan (CT scan) 346
Concerta **224**
Constantino, John 162
context, of communication 244
Coordination Index (Miller Assessment) 136
courses of actions, in reports 249
Covid-19 211
"crack babies" 44
"Crack Cocaine" 44
Cri du Chat syndrome (deletion 5p syndrome) 43
cultural explanation 92
cultural idiom of distress 92
cultural syndrome 92

DAYC-2 (Developmental Assessment of Young Children-2) 140–142
DBC 2 (Developmental Behaviour Checklist 2) 146–147
degenerative 346
deletion syndromes 43, 346
demographic information, in reports 247, **250**
demyelination disorders 347
denial 86–87
"de novo" 44, 346
deoxyribonucleic acid (DNA) 41, 347
depression 88–90

developmental age equivalents 126, 127, 201, 347
Developmental Assessment of Young Children-2 (DAYC-2) 140–142
developmental assessments 117–118, *118*
Developmental Behaviour Checklist 2 (DBC 2) 146–147
developmental coordination disorder 34, 333
"developmental disability" 18
Developmental Profile (DP-4) 140
developmental quotients (DQ) 127, 201, 347
developmental screening tests 139–140
Dewey, John 111
dexamphetamine **224**
diagnosis 227–238, 347; and assessment process 228; of autism spectrum disorder 233–238; considerations in 229, 231, 235; decision in labelling 237; definition of 227; examples of 230–238; expertise and experience 229–230; "from referral to diagnosis to action" flowchart 228; of global developmental delay 231–232, **232**; list of diagnostic conditions 229; process in 227; in reports 248–249; sample reports 269, 271–274, 275–277
Diagnostic and Statistical Manual of Mental Disorders (DSM) 18, 21, 347
Dickens, Charles 59
DiGeorge sequence 54
Dilantin 44
dimethylglycine (DMG) 347
direct skills 116
disability rights: development of 14–16; legislations and acts 16
disability support 97–105
disbelief 86
distress, cultural idiom of 92
DNA (deoxyribonucleic acid) 41, 347
Doll, Edgard 141
dopamine 347
Dowling, C. 2
Down, John Langdon 11, 45
Down, Reginald 11
Down syndrome (trisomy 21 syndrome) 11, 41, 42, 49–52
DP-4 (Developmental Profile) 140
DQ (developmental quotients) 201, 347
DSM (Diagnostic and Statistical Manual of Mental Disorders) 18, 21, 347
"due diligence" 104
duplication 3q syndrome 43, 60
duplication 9p syndrome (trisomy 9p syndrome) 43, 60
duplication 10p syndrome 60
duplication 15q syndrome 43, 60
duplication syndrome 43, 60, 347
dysmorphic characteristics 46, 347
dyspraxia 269, 347

Early Intervention Program for Infants and Children (EIPIC) (Singapore) 101
echolalia 36, 170, 258, 270, 275, 329, 347
EEG (electroencephalogram) 31, 347
Einfeld, Stewart 146
electroencephalogram (EEG) 31, 347
eligibility criteria 104
emerging skills 202–203
Enhanced Pilot for Private Intervention Providers (Enhanced PPIP) (Singapore) 101
environmental agents 44–45, 64–66
epilepsy 31, 347
Epilim **224**
equipment and toys 190–191
ethnic diversity 91, 179, 347
eugenics 14, 347
executive summary, in reports 247
"extreme autistic aloneness" 27

factor score 348
faith 90–94
feedback 216–219; common language in 219; defocusing frame 219; elements of 218; hopeful formulation frame 219; location and timing 217; overview 216; parent-friendly frame 218; to and from parents 231, 235; questions to ask in 219; on therapies and intervention programs 221–225
"feral child" 10
fetal alcohol spectrum syndrome 44, 64–66; diagnostic criteria **65**
fetal dilantin syndrome 44
fetal valproate syndrome 44
fetal warfarin syndrome 44
final summations, in reports *250*
"finding out" 77
fine motor skills 119–120, *120*; development sequence **335–336**
FISH (fluorescence in situ hybridization) 46, 348
"Floating-Harbor syndrome" 45
fluorescence in situ hybridization (FISH) 46, 348
"focus group" research 77
Follow Through 14
follow-up and support 299–301
form, of communication 244
Foundations Index (Miller Assessment) 136
Foundations of Learning subscale 127
fragile x syndrome 60–61
"Framework for the Assessment of Children in Need and their Families (UK)" 100
frontal bossing 245

354 *Index*

GAC (general adaptive composite) score 113, 143, 348
Galton, Francis 11
Gaussian curve 111, *113*
GCI (general cognitive index) 135
gene 41, 348
general adaptive composite (GAC) score 113, 143, 348
general cognitive ability 348
general cognitive index (GCI) 135
general intelligence 11, 348
general mental ability 348
genetic code 41
genetic disorders 40–48
genetic expression 44, 348
genetic mutations 43–44, 60–62, 348
genetic testing 46
Gesell, Arnold 13
Gilberg, Christopher 28
Gilliam Autism Rating Scales, 3rd Edition 164
Gilliam, James E. 164
"global developmental age" 126
global developmental delay 24, 97–98; case summaries 281–288; diagnosis of 231–232; DSM 5 criteria for 326; ICD-11 criteria for 326
Goldstein, Sam 165
Goodenough, Florence 13
Goodenough-Harris "Draw-A-Man" test 13
grief 84–90; acceptance 89–90; anger 87–88; bargaining 88; denial 86; depression 88–89; disbelief 86; guilt 87; shock 85–86
Griffiths III scale 118, 122, 125–129; Avenues of Learning *128*; Baby Scales 125, 127; development age equivalents 126, 127; developmental quotients 127; general quotient 126; history 125–127; practical reasoning subscale 122, 127; predictive validity 202; sample report 260–263, 264–265, 276–277; subscales 127; training 197–198
Griffiths, Ruth 13, 114, 125–126, 202
gross motor skills 119, *120*, 199; sequence of **337–338**
guilt 87

Head Start 14
Henri, Victor 12
High Functioning Individuals CARS 2 HF Rating Booklet 164
histograms 248
humour, learning about 115
Huntley, Michael 127

ICD (International Classification of Diseases) 18, 21, 348
"idiots" 13
"imbeciles" 13
indirect skills 116
infantile autism 25, 28
infantile psychosis 11
initial contact, in assessment process 194
"inquisitive" group 79
intellectual disability (intellectual developmental disorder) 22–23; DSM 5 criteria for **327–328**; ICD-11 criteria for 327
intelligence 12, 348
International Classification of Diseases (ICD) 18, 21, 348
International League of Societies for the Mentally Retarded 15
interpreters 206–207
intrauterine 348
involuntary reflex behaviours 119
Iowa Tests for Young Children 13
IQ 14, 348
Itard, Jean Marc Gaspard 10

jumping, in gross motor developmental stages **337–338**

Kanner, Leo 27
Kessler, David 89–90
Klinefelter, Harry 52
Klinefelter syndrome 42, 52
known aetiology 97
Kubler-Ross, Elizabeth 84, 89–90

Lamp Words for Life 208
language development sequence **339–340**
language disorder 24, 331
Language Scale (Bayley-4) 132
language skills 121
Lansing, Margaret D 168
learning, in young children 114–117
LeCouteur, Ann 167
Lemoine, Paul 64–67
"*Lessons from my Child*" 85
"life lessons" 90
listening skills 121
live streaming 211
"lockdown" 211
Longwell, Sarah Geraldine 141
Lord, Catherine 167, 169
Love, Steven R 163
Luiz, Dolores 127

Magenis, Ellen 45
magnetic resonance imaging (MRI) 9, 30, 348
Marfan syndrome 44
"maternal uniparental disomy" 59
Mbp (megabase pair) 43, 348
McCarthy, Dorothea 135

McCarthy Scales of Children's Abilities 135–136
MECP2 protein 61
medications 223–225; side effects of 224–225
megabase pair (Mbp) 43, 348
melatonin 224, 348
Memory Scale (McCarthy Scale) 135
"mental age" 126
"mental defectives" 13
Merrill-Palmer Scale of Mental Tests 13
metopic ridges 245
microdeletion syndrome 43, 53–58, 281–283
microduplication syndromes 43, 60
mild developmental delay 236
Miller Assessment for Preschoolers 136
Miller, Lucy 136
Minnesota Preschool Scale 13
MMR vaccine 348
mobile phone videos 210
mobility and balance skills 119
"mock attack" 115
Modified checklist for autism in toddlers, revised (M-CHAT-R) 162–163
"mongolism" 11
mosaic Down syndrome 51
mosaicism (47XXy/46XX syndrome) 51, 52, 348
Motor Scale (Bayley-4) 131
Motor Scale (McCarthy Scale) 135
MRI (magnetic resonance imaging) 9, 30, 348
multifactorial inheritance 44, 348
mutations 43–44, 60–62

Naglieri, Jack A. 165
narcolepsy 349
National Disability Insurance Scheme (NDIS) (Australia) 97
Needs Assessment and Service Coordination Organization (New Zealand) 98
neonatal 348
neonatal intensive care units (NICU) 348
neurodevelopmental disorders 21–37, 348; attention deficit/hyperactivity disorder 32–34; autism spectrum disorder 25–27, **26**; definition of 21–22; developmental coordination disorder 34; global developmental delay 24; historical overview 9–19; intellectual disability 23; language disorder 24–25; perinatal causes 18, **19**; pervasive demand avoidance syndrome 35–37; postnatal causes 18, **19**; prenatal causes 18, **19**; stereotypic movement disorder 34–35; tic disorders 35
Newson, Elizabeth 36
New Zealand 98
non-government agencies 187
Nonverbal Index (Miller Assessment) 136

normal population 111, 116
Norway 97

off-site observations 208–210
Olshansky, S. 85
"*On the Origin of Species*" (Darwin) 11
Ortega y Gasset, José 116
Oslo Breakfast program 14

parental experience of assessment 84–94; and faith/spirituality 90–94; finding out 77; grief 84–90; overview 84
parents: inquisitive group 79; passionate group 79
Patau syndrome (trisomy 13 syndrome) 42
PCE (prenatal cocaine exposure) 44
PEP-3 (Psychoeducational Profile, 3rd Edition) 168–171
perceived cause 92
percentile **114**, 200, 349
Perceptual-performance Scale (McCarthy Scale) 135
perinatal 349
persistent complex bereavement disorder 94
pervasive demand avoidance syndrome 35–37
pervasive developmental disorder (not otherwise specified) (PDD-NOS) 29, 36
phenotype 41, 46, 349
phenylketonuria 14, 125
PICs (private intervention centres) 101
"point mutations" 43
"positive illusions" 90
"positive psychology" 90
postural strength 119
"Practical Reasoning" 122
Prader-Willi syndrome (15q11-q13 syndrome) 41, 43, 58–59
Prader-Willi syndrome critical region (PWSCR) 58
pre-assessment preparation 187–192; assessment contexts 187; assessment room 189–190, *190*; equipment and toys 190–191; questionnaires 230, 234; referrals 188–189; scheduling 191–192; settings 187; suggestions 188
pre-assessment questionnaires 230, 234
precocious schizophrenia 11
predictive validity 13, 117–118, 349
prenatal cocaine exposure (PCE) 44
preschool-age children: educational opportunities 116; learning in 116
private intervention centres (PICs) 101
Proloqo2go 208
Psychoeducational Profile, 3rd Edition (PEP3) 168–171
psychologists, career journeys 187

psychometric assessments 111–124; defined 349; developmental assessments 117–118, *118*; generalizations 117–118; gross motor skills 119; overview 111; in reports 248; sample reports 257–263, 274–277; sequence of development 119–124
public hospitals 187
Public Law 94–142 15
Public Law 99–457 15, 16
public laws 15–16
PWSCR (Prader-Willi syndrome critical region) 58

Quantitative Scale (McCarthy Scale) 135
Questionnaire for Parents or Caregivers CARS 2 QPC 164
questionnaires and checklists 138–147; adaptive behaviour questionnaires 141–144; benefits 138; developmental screening tests 139–140; questions to be asked in using 138; special population 145–147
questions, in assessment process 193

Rasch, Georg 349
Rasch model 349
reasoning skills 122
reasons for assessment 96–106; accurate descriptions of what children can and cannot do 105; disability support 96–106; school 105
receptive language 97
"*Recognizable Patterns of Human Malformation*" 46
recommendations, in reports 249
reconstruction 85, 89
referrals 188–189
"reflex" actions 119
Reichler, Robert J. 168
reliability 13, 14, 350
report writing 241–251; audiences 241; common language *245*; as communication 244–245; computer-generated scoring and reporting 245–247; families 242; government departments and other agencies 243; medical practitioners 242; purposes of 241; sections 247–250; therapists 242–243; typical layouts 247–250, *250*
Rett syndrome 44, 61–62
Ritalin **224**
running, in gross motor developmental stages 337
Rutter, Michael 28, 167, 169

sample reports 252–296; background information 252–254, 258, 263, 266–267, 271, 275, 282, 288, 290, 292; behaviour at assessment 263; diagnostic assessment outcomes 257, 269–274, 275; diagnostic report 252–257; executive summary 268, 274, 277, 288; Griffiths III 260–262, 264, 276–277; psychometric assessments 260–262, 276–277; score summary 255–256
scheduling 191–192
schools, eligibility criteria 104
Schopler, Eric 163, 168–171
score summary, in reports 249
scoring 214–215; computer-generated 214–215, 245–247
secretin 31, 349
self-introduction skills 122
semantic-pragmatic disorders 25, 349
sequence of development 119–124; early learning and reasoning skills 122–124; fine motor skills 119–121, *121*; gross motor skills 119, *120*; personal/social development 122; speech, language and communication skills 121
serotonin 30, 349
Sesame Street 14
settings 187–188
"75-25" rule of assessment 197, 199, *200*, 200–210; assessment skills 203–205; emerging skills 202–203; guidelines **206**; information derived from assessments 201–202; interpreters 206–207; mobile phone videos 210; off-site observations 208–210; overview 200–201; qualitative descriptions of test items passed **204**; signing and communication devices 207–208
shock 85–86
SHORT syndrome 45
short-term memory skills 121
Shprintzen, Robert 53
Shprintzen syndrome 53
signing and communication devices 207–208
silent seizures 349
Skype 139, 143, 211
sleep medications 224
Smith, Anne 45, 57
Smith-Magenis Syndrome (17p11.2 syndrome) 41, 43, 45, 46, 57, *57*
social (pragmatic) communication disorder 37, 332
"social competence" 141
"social distancing" 211
Social-Emotional Scale (Bayley-4) 131
social engagement skills 122
social greeting and farewell skills 122, 199
social occasions 170
Social Responsiveness Scale-2 (SRS-2) 162
"sole traders" 187, 188
Spearman, Charles 12

"Special Educational Needs Code of Practice (UK)" 100
special education programs 104, 140
special population questionnaires and checklists 145–146
spectrum disorders 349
speech skills 121
spirituality 90–94
SRS-2 (Social Responsiveness Scale-2) 162
stability 350
standard deviation **114**, 349
standard error of measurement 349
standard scores 114, 201, 349
Standard Version CARS 2 ST Rating Booklet 164
Stanford-Binet scale 114
stanines 201
stereotypic movement disorder 34–35, 333–334
stereotypy 349
stimulant medications 224, 349
suggestions, in assessment process 194–196, 197–199
Supplementary Security Income (SSI) 98
support and follow-up 299–301
Sure Start program 100
symptomatology 350
syndrome 350
"System accountability" 104
Szatmari, Peter 28

telehealth 211–212
"theory of mind" 46, 115, 122, 127, 350
Thomas, B. 2
throwing, in gross motor developmental stages **338**
tic disorders 35, 350
Tonge, Bruce 146
toys 190–191
transition point 104
translocation syndrome 43, 52, 350
Treatment and Education of Autistic and Related Communication Handicapped Children (TEACCH) program 163
trigonocephaly 245

trisomy 42, 350
trisomy 13 syndrome (Patau syndrome) 42
trisomy 21 syndrome (Down syndrome) 11, 42, 49–52
T-score 135, 166, 350
Turner, Henry 53
Turner syndrome 53

unintended neglect 274–277

validity 13, 350
valproate 44
Van Bourgondien, Mary E 163
"velocardiofacial syndrome" 43, 53–56
Verbal Index (Miller Assessment) 136
Verbal Scale (McCarthy Scale) 135
Victor of Aveyron 10
Vineland Adaptive Behavior Scales III (Vineland III) 142–143, **142**
Vineland Social Maturity Scales 13, 141–142
Vineland-3 Adaptive Behavior Scales 132
vocabulary 121
volumetric studies 30, 350

Wakefield, Andrew 31
walking, in gross motor developmental stages **337**
warfarin 44
Wellman, Glenna Janette 163
Weschler scale 114
"Wild Boy of Aveyron" 10
Williams, J. C. P 57
Williams syndrome (Williams-Beurens syndrome) 41, 57–58
Wolf-Hirschhorn Syndrome 43, 59

X chromosome 41
XXX syndrome 42
XXXXX syndrome 42
XXXY syndrome 42

Y chromosome 41

Zoom 139, 143, 211
Z scores 201